Parkinson's Disease in the Older Patient
SECOND EDITION

Edited by

JEREMY PLAYFER
Emeritus Consultant Geriatrician
Royal Liverpool Hospital

and

JOHN HINDLE
Consultant Physician, Care of the Elderly
Llandudno Hospital

Foreword by
ANDREW LEES
Professor
The National Hospital for Neurology and Neurosurgery, London

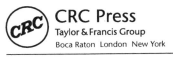

CRC Press
Taylor & Francis Group
Boca Raton London New York

CRC Press is an imprint of the
Taylor & Francis Group, an **informa** business

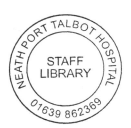

First published 2008 by Radcliffe Publishing

First Edition 2001 published by Arnold.

Published 2016 by CRC Press
Taylor & Francis Group
6000 Broken Sound Parkway NW, Suite 300
Boca Raton, FL 33487-2742

CRC Press is an imprint of Taylor & Francis Group, an Informa business

First issued in paperback 2019

No claim to original U.S. Government works

ISBN 13: 978-0-367-44613-0 (pbk)
ISBN 13: 978-1-84619-114-5 (hbk)

Visit the Taylor & Francis Web site at
http://www.taylorandfrancis.com

and the CRC Press Web site at
http://www.crcpress.com

British Library Cataloguing in Publication Data

A catalogue record for this book is available from the British Library.

Typeset by Pindar New Zealand (Egan Reid), Auckland, New Zealand

Contents

Foreword to second edition

In the late 1970s when I started my neurological training at Queen Square I had the good fortune to be able to seek advice from Macdonald Critchley, who was by then emeritus but still lived in a flat in the square. He was very interested in the neurology of old age and emphasised to me that this remained terra incognita and a fertile hunting ground for new neurological phenomena. He advised me to read his Goulstonian lectures on the topic published in the *Lancet* in 1931 which were to introduce me for the first time to this fascinating and neglected area. A few years later I watched Olivier portray the demented and senile Lear on television with a strained quivering voice, flexed posture and shuffling gait. Kinnier Wilson, Queen Square's Marco Polo of the extrapyramidal system and one of Critchley's teachers wrote, 'Advancing years bring a certain amount of muscular stiffness and loss of elasticity, when the senile gait may turn to a shuffle, the senile voice to a monotone, hence in ascribing such symptoms merely to senescence one may misinterpret the onset of paralysis agitans.' The diagnosis of Parkinson's disease is predicated upon the demonstration of decay in the amplitude of repetitive motor tasks which may present particular challenges in the elderly patient. There remain many unanswered questions relating to Parkinsonism in old age, not least the murky borderland between senile tremor and Parkinson's disease. It has also been intriguingly proposed that the incidence of the malady might actually diminish in the ninth decade and that the clinical picture of Parkinson's disease presenting over 70 differs from the classical form by its greater frequency of axial and bulbar symptoms, early gait disturbance and dementia. These symptoms can occur in old age in the absence of Parkinsonism and the interaction of the biological effects of aging on the primary neurodegenerative process of Parkinson's disease remains an area of very active research. Drs Playfer and Hindle are to be congratulated in putting together a fresh and new version of their highly successful book *Parkinson's Disease in the Older Patient*. This new edition deserves to receive a wide readership and comparable acclaim.

Professor Andrew Lees
The National Hospital for Neurology and Neurosurgery, London
September 2007

Foreword to first edition

I am honoured to have been asked to write the Foreword for *Parkinson's Disease in the Older Patient*, which has been prepared by many healthcare professionals who specialise in the management of this chronic and debilitating neurological condition.

During the past three decades, several changes to society have had implications for people and their families living with Parkinson's disease, which include:

➤ the change in the role of voluntary organisations highlighting the importance of listening to the needs of the customers;
➤ demographic changes resulting in the increase in the number of elderly, frail people;
➤ the change in the roles of women within our society through education and career structure;
➤ the decrease in the availability of informal carers due to a falling birth rate and a change in family structure;
➤ the need to focus more sharply on the needs of the ageing population in order to meet appropriately the needs of the elderly, the customers.

Demographic changes mean that Parkinson's disease is set to become more common with the rise in the number of elderly putting even more pressure on carers. There is an urgent need to focus more sharply on families affected by neurological disorders so that their needs can be met appropriately. People want to participate in the management of their illness.

We need to combine the knowledge and clinical observations of the healthcare professionals with the experiences of those people living with, and impacted by, chronic neurological illnesses on a daily basis. It is only then that it will be possible to achieve an integrated picture of the challenges of managing a chronic neurological illness such as Parkinson's disease.

Parkinson's Disease in the Older Patient concentrates upon the holistic care of people impacted by Parkinson's disease, and stresses the importance of improving standards of care which will improve participation in life.

On behalf of the Parkinson's Disease Society of the United Kingdom, I would like to thank all who have contributed their time and expertise in producing such a valuable resource.

Mary Baker MBE
Chief Executive
Parkinson's Disease Society
February 2001

Preface to second edition

In preparing the second edition of *Parkinson's Disease in the Older Patient* we have been struck by the growth of knowledge and the speed with which the management of Parkinson's disease (PD) changes. We have been extremely lucky to retain most of the authors from the first edition and are grateful for their enormous effort in rewriting their chapters and reviewing the progress that has been achieved. We have carefully tried to retain the spirit and purpose of the book. We feel sure it is right to emphasise the older patient, and with two-thirds of PD patients over 70 years old, the management of the disease is inevitably complex. There is a need to look at all the factors which may lead to disability and loss of quality of life.

PD is more than just a motor disorder. Since the first edition of the book this is more generally accepted. We hope we capture the style and importance of an interdisciplinary approach putting the multidisciplinary team at the centre of PD management. This is essential in any geriatric approach.

All the authors of this book are contributors to the growth of knowledge in PD. They all regularly produce original publications and contribute to learned conferences. We are particularly indebted to the PD section of the British Geriatrics Society. This book arose out of the popular Science to Practice Meeting that the section holds at the Royal College of Physicians (London). It is now in its 11th year. Most of the authors have contributed to this series and we are particularly indebted to Dr Dorothy Robertson who has been inspirational in encouraging a true rehabilitation forum for PD.

Anybody interested in PD will be excited at the progress that is being made in our understanding of the disease. Although this is generally led by basic scientists, it is vital that their results are interpreted and translated by leading clinicians in the field. Many of the insights derive from molecular biology and genetics. The index cases are often younger patients with rare genetic mutations. Nevertheless, the findings can be generalised to have relevance to the disease process in the older patient. Epidemiological research highlights the disease in the elderly and gives clues to aetiology.

Getting the diagnosis right, assessing the needs of patients and being able to focus on the disabling aspects of the disease are the core skills of the geriatrician. The chapters dealing with these topics in Part 2 span both theory and practice and should prove valuable to practitioners of all disciplines.

We have tried to keep the book broadly the same length as the first edition. It is inevitable that certain areas do need expansion. This is particularly so on non-motor aspects of PD where the spotlight has fallen on the neuro-psychiatry of the disease. We have an additional chapter on sleep disturbance.

Part 5 of the book on therapy and management maintains a broad approach from the generality of organising services through drug therapy and rehabilitation and surgery. Throughout the book there is an emphasis on contemporary research findings and evidence-based practice. This has been greatly helped by the publication of the NICE guidelines on the management of PD.

We were very pleased by the success of the first book. Both printings sold out and we were amused that rare copies appeared on e-bay and were offered at well over the list price. People have asked us when the next edition of the book will be published and we are most grateful that Radcliffe Publishing has undertaken this second edition.

Both of us have found that our first edition copies are worn out from frequent use and we hope that the new edition will be practical and well used by the purchasers. We hope it will be of great use to all the disciplines concerned with PD, and will benefit patients.

Jeremy Playfer and John Hindle
September 2007

Preface to first edition

Parkinson's disease (PD) is a chronic progressive neuropsychiatric disorder, which is the second most common cause of chronic neurological disability in the UK. Although PD does occur in younger people, it is predominantly a condition of the elderly.

It is increasingly recognised that PD is not simply a movement disorder, but is a multisystem neurological disorder which affects cognitive processes, emotion and autonomic function. The recent Global Parkinson's Disease Survey found that quality of life depended not only on the stage of disease and medication but also on the level of depression, satisfaction and optimism. At the Sixth International Congress of Parkinson's Disease and Movement Disorders, held in Barcelona in June 2000, many presenters confirmed that the effects of treatment on quality of life are dependent on factors other than the quality of movement. Depression, disability, postural instability and cognitive impairment have the greatest influence on quality of life in PD. PD has a marked effect on quality of life at all stages of the disease, and at all ages. Impaired quality of life and carer strain increase with advancing disease and age, and parallel increasing costs. The economic effects of PD vary according to the stage of the condition. The total costs of the condition increase with advancing age and advancing disease stage. In younger patients the greatest costs are for the drugs and loss of earnings, while in older patients the largest costs are social and long-term institutional care. These cost burdens fall on patients, carers, health and social care agencies.

Neurological services have increasingly recognised the importance of interdisciplinary working in the management of PD. Interdisciplinary working has always been at the centre of the speciality of geriatric medicine, and the importance of the involvement of physiotherapists, occupational therapists, speech therapists and other disciplines in the management of PD is well recognised. The Cochrane Systematic Review has, however, identified the requirement for more rigorous study of physiotherapy, occupational therapy and speech and language therapy in the treatment of PD. The efficacy of the PD nurse specialist in moderate disease severity has been shown in one randomised trial, and the role of these nurses in primary care is expanding.

In the UK there is a relatively small number of neurologists, but there is a large and well-developed geriatric service based on interdisciplinary teams. Geriatricians have always recognised the importance of cognition and depression in the management of many disorders, and this approach is now the focus of neurological practice in the management of PD. In the UK, the majority of patients with PD are cared for through geriatric PD services. Specialists in geriatric medicine have developed a large expertise in the management of PD, focusing particularly on the needs of elderly patients. In this book we have brought together many of the leading experts in the management of PD in the elderly in the UK. The specialist expertise of the contributors to this book is widely recognised through participation at national and international conferences, and the publication of research on aspects of PD in the elderly. In this book we provide a unique insight into the management of elderly patients suffering from PD.

John Hindle and Jeremy Playfer
February 2001

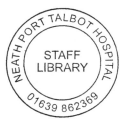

Acknowledgements

In bringing together this book we acknowledge the help and support of the British Geriatrics Society Section on Parkinson's Disease, and of the Parkinson's Disease Society of the United Kingdom. We are very grateful for the help and support given to us by the editorial and production staff at Radcliffe Publishing and for the proof reading by Pindar New Zealand. We thank all the patients and staff at the Llandudno and Liverpool Parkinson's disease clinics for their help and encouragement. We thank especially our secretaries Mrs Pauline Doran and Mrs Christine Ellis for their patience. Finally we would like to thank our families for allowing us space and time, particularly our wives Dr Catherine Hindle and Mrs Elizabeth Playfer for their tolerance.

John Hindle and Jeremy Playfer
September 2007

List of contributors

Ana Aragon
Senior Occupational Therapist
Bath

Dr Richard Brown
Department of Psychology
Institute of Psychiatry, London

Dr K Ray Chaudhuri
Regional Movement Disorders Unit
King's College Hospital, London

Dr Rosanna Cousins
Associate Professor of Health
Deanery of Science and Social Sciences
Liverpool Hope University

Dr Ann Davies
Consultant Lead Clinical Psychologist, Older Adults
Mersey Care NHS Trust;
Senior Research Fellow
School of Psychology, University of Liverpool

Janice Fiske
Guys Hospital, London

Dr Duncan Forsyth
Consultant Geriatrician
Department of Medicine for the Elderly
Addenbrooke's NHS Trust Hospital, Cambridge

Dr Mahendra Gonsalkorale
Emeritus Consultant Geriatrician
Hope Hospital, Salford

Dr Catherine Hindle
General Practitioner
Conwy

Dr John Hindle
Consultant Physician, Care of the Elderly
Llandudno Hospital

Dr Peter Hobson
University Department of Geriatric Medicine
Cardiff University (North Wales)
Glan Clwyd Hospital, Rhyl

Karen Hyland
Senior Dietician
Colindale Hospital, London

Professor Rose Anne Kenny
Head of Medical Gerontology
Trinity College of Neuroscience
University of Dublin

Andreas Kouyialis
Specialist Registrar
The Walton Centre for Neurology and Neurosurgery, Liverpool

Dr Doug MacMahon
Consultant Physician
Camborne–Redruth Hospital

Dr Graeme Macphee
Consultant Physician and Honorary Clinical Senior Lecturer
Movement Disorders Clinic and Department of Medicine for the Elderly
Southern General Hospital, Glasgow

Lizzy Marks
Department of Speech and Language Therapy
University College Hospital, London

Dr Jolyon Meara
Senior Lecturer
University Department of Geriatric Medicine
Cardiff University (North Wales)
Glan Clwyd Hospital, Rhyl

Gay Moore
Superintendent physiotherapist (retired), Bath

Maralyn Moran
Parkinson's Disease Nurse Specialist
Morriston Hospital, Swansea

Elizabeth Morgan
Parkinson's Disease Nurse Specialist
Rookwood Hospital, Llandaff

Professor Desmond O'Neill
Associate Professor
Trinity College, Dublin
Tallaght Hospital, Dublin

Dr Peter Overstall
Department of Geriatric Medicine
Hereford County Hospital

Dr Jeremy Playfer
Emeritus Consultant Geriatrician
Royal Liverpool Hospital

Dr Helen Roberts
Senior Lecturer in Geriatric Medicine
Southampton General Hospital

Dr Dorothy Robertson
Consultant, Older People's Unit
Royal United Hospital, Bath

Dr David Stewart
Consultant Physician
Medicine for the Elderly
Victoria Infirmary, Glasgow

Sue Thomas
Professional Nursing Department
Royal College of Nursing

Dr Christopher Turnbull
Consultant Geriatrician
Arrow Park Hospital, Wirral

Mr Thelekat Varma
Consultant Neurosurgeon
The Walton Centre for Neurology and Neurosurgery, Liverpool

Liz Whelan
Parkinson's Disease Nurse Specialist, Bath

PART 1

Background

A history of Parkinson's disease

JOHN HINDLE

Introduction

Symptoms suggestive of Parkinson's disease (PD) have been described for many centuries, having been found in Egyptian papyrus and Sanskrit texts and other documents in ancient times. PD was first distinguished from other causes of tremor and weakness by Dr James Parkinson in his famous paper of 1817 entitled 'An Essay on the Shaking Palsy'. In this, he defined the condition as 'involuntary tremulous motion, with lessened muscular power, in parts not in action and even when supported; with a propensity to bend the trunk forwards, and to pass from a walking to a running pace: the senses and intellect being uninjured'.[1] The history of the development of

Parkinsonism: clinical features

Unfortunately, over the next 45 years, Parkinson's treatise on the shaking palsy received little attention in England. During this period, however, Wilhelm Von Humboldt, in his letters from 1828 until his death in 1835, gave one of the clearest clinical descriptions of the condition by a patient. He described a resting tremor, akinesia, and was the first to describe micrographia. He called the problems in writing a 'special clumsiness', which he attributed to a disturbance in executing rapid complex movements. He described 'internal tremor not visible by others, which causes a distortion of the continuity of my movements'. He insisted that he was not suffering from a disease, but the effects of accelerated ageing.[9]

It was not until the 1860s that Parkinson's treatise really came to light, when the French neurologists Trousseau and then Charcot and Vulpian, working at the Salpêtrière in Paris, further elucidated the clinical features of the condition.[8] Trousseau described the use of the term *paralysis agitans* as inappropriate since 'there is no paralysis at the commencement of this strange form of chorea'. He confirmed the absence of weakness, described rigidity and proposed explanations for the festinant gait. His description of the condition as 'a strange form of chorea' was, however, wide of the mark.[10] It was Charcot's descriptions which first allowed physicians really to differentiate Parkinson's disease from other neurological disorders. Whilst acknowledging James Parkinson's original description, it is impossible to overestimate Jean–Martin Charcot's contribution to further clarifying the nature of Parkinson's disease. Charcot had difficulty acquiring a copy of Parkinson's 'Essay on the Shaking Palsy', and had his students translate it into French. Charcot referred to Parkinson's essay and stated that 'this is a descriptive and vivid definition that is correct for many cases, most in fact, and will always have the advantage over others of having been the first, but it errs by being too general'. Charcot described tremor by the frequency of movement and action associated with the tremors' greatest intensity, much as in modern neurology. He undertook many famous experiments in his lecture theatre, including one to prove that the head tremor in Parkinson's was only secondary to limb and trunk tremor, in which he tied feathers on rods to patients' heads. He clarified the observation that movement, or support, diminishes limb tremor, clearly demonstrating that he realised the importance of movement in the control of parkinsonian tremor. He also described abnormalities of bradykinesia, stance, posture and gait. Parkinson did not describe rigidity, but Charcot identified it as an important sign and differentiated it from spasticity. This emphasis on the absence of pyramidal weakness was an important advance. Charcot discarded the term *shaking palsy*, realising that there was no paralysis involved, and generously coined the term 'Parkinson's disease'.[11] Paul Richer, who was a student of Charcot's and later the head of the laboratory at the Salpetriere, drew many famous pictures of Charcot's cases (*see* Figure 1.1). He later became the Professor of Creative Anatomy at the school of fine arts, and it is through his work that we can clearly see the accuracy of Charcot's clinical descriptions.[10]

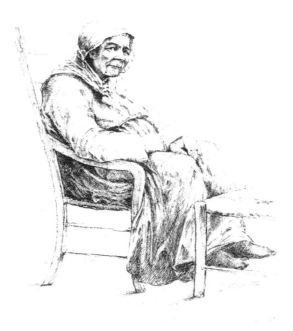

FIGURE 1.1 'Maladie de Parkinson' by Paul Richer. Illustration AP-HP/Phototheque reproduced with permission.

Psychological symptoms

Psychological symptoms were described by Charcot and British neurologists, but were thought not to be an integral part of the disorder (*see* Chapter 6). Benjamin Ball, the first Professor of the new speciality of psychiatry, in Paris, compared the mental slowing in Parkinson's disease to melancholic depression. He stated in 1882 that, 'The psychiatric complication takes the form of depression . . . accompanied by suicidal behaviour, hallucinations and stupor.'[2] Psychiatric phenomena were, however, not accepted as a part of the disorder until the early twentieth century.

Parkinsonism and neurotransmission

The cause of Parkinson's disease was still unclear, but another student of Charcot's, Edouard Brissaud, favoured the 'locus niger' as a site for the condition, based on cases in the literature and other pathological findings. In 1912 Frederick H. Lewy described inclusion bodies in the cells of the striatum and globus pallidus. A worldwide epidemic began in 1916, with some people being struck down by an illness that resembled Parkinson's disease. Constantine Von Economo, who named the disease encephalitis lethargica, recognised this condition to be caused by a virus. In 1919, Tretiakoff further confirmed abnormalities of the substantia nigra by demonstrating inflammatory lesions in encephalitis lethargica. Despite this momentous finding a hundred years after the original description, the site of Parkinson's disease was not universally accepted.[2,12]

The father of British neurology, William Gowers, working in London in 1888 published his standard text of neurology, *A Manual of Diseases of the Nervous System*. He described the symptoms of Parkinson's disease and recommended some interventions, including rest and avoidance of stress. He also recommended the use of morphia and Indian hemp, which helped the symptoms for quite a while, though it was unclear at the time why these chemicals helped.[2,12] Around the same time, in 1887, the Spanish scientist Cajal, carrying on from the work of the Italian scientist Golgi, developed a theory of interconnections between nerves cells functioning across minute spaces, which he later called synapses. Much later, in 1920, a married couple of German pioneers, Cecile and Oscar Vogt, proposed a theory of chemical connections between the striatum and other parts of the brain. In the 1930s, the German pharmacologist Otto Loewi linked these theories by developing a theory of neurotransmission, and this was supported by the British physiologist and pharmacologist Henry Dale, who observed that acetylcholine produced responses in the parasymphathetic nervous system.[12]

Pharmacotherapy: dopa and levodopa

In 1912, Funk discovered dihydroxyphenylalanine (dopa) while synthesising adrenaline. Over many years, the full chain of reactions and formation of adrenaline from tyrosine, dopa, dopamine and noradrenaline was elucidated. Hornykiewicz, working in Vienna in 1959, discovered the importance of dopamine in the basal ganglia, and described a lack of dopamine in the striatum. Working with another Viennese doctor, Walther Birkmayer, Hornykiewicz began a series of investigations into the clinical use of levodopa as a medication for parkinsonism. Together, they realised the importance of levodopa as a precursor to dopamine, and also ascertained the need for the administration of this precursor in order to penetrate through the blood–brain barrier into the brain. In 1961, they described the stunning effects of intravenous administration of levodopa on parkinsonian patients, producing a complete abolition of akinesia. Bedridden patients who were previously unable to sit up could suddenly perform all activities with ease. Difficulties were experienced in establishing correct dosage regimes. Eventually Dr George S. Cotzias, a senior scientist in Brookhaven Laboratory, in the USA, opted for gradually increasing dosages, after acclimatisation, to avoid nausea and other side effects. After reporting, in 1968, moderate to dramatic results of 26 patients, Dr Cotzias was snowed under with appeals for help.[12]

Following publication of the efficacy of levodopa, Dr Oliver Sacks, who was a staff physician at Mount Carmel Hospital in New York, utilised this drug in the treatment of patients with encephalitis lethargica, and in his book *Awakenings*, he tells the moving story of the results of treatment.[13] With increasing use of levodopa it soon became clear that the effects of treatment were not long-lasting, and problems of abnormal involuntary movements developed. Strategies to combat these difficulties included development of drugs to block the breakdown of levodopa in the blood and the use of Benserazide and Carbidopa combined with levodopa. Subsequent developments have tried to improve on the 'gold-standard' effect of levodopa and to minimise the consequence of long-term levodopa treatment.

Neurosurgery

In parallel to all the development in drug therapy, there was increasing interest in functional neurosurgery for Parkinson's disease. The first approach was open functional surgery, which included lesioning of the cortical spinal tracts and trans-ventricular surgery of the basal ganglia, but these procedures were abandoned because of high mortality.[14]

In 1888, Dr Robert H. Clark, who was a graduate from Cambridge and studied medicine at St George's Hospital, and Victor Horsley, from the University College in London, developed pioneering aseptic procedures and a stereotactic apparatus for investigation of cat cerebellum. This apparatus enabled a small probe to reach with absolute precision, by the shortest path, predetermined points within the cranium.[12] Much later in 1947, Wycis and Spiegel developed a stereotactic apparatus based on Clarke's earlier machine. They used their stereo-encephalotome to produce lesions by electrodes. It became clear that most effective lesions for the treatment of Parkinson's disease symptoms were in the thalamus and globus pallidus portion of the basal ganglia. These were replaced at the end of the 1950s by lesions in the venterolateral thalamus. A few surgeons had pioneered lesions of the subthalamic area, with favourable results, and by 1969 the results of more than 37 000 stereotactic operations had been published. Clear criteria for techniques and selection were described, and stereotactic atlases were published. At this time, levodopa became generally available and stereotactic operations declined dramatically. As a result of the shortcomings of levodopa therapy in long-term treatment, thalamotomy gradually regained its place with the reintroduction of pallidotomy by Laitinen in 1992, and then thalamic stimulation for pharmacotherapy-resistant tremor by Benabid and collaborators in 1991.[14]

Modelling the condition

In conjunction with the advances in the drug and surgical treatment of Parkinson's disease, there were major developments in modelling of the functions of the basal ganglia. Hughlings Jackson, in 1868, claimed that instability of activities of the striatum led to choreoform, or overactive, movements. Theories of the interaction between the basal ganglia and production of movement disorders were further developed by many workers, including Ramsay Hunt in the 1920–30s and Denny Brown in the 1960–70s. These led to the theory of the striatum being a clearing-house for the neurological mechanisms of voluntary movements. It became clear that the basal ganglia have an important role in control of posture and locomotion, and a major role in cognition. The single most important development in the study of models of Parkinson's disease was the discovery that methyl-phenyl-tetrahydro-pyridine

Neurochemistry

Depletion of the neurotransmitter dopamine is the main neurochemical abnormality in PD. Other neurotransmitters affected include noradrenaline, serotonin and acetylcholine, but the role of these substances is uncertain.

Almost 80% of brain dopamine is found in the striatonigral complex comprising the putamen, caudate and substantia nigra pars compacta (SNc). The SNc is the principal source of dopaminergic neurones. These project mainly to the putamen and caudate.[1] The extent of dopamine depletion in these structures correlates with neuronal loss in the SNc. In PD dopamine depletion is more evident in the putamen than caudate.[2]

In the brain, dopamine is synthesised from the amino acid tyrosine. The first step is conversion of tyrosine to L-3, 4-dihydroxyphenylalanine (L-Dopa, levodopa), catalysed by the enzyme tyrosine hydroxylase. This is the rate-limiting step in dopamine production. Levels of tyrosine hydroxylase are low in PD, which explains why tyrosine is ineffective as therapy. Levodopa is converted to dopamine by dopa decarboxylase (aromatic amine decarboxylase), and the dopamine is stored in vesicles and released by a calcium-dependent mechanism. After release, dopamine is removed from the synaptic cleft by an active re-uptake mechanism, following which it is available again for vesicular storage. Dopamine is metabolised enzymatically by both intracellular monoamine oxidase (principally MAO-B) and extracellular catechol-O-methyl transferase (COMT).[3] Homovanillic acid is the main metabolite.

Dopamine receptors

Two families of dopamine receptor have been identified: the D1 family which includes D1 and D5 receptors, and the D2 family which includes D2, D3 and D4 receptors. After binding to D1-type receptors dopamine acts via an increase in cyclic AMP, whereas the effect on D2-type receptors is to decrease cyclic AMP.[4] D2 receptors are thought to be important mediators of the therapeutic effects of pharmacological agents, while the role of D1 receptors is less clear.

Physiology of basal ganglia motor control

The defect in PD causes disruption to the dopaminergic nigrostriatal projections and interferes with function of the motor circuit of the basal ganglia. This circuit is involved in the control of both voluntary and involuntary movements. The function of the motor circuit is very complicated, and several subcircuits which interact in a complex manner (and are still poorly understood) are involved.[5] These include the interaction between the globus pallidus externa (GPe) and the subthalamic nucleus (STN), which is thought to be of particular importance. The following is a simplified version of current understanding of how motor activity is influenced by this circuit and how this function is altered in PD.

The key to understanding the function of the basal ganglia in controlling movement is the appreciation of the roles of the globus pallidus interna (GPi) and the venterolateral thalamus (VL). The VL has an excitatory output to the motor cortex and thus facilitates movement. The GPi, along with the substantia nigra pars reticulata (SNr), has an inhibitory output to VL and therefore acts as a 'brake'. This means that the effect of increased output from the GPi/SNr is to inhibit movement.

GPi receives input from the putamen via two pathways – direct and indirect. The direct pathway runs monosynaptically from putamen to GPi and its effects are inhibitory, i.e. to release the brake on movement exerted by GPi. The indirect pathway runs from the putamen via GPe and STN. STN has an excitatory effect on GPi, mediated by glutamate.[6] The effect of the indirect pathway is therefore to increase the braking on movement from GPi.

Normal dopamine release from the SNc acts on both of these pathways, direct and indirect. By acting on dopamine D1 receptors, the direct pathway is stimulated to decrease the braking effect on movement from GPi. By acting on dopamine D2 receptors, the indirect pathway is inhibited, decreasing the stimulus for GPi to exert a braking effect.[7] Normal SNc function therefore results in a low braking effect from GPi to VL and thus allows VL to facilitate movement via its excitatory effects on the motor cortex.

In PD, decreased dopamine release from SNc disrupts this mechanism. Understimulation of the direct pathway and underinhibition of the indirect pathway result in an increased inhibitory ('braking') output from GPi to VL. Thus, the excitatory effects of VL on the motor cortex are diminished and movement inhibited (*see* Figure 2.1). The important consequences of abnormal increased activity of GPi and STN on motor function are the reason these areas are important target sites for neurosurgery whether by ablation or by high-frequency stimulation.

Pathology

The pathological changes of PD include cell loss in a specific distribution, the presence of Lewy bodies in surviving cells, and an undamaged striatum (comprising putamen and caudate).

Cell loss

The main area of cell loss is in the substantia nigra (SN), although cell loss also occurs outside the SN in a widespread but specific pattern. Other areas affected include the noradrenergic locus coeruleus, the thalamus, the hypothalamus, the cholinergic nucleus basalis of Meynert, dopaminergic neurones of the ventral tegmentum, the serotonergic raphe nuclei, the limbic cortex and cerebral neocortex, and the autonomic nervous system (including sympathetic and parasympathetic ganglia and the myenteric plexus in the walls of the oesophagus and colon).[8,9]

The SN is divided into the pars reticulata and the pars compacta (SNc), the latter portion being affected predominantly. Cell loss in excess of 50% of normal levels is required for clinical symptoms to develop.[10] The SNc can be further subdivided into ventral and dorsal tiers. Cells in the dorsal tier contain more neuromelanin compared with the ventral tier. Neuromelanin is derived from the auto-oxidation of dopamine and accumulates throughout life. The increase in neuromelanin in the dorsal tier probably represents more active dopamine turnover compared with the paler ventral cells.[11]

Cell loss in the SNc in PD preferentially affects the ventral tier.[12] By death, about 23% of cells in the SNc remain compared with normal, but the surviving cells are mainly in the dorsal tier.[9] This is in contrast with normal ageing where the dorsal tier is mainly affected, the SNc showing a neuronal loss of approximately 5% per decade after the age of 40 years. The loss is greater in the dorsal tier by a ratio of over 3:1.[10] This is evidence that PD is not simply an exaggeration of the ageing process.

The pathological changes seen in PD are more active that those seen in ageing. An increase is seen in neuronal fragmentation, extraneuronal melanin and gliosis over and above that seen in age-matched controls. Six times as many neurones are being actively phagocytosed compared with controls.[13]

The functional consequence of nigral cell loss is the loss of normal nigrostriatal

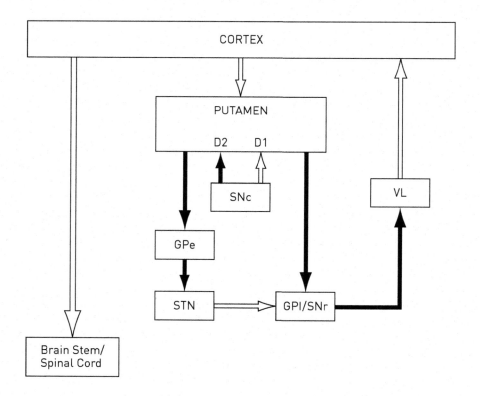

NORMAL

FIGURE 2.1 (A) The normal motor circuit. Open arrows represent excitation; solid arrows indicate inhibition. Key: SNc substantia nigra pars compacta; GPe globus pallidus externa; STN subthalamic nucleus; GPi globus pallidus interna; SNr substantia nigra pars reticulata; VL venterolateral thalamus.

innervation and the clinical features of PD. As much as 80% of dopamine may be lost in the striatum by the time that clinical symptoms emerge. By death, dopamine levels are reduced to 2% of normal in the putamen, and to 16% of normal in the caudate.[9]

The consequences of cell death in other affected areas are less well understood. It is thought that damage in the cerebral cortex, the nucleus basalis of Meynert, and the ventral tegmentum is associated with cognitive dysfunction. Although damage to the autonomic system can be linked to clinical features of autonomic failure, other factors (including antiparkinsonian medication) are relevant. The consequence of damage in other areas including the thalamus, locus coeruleus and raphe nuclei is unknown.

Despite the consequences of abnormal innervation from the SN, it is likely that no cell loss occurs in the striatum. This is in contrast to the marked striatal degeneration seen in other conditions such as multiple system atrophy (striatonigral degeneration), progressive supranuclear palsy, corticobasal degeneration and Huntington's disease.[14]

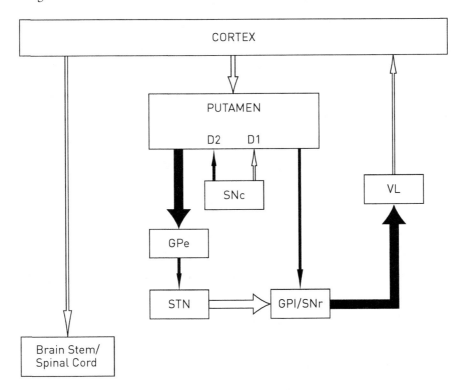

PARKINSON'S DISEASE

FIGURE 2.1 (B) The motor circuit in Parkinson's disease. Open arrows represent excitation; solid arrows indicate inhibition. Key: SNc substantia nigra pars compacta; GPe globus pallidus externa; STN subthalamic nucleus; GPi globus pallidus interna; SNr substantia nigra pars reticulata; VL venterolateral thalamus.

Aetiology

A major problem in defining aetiological factors in PD is the presence of a large amount of preclinical disease. The overall age-adjusted prevalence of ILBD is 5.6% compared with a typical prevalence of clinical PD of 0.2%.[34] ILBD is therefore many times more common than clinical disease. Most individuals with ILBD will never go on to manifest clinical PD, perhaps because they do not live long enough for this to become apparent.[22] It has been postulated that clinical PD represents the youngest 5–10% of a virtual bell-shaped distribution curve of incidence that has a maximum at an age approaching 175 years.[34] Thus, only a small percentage of individuals with PD pathology are open to study in a search for aetiological factors. Furthermore, there might be important differences in these subjects with respect to risk factors compared with the majority with ILBD.

Ageing

Advancing age is the single most important risk factor for developing PD. Prevalence rates for PD in epidemiological studies typically show an exponential increase from 1 per 1000 in the general population to as much as 2% in those over 80 years of age.[35] It is difficult to define what 'normal' ageing of the central nervous system (CNS) is. It is unclear to what extent the changes seen are physiological or represent the accumulated effects of pathological processes. Nonetheless, a number of changes are recognised to occur with ageing. These include a decrease in the numbers of pigmented neurones in the substantia nigra,[36] a decrease in striatal dopamine,[37] a decrease in striatal tyrosine hydroxylase (involved in dopamine synthesis),[38] and a decrease in dopamine receptor density.[39] As previously discussed, however, the distribution of neuronal loss within the substantia nigra is different from that seen in PD. The exact role of ageing in pathogenesis is not clear, but it does not appear that PD is caused by an exaggeration of normal ageing processes. It is likely that age-related changes combine with other pathological mechanisms to produce the clinical syndrome.[40]

Genetics

Genetic studies are difficult to carry out in PD. Evidence for a genetic role in the aetiology of PD has come from a number of sources including twin, family, case-control and epidemiological studies. Each has its problems, mainly due to the absence of a good marker for the condition and the subsequent difficulty in case ascertainment.

Genetic disease can be either single gene and Mendelian or due to a complex interaction of multiple genes in a non–Mendelian manner. The latter almost certainly accounts for the majority of genetic influence on PD, but a number of major advances have taken place in recent years in describing the role of single-gene defects in causing familial PD.

Family studies

Most patients with PD do not have a family history, and it is highly likely that non-genetic factors are important in aetiology. Nonetheless, family history is the next most important risk factor for PD after age. A positive family history can be obtained in 20–30% of patients with PD.[41] This rises to a positive history in 43% versus 9% of controls if a history of tremor alone is included.[42] Case-control studies give conflicting results with the relative risks for a first-degree relative of developing PD varying from 3.5[43] to 1.7 in a recent study.[44] In this study, relatives of younger-onset patients (<=66 years) had an increased relative risk of 2.6 with no increase in relative risk found for relatives of older-onset patients. This provides evidence of a stronger genetic component in younger-onset PD.

Twin studies

Early twin studies in PD failed to demonstrate a significantly increased concordance rate in monozygotic compared with dizygotic twins, and were interpreted as evidence that genetic factors were not relevant. The studies were potentially flawed due to the fact that PD could only be identified if it had become clinically apparent in a sibling and a failure to recognise atypical presentation, e.g. isolated tremor, as a forme fruste of PD. Later, however, the use of PET scans has demonstrated abnormal fluorodopa uptake in apparently unaffected siblings. Concordance rates of 45% in monozygotic versus 29% in dizygotic twins have been reported,[45] but the results were inconclusive. A further study, again using fluorodopa PET scanning to identify asymptomatic disease, has shown concordance rates rising to 75% in monozygotic twins compared with 22% in dizygotic twins over a seven-year follow-up period. Such evidence suggests a significant role for inheritance in the development of sporadic PD.[46] A more recent study from Sweden, however, demonstrated very low concordance rates in twins.[47] It is possible therefore, that heritability is higher for nigrostriatal dysfunction (as demonstrated by PET) but that the subsequent development of symptomatic PD depends on an environmental insult.

Epidemiology

Epidemiological studies have shown that the prevalence of PD is not uniform throughout the world. A number of studies have shown that populations moving from a low-prevalence area to one in which there is a higher prevalence of PD, gradually acquire the same prevalence as is usual in the 'host' country. For example, the prevalence of PD in Nigeria is much lower than among African-Americans in the USA, despite a fairly homogeneous genotype.[48] This is good evidence for an environmental factor in the causation of PD, but such studies must be interpreted with some caution. There are a number of possible sources of error. It is difficult to be sure of the true prevalence in the country of origin, particularly if it has poorly developed medical services. Cases of PD may not be diagnosed reliably, giving a falsely low prevalence. It is also possible that, in some cases, migrants are not typical of the population at large and do not share the same predilection to develop PD.

Single-gene defects as a cause of PD

Over the past few years a number of single-gene defects associated with parkinsonism have been described (*see* Table 2.1). Where known, the protein products of these genes have been shown variously to be associated with abnormal protein accumulation and degradation, oxidative stress and mitochondrial dysfunction. An important mechanism of cellular damage emerging from this work appears to dysfunction of the ubiquitin-proteosome system (UPS). The UPS is essential for the degradation and clearance of misfolded and redundant proteins. Proteins are 'labelled' for degradation by becoming attached to chains of the protein ubiquitin. This is a three-stage enzymatic process. The polyubiquinated protein is then cleaved by the proteosome. The proteosome is a large multi-catalytic protease and is essential for cellular function. It protects the cell against oxidative stress and and prevents the accumulation of damaged or toxic proteins.

TABLE 2.1 Single gene defects causing PD

Gene locus	Inheritance	Pathology/pathogenesis	Clinical features
PARK 1	Dominant	Alpha-synuclein mutation resulting in protein aggregation	Young onset, rapid progression. Good response to L-Dopa
PARK 2	Recessive	Parkin (ubiquitin ligase) dysfunction causes impaired protein clearance	Early onset. Mild PD symptoms
PARK 3	Dominant	Unknown	Onset in 60s
PARK 4	Dominant	Alpha-synuclein over-expression resulting in protein aggregation	Young onset, rapid progression. Typical response to L-Dopa
PARK 5	Dominant	Ubiquitin C-terminal hydrolase-L1 dysfunction causes impaired protein clearance	Typical PD phenotype with good L-Dopa response
PARK 6	Recessive	PINK 1 enzyme dysfunction leads to oxidative stress	Young onset, slow progression. Good L-Dopa response
PARK 7	Recessive	Reduced levels of DJ-1 protein increase oxidative stress	Early onset, slow progression
PARK 8	Dominant	LRRK-2 enzyme dysfunction causes impaired mitochondrial function	Most closely resembles sporadic PD
PARK 10	Dominant	Unknown	Onset 50–60 years
PARK 11	Dominant	Unknown	Late onset

In 1990, the pedigree of an Italian American family was described in which parkinsonism was inherited as an autosomal-dominant condition.[49] Clinically, the disease was consistent with idiopathic PD, but there was a tendency for an earlier age of onset and a rather more aggressive course than usual. Post-mortem studies have confirmed the presence of typical pathology with Lewy bodies. Subsequent investigations showed that the problem lay in a mutation of the α-synuclein gene on chromosome 4 [PARK 1].[50] The same mutation has subsequently been identified in three Greek families, and a second mutation in a German family.[51] The biological role of α-synuclein is unknown but it is involved in the regulation of dopamine metabolism.[52] It has been postulated that the mutation results in an abnormality in folding of the protein, causing it to accumulate.[53]

Since the report of this gene mutation, a number of groups have searched for its occurrence in kindred with familial PD. No other cases have been found in either a large European study of familial PD[54] or in a British study of sporadic PD.[55] and it is clear that the α-synuclein mutation is a very rare cause of PD.

PARK 2 is a mutation involving the gene for parkin, an ubiquitin ligase involved in the UPS. This leads to the accumulation of cellular proteins and is associated with an early-onset PD without Lewy bodies.[56] This suggests that ubiquitinisation has an important role in the formation of Lewy bodies. Other single-gene causes of PD are summarised in Table 2.1. In general terms, the recessive forms cause earlier-onset disease (typically before 40 years of age) and are more slowly progressive.[57] Of the dominant forms, the recently described PARK 8 is a mutation of the LRRK-2 gene which codes for a protein named dardarin.[58,59] It most closely resembles sporadic PD in age of onset and clinical features and appears to be the most common cause of autosomal-dominant PD yet discovered.[60]

'Candidate' gene studies

The developments in describing single-gene defects as a cause of PD have been exciting and valuable in providing clues to pathophysiology. These single-gene defects, however, do not account for the majority of sporadic cases of PD since inheritance is likely to be determined by a number of genes interacting in a complex manner. Rather than search randomly in the genome for genes associated with PD, a more rapid approach may be to use our knowledge of the pathology and factors involved in pathophysiology of PD and to target genes known to have a biological action which might be relevant – so-called 'candidate' studies. Genes involved in dopamine metabolism, oxidation reactions, detoxification, mitochondrial function, and iron metabolism have been examined, amongst others.[61] Results have been variable and no clear linkage with PD has been demonstrated.

Environmental factors

A great deal of effort has been made to identify environmental factors causing PD. Toxic substances have been found which cause a parkinsonian syndrome that is similar, but not identical, to idiopathic PD. A number of factors that appear to be associated with an increased risk of PD have also been described. It is likely that the less 'genetic' the susceptibility to PD, the more age and environment need to contribute to the development of disease.[62]

Specific toxins

Manganese causes an akinetic rigid syndrome in man, predominantly due to a toxic effect on the globus pallidum and striatum. The mechanism of this toxic action is unknown. There are clear clinical differences, however, from PD.[63] Other metals (including copper and iron) have been shown to be increased in the substantia nigra, but this is probable a secondary phenomenon and not the primary cause of PD.[41] In survivors of poisoning, carbon monoxide causes parkinsonism to develop after a few days or weeks by necrosis of the globus pallidum.[64]

The discovery that the 'designer drug' contaminant 1-methyl-4-phenyl 1, 2, 3, 6-tetrahydropyridine (MPTP) could cause an acute parkinsonian syndrome has proven to be an extremely valuable clue as to the pathogenesis of PD.[65] A number of individuals who repeatedly injected themselves with this agent developed an akinetic rigid syndrome within days, the clinical syndrome being very similar to idiopathic PD. There is a response to levodopa and typical complications of therapy (including fluctuations and dyskinesias) develop.[66] Lewy body pathology is not seen, however, and the syndrome cannot therefore be regarded as identical to idiopathic disease. MPTP is a protoxin; it is converted to the toxic metabolite 1-methyl-4-phenylpyridium ion (MPP+). This compound is taken up actively by the dopamine re-uptake system and concentrated in dopaminergic neurones. Once in the cells, MPP+ interferes with mitochondrial function and thus cellular energy production. The specific site of action is Complex 1 of the mitochondrial respiratory chain. MPP+ is also a generator of free radicals – another mechanism for neurotoxicity.[64] MPTP causes acute parkinsonism in other primates, and has permitted the development of animal models for PD.

The discovery of MPTP stimulated a search for other toxic substances in the environment as possible causes of idiopathic disease. High on the list of suspects have been pesticides and herbicides, particularly as MPP+ is chemically related to paraquat, a previously commonly used herbicide. This hypothesis would fit well with a reported increase in PD in association with rural living (see below). Against this, however, is the fact that the prevalence of PD has not risen since the widespread introduction of these chemicals.[41]

Other risk factors

A number of studies have described a relationship between rural living and the development of PD.[67,68] The evidence is contradictory, however, with other studies showing no such association.[69] A number of factors have been suggested to explain this, including well-water drinking and exposure to agricultural chemicals.

The possibility that oxidative mechanisms are relevant for the pathogenesis of PD (see below) has prompted examination of dietary factors, and an association with increased animal fat consumption has been described.[70] Antioxidants including vitamins E and C have been examined for a potentially protective role, but no clear consensus has emerged. Vitamin E supplementation is likely to have no effect on the progression of PD.[71]

Cigarette smoking has been shown repeatedly to be associated with a decreased risk of developing PD,[41] with non-smokers having generally been shown to be twice as likely to develop the disease. This effect remains even after allowing for differences in mortality. Suggested mechanisms include the fact that nicotine causes dopamine release and up-regulation of dopamine receptors, potentially masking signs of early or mild disease. Cigarette smoke contains a monoamine oxidase B (MAO-B) inhibitor.[72] This might be relevant for a number of reasons: MAO-B inhibition decreases dopamine breakdown and could therefore boost levels in the brain. Reduced free radical production associated with this action on dopamine could also protect against oxidative stress. Finally, MPTP-induced parkinsonism may be ameliorated by MAO-B inhibition by preventing conversion to MPP+.[72]

Not all studies have confirmed the protective effect of smoking. There is some doubt as to whether there is a true dose-response relationship; indeed, it has been suggested that the relationship may be the other way round, i.e. that PD might reduce smoking, perhaps due to psychological factors.[42]

Coffee drinking has also been shown to be associated with a reduced risk of developing PD.[73] The mechanism is unknown.

Pathogenesis

Apoptosis

Whatever the cause or causes of PD, it is likely that nigral cell loss occurs via a common pathophysiological pathway, leading to apoptosis (programmed cell death). Cells can die either by necrosis or apoptosis. In necrosis, an external insult is responsible for death, whereas in apoptosis cell death occurs as a result of an intracellular process regulated by genes. Apoptosis is well documented as a normal physiological process in the development of the nervous system.[74] More recently, its pathological role in neurodegenerative disorders has been recognised. The identification of apoptosis depends on finding specific morphological changes, including chromatin clumping.[75] This is technically difficult and there some controversy remains over whether apoptosis is important in PD.[76,77] There is, however, a developing consensus that changes of apoptosis can be identified in the SNc at post-mortem examination. The number of apoptotic nuclei in the SNc in PD at 2% is approximately 10-fold that seen in normal ageing.[62]

A number of processes interact to cause apoptotic cell death in the SNc in PD, including oxidative stress, mitochondrial dysfunction and excitotoxicity.

Oxidative stress

The cells of the SNc are particularly vulnerable to oxidative damage due to the presence of dopamine, neuromelanin, and high levels of iron.[62,64] Dopamine undergoes oxidative deamination (mediated by monoamine oxidase); in addition, dopamine is prone to auto-oxidation. These processes yield metabolites including hydrogen peroxide. Neuromelanin binds ferric iron, and can reduce it to its reactive ferrous form – a process which facilitates the conversion of hydrogen peroxide to oxyradicals, including the highly toxic hydroxyl radical. Other products of dopamine auto-oxidation include the superoxide radical (*see* Figure 2.2).

Increased iron levels also occur in other neurodegenerative diseases including multiple system atrophy and progressive supranuclear palsy. These conditions are also associated with cell loss in the basal ganglia. Increased iron is not seen in ILBD;

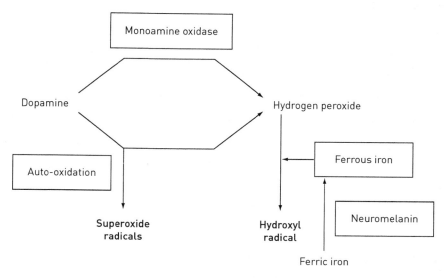

FIGURE 2.2 Oxidative mechanisms and free-radical production.

it is probable therefore that this is a secondary and late phenomenon. Nonetheless, it is might still be of importance as it could form part of the cascade leading to cell death.[64,78]

In normal cells there are a number of defence mechanisms to protect against oxidative damage, including the scavenger enzymes catalase and peroxidase. Important in this process is the presence of reduced glutathione (GSH), levels of which have been shown to be low in the substantia nigra in PD, suggesting increased free-radical generation. Low nigral glutathione levels are also found in ILBD but not in other parts of the brain or in other neurodegenerative diseases. It is possible therefore that this is an important mechanism early in the development of PD.[57,71]

There is direct evidence for oxidative damage in the substantia nigra in PD. Levels of malondialdehyde are increased, indicating increased lipid peroxidation.[79] In addition, 8-hydroxy-2-deoxyguanosine is increased, indicating oxidative damage to DNA.[80]

Mitochondrial dysfunction

Mitochondria play a crucial role in cellular energy production by generating ATP in the process of oxidative phosphorylation. The mitochondrial respiratory chain consists of five protein complexes. Complex 1 is deficient in the substantia nigra in PD by approximately 35%.[64] The deficiency is specific to Complex 1, with other proteins in the respiratory chain being unaffected. The deficiency is also site- and disease-specific; other parts of the brain appear to be unaffected and the deficiency is not found in other degenerative diseases such as multiple system atrophy which show a similar nigral cell loss.[62] A modest (20–25%) reduction in Complex 1 activity can also be demonstrated in the platelets of patients with PD,[81] though this is not sufficiently sensitive to be used as a biological marker for the condition.

It has been suggested that mitochondria may have a critical role in the sequence of events leading to apoptosis. A decrease in mitochondrial membrane potential and increased intramitochondrial calcium appear to be important early events in this process. These lead to the opening of a mitochondrial pore and the release of apoptosis-initiating factors.[62]

Mitochondrial dysfunction and oxidative stress may interact to reinforce the toxic effects of each. It is postulated that Complex-1 deficiency is associated with superoxide ion generation, increasing oxidative stress. This in turn might worsen the Complex-1 defect in a vicious spiral of toxicity.[64]

In addition, it has been noted that degradation of proteins by the ubiquitin-proteosome system (see above) requires a series of ATP-dependent peptidases. A mitochondrial respiratory chain defect will therefore impair this process.[82]

Inflammation

Inflammatory processes have also been implicated in the pathophysiology of PD with increased levels of inflammatory mediators (interleukins and TNF-α) found.[83] These stimulate the activation of microglial cells and increase nitric oxide (NO) production which further increases oxidative stress and exacerbates cellular damage. Anti-inflammatory agents are also being tested in pre-clinical studies as potential future treatments.

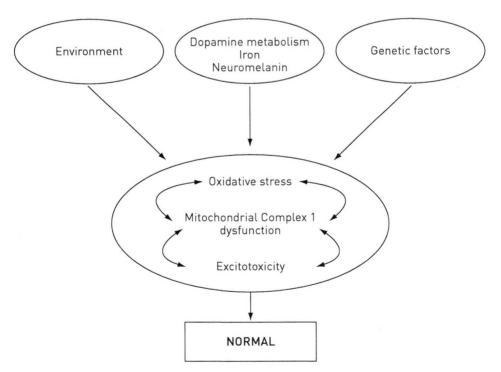

FIGURE 2.3 Pathogenesis of Parkinson's disease.

Excitotoxicity

The striatum contains widespread glutaminergic projections acting on N-methyl-D-aspartate (NMDA) receptors. Glutamate is an excitatory neurotransmitter with the potential to cause cell damage via excitotoxicity. Glutaminergic stimulation is mediated by an influx of calcium ions into the cell. If excessive, this can cause toxicity via activation of a variety of enzyme systems.[80] Normally, excessive calcium influx is blocked by magnesium ions within the receptor ion channel, this blockade being dependent on the ability of the cell to maintain a normal membrane electrical potential. This in turn is dependent on mitochondrial ATP production. Thus, mitochondrial dysfunction in PD may lead to decreased magnesium blockade and expose the nigral cells to excitotoxicity from excessive calcium influx.[84] In PD, physiological levels of glutamate stimulating the NMDA receptors might be toxic, further increasing mitochondrial damage and oxidative stress[62] (*see* Figure 2.3).

Conclusion

Ageing is an important aetiological factor which interacts with a genetic predisposition, environmental factors and pathological processes to increase a person's liability to develop PD.

REFERENCES

1 Graybiel AM, Hirsch EC, Agid Y. The nigrostriatal system in Parkinson's disease. *Adv Neurol.* 1990; **53**: 17–29.

2 Agid Y, Cervera P, Hirsch E, *et al.* Biochemistry of Parkinson's disease 28 years later: a critical review. *Mov Disord.* 1989; **4**(S): 126–44.

3 Goldstein M, Lieberman A. The role of the regulatory enzymes of chatecholamine synthesis in Parkinson's disease. *Neurology.* 1992; **42**: 8–12.

4 Calne DB. Treatment of Parkinson's disease. *N Eng J Med.* 1993; **329**(14): 1021–7.

5 Wichmann T. Physiology of the basal ganglia and pathophysiology of movement disorders of basal ganglia origin. In: Watts RL, Koller WC, editors. *Movement Disorders: neurological principles and practice.* New York: McGraw-Hill; 1997: 87–97.

6 Greenberg DA. Glutamate and Parkinson's disease. *Ann Neurol.* 1994; **35**: 639.

7 Gerfen CR, Engber TM, Mahan LC, *et al.* D1 and D2 dopamine receptor-regulated gene expression of striatonigral and striatopallidal neurons. *Science.* 1990; **250**(4986): 1429–32.

8 Gibb WRG, Lees AJ. Pathological clues to the cause of Parkinson's disease. In: Marsden CD, Fahn S, editors. *Movement Disorders.* Oxford: Butterworth-Heinemann; 1994: 147–66.

9 Gibb WRG. Functional neuropathology in Parkinson's disease. *Eur Neurol.* 1997; **38**(Suppl 2): 21–5.

10 Fearnley JM, Lees AJ. Aging and Parkinson's disease: substantia nigra regional selectivity. *Brain.* 1991; **114**: 2283–301.

11 Gibb WRG. Neuropathology of the substantia nigra. *Eur Neurol.* 1991; **31**(Suppl 1): 48–59.

12 Gibb WRG, Lees AJ. Anatomy, pigmentation, ventral and dorsal subpopulations of the substantia nigra, and differential cell death in Parkinson's disease. *J Neurol Neurosurg Psychiatry.* 1991; **54**: 388–96.

13 McGeer PL, Itgaki S, Akiyama H, *et al.* Rate of cell death in parkinsonism indicates active neuropathological process. *Ann Neurol.* 1988; **24**: 574–6.

14 Oertel WH, Hartmann A. The pathology of Parkinson's disease and its differentiation from other parkinsonian disorders. In: LeWitt PA, Oertel WH, editors. *Parkinson's Disease: the treatment options.* London: Martin Dunitz; 1999: 11–20.

15 Braak H, Del Tredici K, Rub U, *et al.* Staging of brain pathology related to sporadic Parkinson's disease. *Neurobiol Aging.* 2003; **24**(2): 197–211.

16 Ponsen MM, Stoffers D, Booij J, *et al.* Idiopathic hyposmia as a preclinical sign of Parkinson's disease. [See comment]. *Ann Neurol.* 2004; **56**(2): 173–81.

17 Braak H, Rub U, Jansen Steur EN, *et al.* Cognitive status correlates with neuropathologic stage in Parkinson disease. *Neurology.* 2005; **64**(8): 1404–10.

18 Lennox GG, Lowe JS. Dementia with Lewy bodies. In: Quinn NP, editor. *Bailliere's Clinical Neurology: Parkinsonism.* London: Bailliere Tindall; 1997: 147–66.

19 Spillantini MG, Crowther RA, Jakes R, *et al.* Alpha-Synuclein in filamentous inclusions of Lewy bodies and Lewy neurites from Parkinson's disease and dementia with Lewy bodies. *Proc Natl Acad Sci USA.* 1998; **95**(11): 6469–73.

20 Lowe JS. Lewy bodies. In: Calne DB, editor. *Neurodegerative Diseases.* Philadelphia: WB Saunders; 1994: 51–69.

21 Harrower TP, Michell AW, Barker RA. Lewy bodies in Parkinson's disease: protectors or perpetrators? [comment]. *Exp Neurol.* 2005; **195**(1): 1–6.

22 Gibb WRG, Lees AJ. The relevance of the Lewy body to the pathogenesis of idiopathic Parkinson's disease. *J Neurol Neurosurg Psychiatry.* 1988; **51**: 745–52.

23 McKeith I, Mintzer J, Aarsland D, *et al.* Dementia with Lewy bodies. *Lancet Neurol.* 2004; **3**(1): 19–28.

24 Perl DP, Olanow CW, Calne DB. Alzheimer's disease and Parkinson's disease: distinct entities or extremes of a spectrum of neurodegeneration? *Ann Neurol.* 1998; **44**(Suppl 1): S19–S31.

25 Aarsland D, Tandberg E, Larsen JP, *et al.* Frequency of dementia in Parkinson's disease. *Arch Neurol.* 1996; **53**: 538–42.

26 Lieberman A, Dziatolowsky M, Kupersmith M, *et al.* Dementia in Parkinson disease. *Ann Neurol.* 1979; **6**(4): 335–9.

27 Molsa PK, Martilla RJ, Rinne UK. Extrapyramidal signs in Alzheimer's disease. *Neurology.* 1984; **34**: 1114–6.

28 Boller F, Mizutani T, Roessmann U, *et al.* Parkinson disease, dementia and Alzheimer disease: clinicopathological correlations. *Ann Neurol.* 1980; **7**(329): 335.

29 Hakim AM, Mathieson G. Dementia in Parkinson disease: a neuropathologic study. *Neurology.* 1979; **29**: 1209–14.

30 Hulette C, Mirra S, Wilkinson W, *et al.* The consortium to establish a registry for Alzheimer's disease (CERAD). Part IX. A prospective cliniconeuropathologic study of Parkinson's features in Alzheimer's disease. *Neurology.* 1995; **45**: 1991–5.

31 Leverenz J, Sumi SM. Parkinson's disease in patients with Alzheimer's disease. *Arch Neurol.* 1986; **43**: 662–4.

32 Rajput AH, Uitti RJ, Sudhakar S, *et al.* Parkinsonism and neurofibrillary tangle pathology in pigmented nuclei. *Ann Neurol.* 1989; **25**: 602–6.

33 Giasson BI, Forman MS, Higuchi M, *et al.* Initiation and synergistic fibrillization of tau and alpha-synuclein. *Science.* 2003; **300**(5619): 636–40.

34 Golbe LI. The epidemiology of Parkinson's disease. In: LeWitt PA, Oertel WH, editors. *Parkinson's Disease: the treatment options.* London: Martin Dunitz; 1999: 63–78.

35 Mutch WJ, Dingwall-Fordyce I, Downie AW, *et al.* Parkinson's disease in a Scottish city. *BMJ.* 1986; **292**: 534–6.

36 McGeer PL, McGeer EG, Suzuki JS. Aging and extrapyramidal function. *Arch Neurol.* 1977; **34**: 33–5.

37 Kish SJ, Shannak K, Rajput A, *et al*. Aging produces a specific pattern of striatal dopamine loss: implications for the etiology of idiopathic Parkinson's disease. *J Neurochem*. 1992; **58**(2): 642–8.
38 Cote LJ, Kremzner LT. Biochemical changes in normal aging in human brain. In: Mayeux R, Rosen WG, editors. *The Dementias*. Advances in Neurology, Vol. 38. New York: Raven Press; 1983: 19–30.
39 Wagner HN. Quantitative imaging of neuroreceptors in the living human brain. *Semin Nucl Med*. 1986; **16**: 51–62.
40 Samii A, Calne DB. Research into the etiology of Parkinson's disease. In: LeWitt PA, Oertel WH, editors. *Parkinson's Disease: the treatment options*. London: Martin Dunitz; 1999: 229–43.
41 Veldman BAJ, Wijn AM, Knoers N, *et al*. Genetic and environmental risk factors in Parkinson's disease. *Clin Neurol Neurosurg*. 1998; **100**(1): 15–26.
42 Bonifati V, Fabrizio E, Vanacore N, *et al*. Familial Parkinson's disease: a clinical genetic analysis. *Can J Neurol Sci*. 1995; **22**(4): 272–9.
43 Wood N. Genetic aspects of parkinsonism. In: Quinn NP, editor. *Bailliere's Clinical Neurology: Parkinsonism*. London: Bailliere Tindall; 1997: 37–53.
44 Rocca WA, McDonnell SK, Strain KJ, *et al*. Familial aggregation of Parkinson's disease: the Mayo Clinic family study. *Ann Neurol*. 2004; **56**(4): 495–502.
45 Burn DJ, Mark MH, Playford ED, *et al*. Parkinson's disease in twins studied with 18F-DOPA and positron emission tomography. *Neurology*. 1992; **42**(10): 1894–1900.
46 Piccini P, Burn DJ, Ceravolo R, *et al*. The role of inheritance in sporadic Parkinson's disease: evidence from a longitudinal study of dopaminergic function in twins. *Ann Neurol*. 1999; **45**: 577–82.
47 Wirdefeldt K, Gatz M, Schalling M, *et al*. No evidence for heritability of Parkinson disease in Swedish twins. [See comment]. *Neurology*. 2004; **63**(2): 305–11.
48 Schoenberg BS, Osuntokun BO, Adeuja AO, *et al*. Comparison of the prevalence of Parkinson's disease in black populations in the rural United States and in rural Nigeria: door-to-door community studies. *Neurology*. 1988; **38**: 645–6.
49 Golbe LI, Di Iorio G, Bonavita V, *et al*. A large kindred with autosomal dominant Parkinson's disease. *Ann Neurol*. 1990; **27**(3): 276–82.
50 Polymeropoulis MH, Lavedan C, Leroy E, *et al*. Mutation in the α-synuclein gene identified in families with Parkinson's disease. *Science*. 1997; **276**(5321): 2045–7.
51 Krüger R, Kuhn W, Müller T, *et al*. Ala30Pro mutation in the gene encoding α-synuclein in Parkinson's disease. *Nat Genet*. 1998; **18**(2): 106–8.
52 Perez RG, Waymire JC, Lin E, *et al*. A role for alpha-synuclein in the regulation of dopamine biosynthesis. *J Neurosci*. 2002; **22**(8): 3090–9. [Erratum appears in *J Neurosci*. 2002; **22**(20): 9142].
53 Spillantini MG, Schmidt ML, Lee VM-Y, *et al*. α-Synuclein in Lewy bodies. *Nature*. 1997; **388**: 839–40.
54 Vaughan J, Durr A, Tassin J, *et al*. The alpha-synuclein Ala53Thr mutation is not a common cause of familial Parkinson's disease: a study of 230 European cases. European Consortium on Genetic Susceptibility in Parkinson's Disease. *Ann Neurol*. 1998; **44**(2): 270–3.
55 Warner TT, Schapira AHV. The role of the α-synuclein gene mutation in patients with sporadic Parkinson's disease in the United Kingdom. *J Neurol Neurosurg Psychiatry*. 1998; **65**: 378–9.
56 Hofer A, Gasser T. New aspects of genetic contributions to Parkinson's disease. *Journal of Molecular Neuroscience*. 2004; **24**(3): 417–24.
57 Gasser T. Genetics of Parkinson's disease. [Review] [67 refs]. *Curr Opin Neurol*. 2005; **18**(4): 363–9.
58 Zimprich A, Biskup S, Leitner P, *et al*. Mutations in LRRK2 cause autosomal-dominant parkinsonism with pleomorphic pathology. [See comment]. *Neuron*. 2004; **44**(4): 601–7.
59 Paisan-Ruiz C, Jain S, Evans EW, *et al*. Cloning of the gene containing mutations that cause PARK8-linked Parkinson's disease. [See comment]. *Neuron*. 2004; **44**(4): 595–600.

60 Gilks WP, Abou-Sleiman PM, Gandhi S, *et al.* A common LRRK2 mutation in idiopathic Parkinson's disease. [See comment]. *Lancet.* 2005; **365**(9457): 415–6.

61 Huang Y, Cheung L, Rowe D, *et al.* Genetic contributions to Parkinson's disease. [Review] [300 refs]. *Brain Res Brain Res Rev.* 2004; **46**(1): 44–70.

62 Marsden CD, Olanow CW. The causes of Parkinson's disease are being unraveled and rational neuroprotective therapy is close to reality. *Ann Neurol.* 1998; **44**(Suppl 1): S189–S196.

63 Calne DB, Chu NS, Huang CC, *et al.* Manganism and idiopathic Parkinsonism: similarities and differences. *Neurology.* 1994; **44**: 1583–6.

64 Schapira AHV. Pathogenesis of Parkinson's disease. In: Quinn NP, editor. *Bailliere's Clinical Neurology: Parkinsonism.* London: Bailliere Tindall; 1997: 15–36.

65 Langston JW, Ballard P, Tetud JW, *et al.* Chronic parkinsonism in humans due to a product of meperidine analog synthesis. *Science.* 1983; **219**: 979–80.

66 Langston JW, Ballard P. Parkinsonism induced by 1-methyl-4-phenyl 1, 2, 3, 6 tetrahydropyridine: implications for treatment and the pathophysiology of Parkinson's disease. *Can J Neurol Sci.* 1999; **11**: 160–5.

67 Rajput AH, Uitti RJ, Stern W, *et al.* Geography, drinking water, chemistry, pesticides and herbicides and the etiology of Parkinson's disease. *Can J Neurol Sci.* 1987; **14**: 414–8.

68 Svenson LW, Platt GH, Woodhead SE. Geographic variations in the prevalence rates of Parkinson's disease in Alberta. *Can J Neurol Sci.* 1993; **20**: 307–11.

69 Jimenez-Jimenez FJ, Mateo D, Gimenez-Roldan S. Exposure to well water and pesticides in Parkinson's disease: a case control study in the Madrid area. *Mov Disord.* 1992; **7**: 149–52.

70 Logroscino G, Marder K, Cote L, *et al.* Dietary lipids and antioxidants in Parkinson's disease: a population-based case-control study. *Ann Neurol.* 1996; **39**: 89–94.

71 Parkinson Study Group. Effects of tocopherol and deprenyl on the progression of disablity in early Parkinson's disease. *N Eng J Med.* 1993; **328**: 176–83.

72 Yong VW, Perry TL. Monoamine oxidase B, smoking and Parkinson's disease. *J Neurol Sci.* 1986; **72**: 265–72.

73 Ascherio A, Zhang SM, Hernan MA, *et al.* Prospective study of caffeine consumption and risk of Parkinson's disease in men and women. *Ann Neurol.* 2001; **50**(1): 56–63.

74 Raff MC, Barres BA, Burne JF, *et al.* Programmed cell death and the control of cell survival: lessons from the nervous system. *Science.* 1993; **262**(5134): 695–700.

75 Burke RE. Programmed cell death and Parkinson's disease. *Mov Disord.* 1998; **13**(Suppl 1): 17–23.

76 Hirsch E, Hunot S, Faucheux B, *et al.* Dopaminergic neurons degenerate by apoptosis in Parkinson's disease. *Mov Disord.* 1998; **2**: 383–4.

77 Banati RB, Blunt S, Graeber MB. What does apoptosis have to do with Parkinson's disease? *Mov Disord.* 1998; **2**: 384–5.

78 Jenner P. Oxidative mechanisms in nigral cell death in Parkinson's disease. *Mov Disord.* 1998; **13**(Suppl 1): 24–34.

79 Dexter DT, Carter CJ, Wells FR, *et al.* Basal lipid peroxidation in substantia nigra is increased in Parkinson's disease. *J Neurochem.* 1989; **52**: 381–9.

80 Ahlskog JE. Neuroprotective strategies in the treatment of Parkinson's disease: clinical evidence. In: LeWitt PA, Oertel WH, editors. *Parkinson's Disease: the treatment options.* London: Martin Dunitz; 1999: 93–115.

81 Schapira AHV. Evidence for mitochondrial dysfunction in Parkinson's disease: a critical appraisal. *Mov Disord.* 1994; **9**: 125–38.

82 Schapira AH. Disease modification in Parkinson's disease. *Lancet Neurol.* 2004; **3**(6): 362–8.

83 Hong JS. Inflammation in the pathogenesis of Parkinson's disease: models, mechanisms and therapeutic interventions. *Ann NY Acad Sci.* 2005; **1053**(1): 151–2.

84 Beal MF. Does impairment of energy metabolism result in excitotoxic neuronal death in neurodegenerative illness? *Ann Neurol.* 1992; **31**: 119–30.

3

Epidemiology of Parkinson's disease

JOLYON MEARA AND PETER HOBSON

Introduction

Parkinson's disease (PD) is the second commonest neurodegenerative disorder and very much a disease of older age. There are several features of PD that limit the usefulness of a traditional epidemiological approach to this condition. Firstly, PD is a rare sporadic disorder, at least outside the extremes of old age, with a long pre-clinical stage and often a lengthy clinical stage of mild disease before medical presentation. Secondly, there is no diagnostic test for PD and accurate classification still relies on clinical examination to determine a state of clinically probable PD and ultimately neuropathological examination of the brain to make a diagnosis of clinically confirmed PD. Very few clinico-pathological studies have been published and there is even debate about whether a gold-standard neuropathology for PD actually exists. The situation is further complicated by the fact that PD is much more likely to be a syndrome than a disease. The causes of PD remain unknown though the disease probably results from an interaction involving environmental exposures, the ageing brain and susceptibility genes. Potentially valuable insights into the mechanisms behind PD (mitochondrial dysfunction, oxidative stress, protein mishandling) will, it is hoped, emerge from large prospective cohort studies linking relevant environmental exposures to known genetic profiles.

Diagnosis of PD

The diagnosis of PD relies on the clinical history and examination. Most modern epidemiological studies now employ the PD Brain Bank Clinical Diagnostic Criteria to diagnose PD.[1,2] Diagnosis based on these criteria requires the presence of at least two or more of the cardinal signs of parkinsonism (akinesia, tremor, rigidity and postural imbalance), the absence of clinical features suggesting a different type of parkinsonism (exclusion criteria), and the presence of positive supportive clinical features for the diagnosis of PD. An asymmetric onset of parkinsonism, the presence of a typical pill-rolling tremor in the hand and an excellent response to levodopa treatment are still the best indications that PD is the correct diagnosis. The response to levodopa treatment is not always easy to ascertain even from clinical observation, let alone case note analysis and, of course, requires a period of time to determine. The assessment of levodopa responsiveness may also necessitate drug withdrawal and subsequent re-examination, all of which is time consuming and raises many practical and ethical issues for epidemiological study.

The diagnostic accuracy of clinical criteria based on clinico-pathological studies depends critically on the expertise of the individual applying the criteria, the type of population studied (specialised clinics and services will tend to attract clinically atypical cases), and the sensitivity and specificity of the criteria employed. In expert hands, studies indicate that at death a diagnosis of PD is confirmed pathologically in around 80–90% of cases.[2] As diagnostic criteria become more complicated and precise, specificity is improved at the expense of sensitivity, as true but atypical cases will be misclassified. How well clinical diagnostic criteria perform in large populations at clinical presentation, in early disease or in subjects detected by screening but not previously medically diagnosed is unknown. At the time of diagnosis, diagnostic accuracy will be much less than later after some years of clinical history is available. Long-term prospective studies will enable the presumed initial diagnosis to be regularly reviewed. Neuroimaging with single-photon emission CT (SPECT) scanning is now useful to diagnose neurodegeneration of the nigrostriatal tract though is still too expensive, invasive and time consuming to be useful in large epidemiological studies.[3] Imaging with magnetic resonance scans and positron emission tomography can also help to differentiate PD from other forms of parkinsonism though again this approach has little current application in epidemiological studies.[4]

Descriptive epidemiology of PD

The descriptive epidemiology of PD is now fairly well established in many populations around the world.[5,6] Differences between study populations, case-finding techniques and the diagnostic criteria employed make the comparison of many published studies very difficult. Recent studies have tended to minimise these difficulties by using a more standardised methodology. Community populations are generally preferred, in-person screening is used and results are reported standardised to a 'reference' population.

The prevalence of PD, which reflects incidence as well as differential survival, appears to be fairly uniform around the world.[5] The reported lower prevalence in Africa[7] and the Far East[5] may be due to differences in demographic structure and methodology between studies. The EUROPARKINSON study showed that the prevalence of PD was very similar across Europe with rates of 0.6% for those aged 65–69 years of age, 3.5% for those aged 85–89, giving an overall prevalence rate of 1.6% for those over 65 years of age.[6] Some studies report a slightly higher prevalence in men, which may be attributable to a neuroprotective effect of oestrogen, but could simply reflect survival and diagnostic bias. Prevalence rates are highest in door-to-door screening studies using in-person examination as around 20–40% of cases of prevalent PD are medically undiagnosed.[8,9,10] Prevalence studies using other methods of case ascertainment are subject to bias as a result of selective mortality and poor access to health services delaying or preventing diagnosis. Such factors may account for the apparent lower prevalence of PD in certain ethnic groups.[11] Geographical variation in the prevalence of PD in terms of urban vs. rural living may again reflect methodological bias.[12,13]

In terms of case ascertainment, screening questionnaires are undoubtedly useful as a first-stage procedure in large population studies.[14,15] However, the use of anti-parkinsonian drug prescription[16,17] and death certification alone do not appear to be sound methods of case ascertainment.[18] Self-report of PD as a case-finding technique in large prospective cohorts may be useful as a screening tool but on its own is poorly specific for a neuropathological diagnosis of PD.[19]

Incidence studies are hard and laborious to undertake but provide much better information than prevalence rates on the occurrence and risk of PD. Age-specific incidence of PD again shows a very strong age-associated risk that increases into extreme old age in studies that have used community based in-person screening methodologies.[20] Incidence rates for PD are between 8 and 18 per 100 000 person years and tend to be higher in men than women.[21,22] The incidence of PD does not appear to have altered much over time.[23]

Mortality is increased by PD and may be particularly evident for late-onset disease with reported mortality hazard ratios of between 1.5 and 2.7.[24,25] Reduced life expectancy appears to be strongly linked to the development of dementia.[26,27] Our own prospective study of a community-based cohort of PD patients compared with age- and sex-matched controls clearly demonstrates that despite best modern treatment, mortality in PD is greater than in a control group[27] (see Figure 3.1). In this study dementia was a strongly predictive risk factor for mortality, as were age and disease severity. The effect of dementia can be seen by comparing the survival curves of patients with and without dementia at baseline (see Figures 3.1 and 3.2).

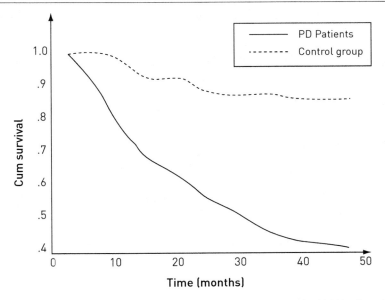

FIGURE 3.1 Kaplan–Meier survival estimates for PD patients (solid line) and controls (broken line) at baseline (PD n =166; controls n = 106).

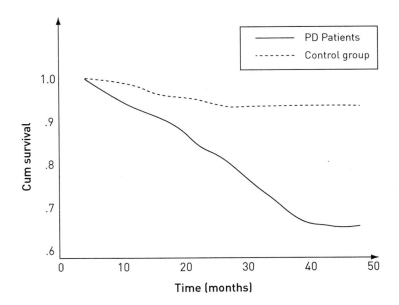

FIGURE 3.2 Kaplan–Meier survival estimates for PD patients who were not demented at baseline (solid line) and controls (broken line) (PD n =86; controls n = 102).

Comorbidity is an important aspect of PD especially for geriatricians and has been evaluated in a small number of studies.[28,29,30] The causes of hospitalisation in a large cohort of subjects with parkinsonism indicate the burden of respiratory infection, psychosis, hip fractures and urinary tract infections.[31]

Risk factors for PD

Generally, sporadic PD is now thought to result from the interaction of critical exposure to environmental agents with susceptibility genes present in individuals at increased risk of the disease. Increased age is the most powerful risk factor for PD. How this is expressed in terms of disease causation is unknown, though clearly may involve ageing processes in the nervous system, increased action of susceptibility genes and longer exposure to environmental agents. The other known risk factors, both genetic and environmental, are likely to explain only a very small proportion of sporadic PD.

Environmental risk factors

Effective evaluation of risk factors requires an approach based on large cohort studies followed up over long periods of time to allow for a significant number of incident cases to be recorded with many person years of follow-up. The measurement of exposure to relevant factors in the diet or environment is a complex issue. The 'window' of exposure to certain factors may be critical in terms of developing disease. It is assumed that the start of nigrostriatal cell death is at least six years before clinical signs develop and therefore exposure to putative risk factors may need to be considered some time before this. How exposure to risk factors is best assessed is also complex and may need to include measures of the total, the duration and the intensity of exposure. Biological models of animal disease, particularly the zebrafish, can help test hypotheses of disease causation that can subsequently be investigated in such studies. This has still to be achieved for PD and most evidence on risk factors is based on small, often retrospective case-control studies.

The most robust finding relating to risk factors in PD appears to be the protective effect of smoking. A large meta-analysis of case-control and cohort studies has shown a relative risk of PD of 0.51 in ever smokers and 0.35 for current smokers.[32] The effect of smoking is likely to be due either to nicotine enhancing dopaminergic transmission or to reduced addictive behaviour seen in PD due to brain dopamine deficiency. Coffee drinking, particularly in men, may also be protective against developing PD (relative risk 0.45–0.89 in five population-based studies), reflecting the dopaminergic effects of caffeine.[33]

Following from the MPTP story, intense efforts were made to link pesticide exposure to increased risk of PD. Subsequently several, but not all, case-control studies showed an increased risk of PD in subjects handling pesticides and this was confirmed by a meta-analysis.[34] Other occupational risks such as manganese exposure in welders is currently under investigation.[35] Dietary factors have been investigated in case-control studies though no clear-cut picture has yet emerged. Dietary intake, not to mention subsequent absorption of nutrients, is difficult to assess accurately. The classic dietary antioxidants have not shown any particularly protective effect in prospective studies.[36]

Genetic risk factors

Although comparisons of concordance rates in mono- and dizygotic twin studies appeared to indicate little genetic risk for PD, these studies were flawed and inconclusive.[37,38] A more recent twin study has shown significant increased genetic risk of developing early-onset PD before the age of 50 years.[39] Studies based on community populations have shown an elevated risk of PD of around three times in those with a first-degree relative affected by the condition.[40,41] These studies are probably identifying the effect of susceptibility genes, which today are largely still unknown. A considerable number of genes and polymorphisms have been evaluated in small studies of PD patients and controls looking for significant associations but to date these have been inconclusive.

Monogenic mutations in several genes have been described that lead to autosomal-dominant and recessive parkinsonism (and other neurological features in some cases) and a nomenclature of the PARK genes (PARK1 to PARK12) has been developed. Three excellent reviews have recently been published in this field.[42,43,44] Generally, gene mutations lead to early-onset parkinsonism with variable rates of progression and levodopa responsiveness. Some mutations, particularly PARK1 (alpha-synuclein), PARK3, PARK5, PARK6 (PINK1), PARK8 (LLRK2) and PARK10, clinically resemble sporadic PD though of the gene mutations for which the neuropathology has been reported thus far, Lewy bodies have only been found in PARK1 and PARK3. The PARK8 mutation, which can lead to late-onset levodopa-responsive parkinsonism, is caused by nigral degeneration with variable presence of Lewy bodies. The PARK2 (parkin) mutation leads to early onset, slowly progressive disease with dystonia. Around 10% of apparently sporadic PD, especially if of early onset, may be due to monogenic causes. What is unknown is how these genes relate to the usual later-onset sporadic PD. Lewy bodies are found in all cases of PARK1 and variably in PARK2 and PARK8. Sporadic PD is most likely, if at all related to these genes, to be linked with the dominant genes PARK 1 and PARK8, the protein products being alpha-synuclein and dardarin respectively. A final common pathway for various forms of PD may be a failure of the ubiquitin-proteasome system.[45] Interestingly, not all subjects with PARK mutations develop parkinsonism, indicating that these mutations are necessary but not always sufficient for the development of familial parkinsonism. Other factors, possibly both genetic and environmental appear to be important in the pathogenesis of familial parkinsonism in some situations.

Conclusion

PD is clearly a heterogeneous condition that is distributed widely throughout the world. Age is the most significant risk factor with perhaps as many as 4% of very elderly people developing parkinsonism. Differences in prevalence and incidence based on geography and ethnicity may be more artificial than real. Mortality is significantly increased in older subjects and appears to be linked to the development of dementia. There is a considerable burden of co-morbidity in older people with PD. Apart from age, smoking, caffeine consumption and exposure to pesticides other risk factors have not yet been described. Genetic factors in the form of susceptibility genes are important in the aetiology of PD and monogenetic forms of familial parkinsonism may be relevant to a minority of early-onset PD. Although some way in the future, the study of the function of alpha-synuclein and dardarin may lead to a better understanding of the cause of PD and to novel therapeutic advances.

REFERENCES

1 Hughes AJ, Daniel SE, Blankson S, *et al*. Accuracy of clinical diagnosis of idiopathic Parkinson's disease: a clinicopathological study of 100 cases. *J Neurol Neurosurg Psychiatry*. 1992; **55**: 181–4.

2 Litvan I, Bhatia KP, Burn DJ, *et al*. Movement Disorders Society Scientific Issues Committee report: SIC Task Force appraisal of clinical diagnostic criteria for Parkinsonian disorders. *Mov Disord*. 2003; **18**: 467–86.

3 Benamer TS, Patterson J, Grosset DG, *et al*. Accurate differentiation of parkinsonism and essential tremor using visual assessment of I123-FP-CIT SPECT imaging: the I123-FP-CIT study group. *Mov Disord*. 2000; **15**: 503–10.

4 Piccini P, Brooks DJ. New developments of brain imaging for Parkinson's disease and related disorders. *Mov Disord*. 2006; **12**: 2035–41.

5 Zhang Z-X, Roman GC. Worldwide occurrence of Parkinson's disease: an updated review. *Neuroepidemiol*. 1993; **12**: 195–08.

6 de Rijk MC, Tzourio C, Breteler MM, *et al*. Prevalence of parkinsonism and Parkinson's disease in Europe: the EUROPARKINSON Collaborative Study. *J Neurol Neurosurg Psychiatry*. 1997; **62**: 10–15.

7 Okubadejo NU, Bower JH, Rocca WA, *et al*. Parkinson's disease in Africa: a systematic review of epidemiologic and genetic studies. *Mov Disord*. 2006; **21**: 2150–6.

8 Tison F, Dartigues JF, Dubes L, *et al*. Prevalence of Parkinson's disease in the elderly: a population study in Gironde, France. *Acta Neurol Scand*. 1994; **90**: 111–5.

9 Morgante L, Rocca WA, Di Rosa AE, *et al*. Prevalence of Parkinson's disease and other types of parkinsonism: a door-to-door survey in three Sicilian municipalities. *Neurology*. 1992; **42**: 1901–7.

10 Claveria LE, Duarte J, Sevillano MD, *et al*. Prevalence of Parkinson's disease in Cantalejo Spain: a door-to-door survey. *Mov Disord*. 2002; **17**: 242–9.

11 Mayeux R, Marder K, Cote LJ, *et al*. The frequency of idiopathic Parkinson's disease by age, ethnic group, and sex in northern Manhatten, 1988–1993. *Am J Epidemiol*. 1995; **142**: 820–7.

12 Shrag A, Ben-Shlomo Y, Quinn N. How valid is the clinical diagnosis of Parkinson's disease in the community? *J Neurol Neurosurg Psychiatry*. 2002; **73**: 529–34

13 Hobson JP, Gallagher J, Meara RJ. A cross-sectional survey of Parkinson's disease and parkinsonism in a rural area of the United Kingdom. *Mov Disord*. 2005; **20**: 995–8.

14 Mutch WJ, Dingwall-Fordyce I, Downie AW, *et al*. Parkinson's disease in a Scottish city. *BMJ*. 1986; **292**: 534–6.

15 Meara RJ, Bisarya S, Hobson JP. Screening in primary health care for undiagnosed tremor in an elderly population in Wales. *J Epid Comm Health*. 1997; **51**: 574–5.

16 Meara RJ, Bhowmick BK, Hobson JP. Accuracy of diagnosis in patients with presumed Parkinson's disease in a community-based register. *Age and Ageing*. 1999; **28**: 99–102.

17 Bertoni JM, Sprenkle PM, Strickland D, *et al.* Evaluation of Parkinson's disease in entrants on the Nebraska State Parkinson's Disease Registry. *Mov Disord.* 2006; **10**: 1623–6.

18 Pressley JC, Tang MX, Marder K, *et al.* Disparities in the recording of Parkinson's disease on death certificates. *Mov Disord.* 2005; **20**: 315–21.

19 Foltynie T, Matthews FE, Ishihara L, *et al.* The frequency and validity of self-reported diagnosis of Parkinson's disease in the UK elderly: MRC CFAS cohort. *BMC Neurology.* 2006; **6**: 29.

20 de Lau LM, Giesbergen PC, de Rijk MC, *et al.* Incidence of parkinsonism and Parkinson disease in a general population: the Rotterdam Study. *Neurology.* 2004; **63**: 1240–4.

21 Benito-Leon J, Bermejo-Pareja F, Morales-Gonzalez JM, *et al.* Incidence of Parkinson disease and parkinsonism in three elderly populations in central Spain. *Neurology.* 2004; **62**: 734–41.

22 Twelves D, Perkins KSM, Counsell C. Systematic review of incidence studies of Parkinson's disease. *Mov Disord.* 2003; **18**: 19–31.

23 Rajput AH, Offord KP, Beard CM, *et al.* Epidemiology of parkinsonism: incidence, classification, and mortality. *Ann Neurol.* 1984; **16**: 278–82.

24 Hely MA, Morris JG, Traficante R, *et al.* The Sydney multicentre study of Parkinson's disease: progression and mortality at 10 years. *J Neurol Neurosurg Psychiatry.* 1999; **67**: 300–07.

25 Guttmann M, Slaughter PM, Theriault ME, *et al.* Parkinsonism in Ontario: increased mortality compared with controls in a large cohort study. *Neurology.* 2001; **57**: 2278–82.

26 de Lau LM, Schipper CMA, Hofman A, *et al.* Prognosis of Parkinson disease: risk of dementia and mortality: the Rotterdam Study. *Arch Neurol.* 2005; **62**: 1265–9.

27 Hobson JP, Meara RJ. Survival in a community-based cohort of Parkinson's disease patients compared to age/sex matched controls. *Age and Ageing.* 2006; **35** suppl 3: i57 (e-pub).

28 Ben-Shlomo Y, Marmot MG. Survival and cause of death in a cohort of patients with parkinsonism: possible clues to aetiology? *J Neurol Neurosurg Psychiatry.* 1995; **58**: 293–9.

29 Gorell JM, Johnson CC, Rybicki BA. Parkinson's disease and its comorbid disorders: an analysis of Michigan mortality data, 1970 to 1990. *Neurology.* 1994; **44**: 1865–8.

30 West AB, Dawson VL, Dawson TM. To die or grow: Parkinson's disease and cancer. *Trends Neurosci.* 2005; **28**: 348–52.

31 Guttmann M, Slaughter PM, Theriault M-E, *et al.* Parkinsonism in Ontario: comorbidity associated with hospitalization in a large cohort. *Mov Disord.* 2004; **19**: 49–53.

32 Allam FM, Campbell MJ, Hofman A, *et al.* Smoking and Parkinson's disease: systematic review of prospective studies. *Mov Disord.* 2004; **19**: 614–21.

33 Hernan MA, Takkouche B, Caamano-Isorna F, *et al.* A meta-analysis of coffee drinking, cigarette smoking, and the risk of Parkinson's disease. *Ann Neurol.* 2002; **52**: 276–84.

34 Priyadarshi A, Khuder SA, Schaub EA, *et al.* A meta-analysis of Parkinson's disease and exposure to pesticides. *Neurotoxicology.* 2000; **21**: 435–40.

35 Jankovic J. Searching for a relationship between manganese and welding and Parkinson's disease. *Neurology.* 2005; **64**: 2021–8.

36 Zhang SM, Hernan MA, Chen H, *et al.* Intakes of vitamins E and C, carotenoids, vitamin supplements, and PD risk. *Neurology.* 2002; **59**: 1161–9.

37 Ward CD, Duvoisin RC, Ince SE, *et al.* Parkinson's disease in 65 pairs of twins and in a set of quadruplets. *Neurology.* 1983; **33**: 815–24.

38 Johnson WG, Hodge SE, Duvoisin R. Twin studies and the genetics of Parkinson's disease – a reappraisal. *Mov Disord.* 1990; **5**: 187–94.

39 Tanner CM, Ottman R, Goldman SM, *et al.* Parkinson disease in twins: an etiologic study. *JAMA.* 1999; **281**: 341–6.

40 Marder K, Tang MX, Mejia H, *et al.* Risk of Parkinson's disease among first-degree relatives: a community-based study. *Neurology.* 1996; **47**: 155–60.

41 Payami H, Larsen K, Bernard S, *et al.* Increased risk of Parkinson's disease in parents and siblings of patients. *Ann Neuro.* 1994; **36**: 659–61.

42 McInerney-Leo A, Hadley DW, Gwinn-Hardy K, *et al.* Genetic testing in Parkinson's disease. *Mov Disord.* 2005; **20**: 1–10.

43 Kubo S, Hattori N, Mizuno Y. Recessive Parkinson's disease. *Mov Disord.* 2006; **21**: 885–93.
44 Hardy J, Cai H, Cookson MR, *et al.* Genetics of Parkinson's disease and parkinsonism. *Ann Neurol.* 2006; **60**: 389–98.
45 Olanow CW, McNaught KSP. Ubiquitin-proteasome system and Parkinson's disease. *Mov Disord.* 2006; **11**: 1806–23.

PART 2

Diagnosis and assessment

4

Diagnosis and differential diagnosis of Parkinson's disease

GRAEME MACPHEE

Introduction: diagnosis

Parkinsonism is a clinical syndrome with three cardinal features: akinesia, rigidity and tremor. Akinesia is a requisite sign for diagnosis and is usually accompanied by rigidity: tremor is a variable finding.

It is now recognised that James Parkinson's essay of 1817 was a description of the syndrome of parkinsonism and that idiopathic Parkinson's disease (IPD) has many imitators. The causes of parkinsonism can be classified into three major groups: (1) idiopathic Parkinson's Disease (IPD); (2) atypical parkinsonian syndromes (parkinsonism plus) and other neurodegenerative disorders, and (3) secondary or symptomatic causes (see Table 4.1). Other aetiologies are increasingly reported for akinetic rigid syndromes[1] and the table is not exhaustive.

TABLE 4.1 Differential diagnosis of parkinsonism

(1) **Idiopathic Parkinson's disease

(2) Parkinsonism associated with neurodegenerative disorders

*Parkinsonism plus or atypical parkinsonian syndromes

- Progressive supranuclear palsy
- Multiple system atrophy
- Corticobasal degeneration

*Parkinsonism associated with other neurodegenerative disease

- *Dementia with Lewy bodies
- *Alzheimer's disease
- Pick's disease
- Amyotrophic lateral sclerosis
- Frontotemporal dementia

(3) Secondary or symptomatic causes

*Drug-induced parkinsonism

- Neuroleptics
- Calcium channel blockers
- Other drugs (e.g. valproate, lithium, amiodarone)

*Parkinsonism associated with cerebrovascular disease

Parkinsonism associated with hydrocephalus

Parkinsonism associated with infections

- Post-encephalitic parkinsonism
- AIDS-associated, e.g. HIV, cryptococcus, toxoplasmosis
- Viral encephalitides
- Neuroborreliosis
- Mycoplasma
- Prion diseases, e.g. Creutzfeld-Jacob disease
- Whipple's disease

Parkinsonism associated with toxic or metabolic disorders

- MPTP (1-methyl-4-phenyl-1, 2, 3, 6-tetrahydropyridine), carbon monoxide, carbon disulphide, methanol, manganese
- Symptomatic massive basal ganglia calcification

Parkinsonism associated with head injury

- Dementia pugilistica (punch-drunk syndrome)

Parkinsonism associated with miscellaneous conditions

- Tumour, e.g. frontal meningioma
- Chronic subdural haematoma
- Dentatorubropallidoluysian atrophy
- Psychogenic

Parkinsonism associated with inherited degenerative disease (usually young onset but rare cases mid- to late-life onset)
Wilson's disease, Huntington's disease, neuroacanthocytosis
Hallervorden-Spatz disease, Spinocerebellar ataxia (SCA) mutations (SCA-2, SCA-3, SCA-17), neuroferritinopathy

Most common cause (**)

Other main causes (*) in elderly

Diagnosis of IPD presents a considerable challenge in older patients. Although IPD is the commonest cause of parkinsonism at all ages, the prevalence of the atypical syndromes, drug-induced parkinsonism and tremor disorders, particularly non-specific 'shaking',[2] also increases with advancing years. Age-associated changes in gait and station, often caused by cryptic neurodegenerative and cerebrovascular disease[3] may cause diagnostic confusion with early parkinsonism.

Extra pyramidal signs (EPS) are common in elderly persons: EPS of variable severity were reported in 15% of community-based subjects who were 65 to 74 years old and in 52% of those over 85 years of age.[4] Clinically evident parkinsonism (two or more of the cardinal motor signs) in a similar population is lower, at around 3%.[5] This suggests a significant reservoir of subtle signs of parkinsonism in elderly subjects, who may or may not go on to develop IPD or another disorder. Parkinsonian signs may occur in association with mild cognitive impairment without evidence of overt neurological disorder[6] and may predict incident dementia.[7] Parkinsonism occurring in the context of dementia becomes increasingly common in the ninth decade.[8]

Making a correct diagnosis of IPD is vital in establishing the prognosis for patient and family and initiating correct management. Equally important, IPD should be distinguished from imitators since outlook and management differ. Misdiagnosis may result in fruitless treatment with dopaminergic drugs, which may produce neuropsychiatric side effects in susceptible older subjects. Accurate diagnosis is also important for epidemiologic and therapeutic research. For these reasons, all elderly persons with suspected parkinsonism should have specialist assessment.

This chapter will discuss the diagnosis of IPD and briefly review the conditions that most commonly mimic IPD with particular emphasis on the atypical or 'parkinsonism plus' syndromes (progressive supranuclear palsy, multiple system atrophy and corticobasal degeneration).

Diagnostic problems

Clinicopathological studies have suggested that the ante-mortem diagnosis of IPD, made by neurologists or geriatricians with a specific interest in parkinsonism is erroneous in 24% of cases;[9,10] This is principally because the cardinal signs occur in conditions other than IPD. The main alternative diagnoses in the UK Brain Bank series of 100 cases were six cases of progressive supranuclear palsy (PSP), five of multiple system atrophy (MSA) and six of Alzheimer pathology.[9] More recent studies suggest an improvement in diagnostic accuracy by specialists. Hughes *et al.* report that dedicated movement disorders specialists achieve a sensitivity of clinical diagnosis of 91%, a specificity of 98% and a positive predictive value of 99%.[11] The method of pattern recognition utilised by experts beyond formal diagnostic criteria was emphasised. In the large DATATOP study, diagnosis was revised by movement disorder specialists in 8% of participants by six years mean follow up.[12]

The diagnostic error rate is highest at disease onset and will fall over time, if the clinician is vigilant for the emergence of atypical features or 'red flags'[13] suggesting alternative diagnoses (*see* Table 4.2). Only 65% of patients with an initial diagnosis of IPD had confirmatory pathology at autopsy in one series[10] but diagnostic accuracy had improved to 76% at five years.

TABLE 4.2 Atypical features in idiopathic Parkinson's disease

Early or prominent feature	Possible alternative diagnosis
Autonomic failure	MSA
Atypical levodopa dyskinesia	MSA
Atypical tremor	ET, DT, CBD, MSA
Minimal or absent tremor	MSA, PSP, VP, NPH
Early postural instability or falls	PSP > MSA, VP, NPH
Pyramidal signs	MSA, VP, PSP, NPH, CBD
Early dementia	DLB, AD, MID, PSP,CJD
Supranuclear gaze palsy	PSP > MSA, CBD
Marked asymmetry of motor signs	CBD
Myoclonus	CBD, MSA, DLB, CJD
Alien limb	CBD
Focal cortical signs	CBD
Palilalia or palilogia	PSP
Severe early dysarthria or dysphagia	PSP, MSA
Stridor, cold hands, marked antecollis	MSA
Wheelchair dependence	MSA

AD = Alzheimer's disease; CBD = corticobasal degeneration; CJD = Creutzfeld-Jacob disease; DT = dystonic tremor; ET = essential tremor; MID = multi infarct dementia; MSA = multiple system atrophy; NPH = normal pressure hydrocephalus; PSP = progressive supranuclear palsy; VP = vascular parkinsonism

Nearly 25% of subjects treated in general practice for Parkinson's disease have no evidence of true parkinsonism,[14] suggesting greater diagnostic error among non-specialists. Common misdiagnoses were essential tremor, ischaemic cerebrovascular disease, and extrapyramidal signs in Alzheimer's disease. Community-based studies in prevalent populations have similarly demonstrated that 15% of patients with the diagnosis of IPD do not meet strict clinical criteria for the disease while around 20% of patients with IPD remain undiagnosed.[15]

Clinical diagnosis

The diagnosis of IPD remains entirely clinical at present since there are no specific biological markers. Some investigations are useful in recognising other causes of parkinsonism. Establishing a diagnosis of IPD (or other parkinsonian syndrome) is a two-step process:
1. confirm the presence of true parkinsonism by clinical examination
2. consider the likely cause based on clinical features, progression of disease and response to treatment. This requires regular clinical review of the patient.

Cardinal features of parkinsonism

Akinesia

Akinesia is the core feature of parkinsonism and must be present if the diagnosis is to be sustained. Akinesia is a symptom complex, comprising some or all of the following features: slowness (bradykinesia); poverty or lack of movement (hypokinesia); progressive early fatiguing and reduction in amplitude of repeated movements; impairment of sequencing or difficulty performing simultaneous motor actions Both programming and execution of movements are impaired, although the latter is usually more severely affected. Fatiguing on repetitive motor tasks is a crucial finding since pyramidal tract lesions may also cause slowness of movement. Absence or poverty of movement is often best detected by casual observation, including features such as decreased blink rate, paucity of facial expression, lack of fidgeting and reduced arm swing when walking. Confirmation of akinesia in the arms and face is important in supporting a diagnosis of IPD since 'lower-body parkinsonism' suggests cerebrovascular disease.

Formal tests for akinesia include asking the patient to tap the tip of the index finger regularly and rapidly on the distal thumb. In parkinsonism, the rhythm is ill sustained and subject to periods of arrest followed by speeding up or complete breakdown of movement. Asking the patient to rapidly pronate and supinate the outstretched arms, rapidly open a clenched fist or tapping the heel on the floor may reveal similar motor timing difficulties. In the presence of tremor, large-amplitude movements may be more reliable in assessing akinesia.

Mirror movements are involuntary movements occurring in similar muscle groups on the opposite side of the body that may emerge during repetitive upper-limb movements and may be a clinical feature of the less affected side in early mild parkinsonism.[16]

Watching the patient write may show disruption in a smooth flow of the pen and the letters may progressively shrink in size. Handwriting may be small (micrographia) when compared with previous correspondence.

Some pitfalls exist in assessing akinesia in the elderly. Slowing of motor performance and reduction in diurnal activity are recognised with advancing age.[17,18] In contrast to the asymmetry which is characteristic of early IPD, age-related slowing is usually symmetrical and does not show the marked fatiguability that defines true akinesia. Careful assessment of sensory function, tone, muscle power and reflexes should identify other diseases of both the peripheral and the central nervous system, which slow motor performance. Focal pathology such as arthritis may also simulate bradykinesia.

The psychomotor retardation of depression may be mistaken for bradykinesia but depression itself is common in early IPD. Meticulous clinical assessment remains the principal tool in distinguishing imitators from early parkinsonism.

Rigidity

Rigidity is recognised as an increase in resistance to passive movements around a joint. It is described as plastic or 'lead pipe' when smooth, or 'cogwheel' when a ratchety feeling of fluctuating resistance occurs in the presence of a tremor which may or may not be clinically evident. Such resistance remains broadly constant throughout the range of excursion, independent of speed of movement. In contrast to rigidity, increased tone in spasticity is velocity dependent. During slow movements, little resistance may be felt; with swift movements a rapid rise in resistance is followed by resolution of resistance, the 'spastic catch'. Gegenhalten or paratonia is an uneven and often progressively increasing resistance to passive movement. Gegenhalten is associated with diffuse cerebral disease or cognitive dysfunction and may be mistaken for cogwheel rigidity.

Froment's manoeuvre may be useful in unmasking rigidity or cogwheeling, which is undetectable on routine testing. Increased tone may be found when the contra-lateral limb is activated (e.g. making a fist; drawing a circle in the air). Caution in interpretation is necessary since a mild increase in tone may be a non-specific response in healthy older persons. Asymmetrical augmentation of tone with cogwheeling is suggestive of IPD.

Tremor

Tremor is an involuntary rhythmic oscillatory movement of a body part. Action tremor is any tremor that is present during voluntary contraction of muscle and includes postural and kinetic tremor. Postural tremor is seen with a sustained posture against gravity, e.g. arms outstretched. Kinetic tremor occurs during any movement. Intention tremor is a form of kinetic tremor and occurs when amplitude of tremor increases during visually guided movements towards a target at the termination of the movement. Resting tremor emerges maximally when a body part is not voluntarily activated and may be seen when a hand rests in the lap or dangles over an armrest. To be certain a tremulous limb is completely supported against gravity, the examiner may need to rest the patient on a bed or couch.

Postural instability and gait disturbance

Postural instability is often included as a fourth cardinal sign of parkinsonism but has limited diagnostic specificity in the elderly. It may result from numerous other disorders affecting afferent and efferent neuronal pathways as well as central processing and musculoskeletal function.

Postural instability is usually the last cardinal feature to appear (by definition, Stage 3 Hoehn and Yahr) but may occur prematurely in older patients.[19,20] The presence of falls early in the clinical course of parkinsonism usually suggests one of the atypical parkinsonian disorders (*see* Table 4.2).

Postural stability is tested by the examiner standing behind the patient who should be asked to broaden the stance. Following explanation, the examiner should pull backwards on the shoulders – the 'pull test'[21] – and be prepared to catch the patient. A normal response is resistance or recovery within one or two steps: the parkinsonian patient may take several steps to recover or begin to fall with retropulsion.

Reduced arm swing is often the first sign of gait disturbance in IPD followed by short-paced, shuffling steps. Breadth of base may be widened early in the disorder as a result of flexed posture but then narrows as a result of commanding rigidity.[22] Gait initiation may be troublesome and turns may only be achieved 'en bloc' with loss of truncal rotation. As the disease progresses, impaired postural reflexes and flexed station may result in festination, where acceleration occurs in an attempt to retain balance. Falls may ensue if a wall or other object is not available for braking. Marked axial rigidity with modest distal parkinsonism and backward falls early in the disease course suggests progressive supranuclear palsy.

Freezing may occur on starting to walk (start hesitation), while trying to turn or when approaching doorways. It is usually a feature of advanced IPD after significant duration of levodopa treatment. Freezing as an isolated or early feature may indicate subcortical cerebrovascular disease, normal pressure hydrocephalus or, rarely, PSP. Camptocormia is an abnormal posture associated with marked flexion of the spine leading to severe stooping that abates on recumbency. It is increasingly recognised in IPD and other parkinsonian and dystonic disorders.

Idiopathic Parkinson's disease

Definitions

Idiopathic Parkinson's disease (IPD) is recognised as a levodopa-responsive parkinsonism with characteristic clinical features and natural history. At autopsy, the brain typically shows Lewy body degeneration of pigmented and other brainstem nuclei. While IPD is traditionally regarded as a sporadic neurodegenerative disorder, an increasing number of genetic loci (PARK 1–11) have been linked to familial parkinsonism, particularly in younger patients. Parkin (PARK2) and LRKK (PARK8) are the two most common mutations and both may produce a clinical syndrome akin to IPD. Interestingly, PARK2 patients demonstrate nigrostriatal degeneration without Lewy bodies while PARK8 patients manifest pleomorphic neuropathology with and without Lewy bodies. The conventional definition of IPD based on clinico-pathological criteria is therefore being challenged.[23] Aetiology based on molecular biology will add precision to diagnostic definition.

A precise clinical definition of IPD is not established but most experts consider the presence of two or more cardinal motor signs (one of which must include bradykinesia) and a consistent response to levodopa with the development of typical levodopa-induced dyskinesia indicative of IPD. Asymmetric onset[24] is a strong indicator of IPD, but anomalies in symmetry and unusual patterns are described.[25]

Strict diagnostic criteria are discussed later. Most require pathological confirmation for definite IPD. Calne's clinical classification[26] is less rigid. It has the merit of defining clinically definite IPD but the earlier caveats relating to postural instability as a cardinal feature in the elderly apply (*see* Table 4.3).

TABLE 4.3 Calne classification (Calne *et al.*[26])

- CLINICALLY POSSIBLE IPD. One of the following: tremor (rest or postural), rigidity, or bradykinesia.

- CLINICALLY PROBABLE IPD. Two of the following cardinal features: resting tremor, rigidity, bradykinesia or postural instability *or* if resting tremor, rigidity, or bradykinesia are asymmetric.

- CLINICALLY DEFINITE IPD. Three of the cardinal features *or* two cardinal features with one of the first three presenting asymmetrically.

Early features of IPD

Pathological changes and cell loss develop gradually in IPD during an unknown period of time. This preclinical period progresses until the symptomatic threshold of nigral cell loss is reached. A period of delay usually follows before diagnosis is suspected with the onset of classical motor symptoms. Prodromal features include non-motor features of mood or personality changes, depression, anxiety, apathy, impaired olfaction, limb pain and paresthesiae, constipation, REM sleep behaviour disorder and seborrheic dermatitis.[27] Unexplained fatigue may be prominent. Difficulty turning in bed is an early motor problem. Other common symptoms and signs of motor dysfunction in early parkinsonism are shown in Table 4.4.

TABLE 4.4 Common symptoms and signs in early parkinsonism

Face	Reduced facial expression (hypomimia)
Speech	Softer, less distinct, 'boring' with lack of intonation
Postural	Difficulty turning in bed and getting out of chairs and cars
Fine motor tasks	Difficulties with handwriting, doing and undoing buttons, grooming and shaving, using kitchen utensils and tools
Gait	Slowing, dragging of one leg, lack of arm swing
Sensory	Stiffness, pain or discomfort in a limb. May present as 'frozen shoulder'

Tremor in IPD

Tremor is present in 75% of patients at presentation. Most patients with IPD develop tremor but some may not.[28] Tremor usually begins unilaterally and distally in a limb – most commonly the arm, but may commence in the leg or a single finger. Tremor often spreads proximally in the arm, before involving the ipsilateral leg and finally crossing to the contralateral limbs. Several types of tremor are recognised in IPD.[29]

➤ Classical 4–6 Hz resting tremor. (Higher-frequency tremor up to 9 Hz may be found, particularly in the early stages).

➤ Postural/kinetic tremor may occur in addition to resting tremor. This may have a similar frequency to rest tremor but can be faster, >1.5 Hz. The higher-frequency tremor may be disabling.

➤ Isolated postural/kinetic tremor with frequency between 4 and 9 Hz may occur in the absence of rest tremor.

The characteristic 'pill-rolling' rest tremor, often coupled with flexion extension movements of the fingers and arms is highly suggestive of IPD or drug-induced parkinsonism.[30] Such tremor will usually diminish on movement and during sleep but is enhanced by stress, anxiety and fatigue. As tremor decreases with voluntary movement, it may increase asynchronously in the opposite hand. Asking the patient to count backwards will often reveal latent resting tremor. In some cases, the typical pill-rolling resting tremor of IPD is seen only during walking.

Rest tremor in IPD is usually accompanied by akinesia but a monosymptomatic rest tremor may occur. There may be mild concurrent extra pyramidal signs such as reduced arm swing and facial expression but other cardinal signs of PD are absent or uncertain. This variant has been labelled 'benign tremulous Parkinson's disease' since little or no progression may occur over a number of years. Functional neuro-imaging demonstrates a dopaminergic deficit suggestive of IPD in the majority of such cases.[31]

Differential diagnosis of tremor

Essential tremor is frequently confused for IPD.[13,14] Like IPD, it becomes increasingly common in old age but is 10 times more common, with prevalence estimates ranging from 13 to 50 cases per 1000 persons over 60 years of age.[32]

ET is a 6–12 Hz bilateral, generally symmetrical, postural and kinetic tremor maximal in hands and forearms. There is often a positive family history with autosomal-dominant inheritance and a high rate of penetrance, usually before 65 years of age.[33] Sporadic cases are increasingly recognised which have been linked to putative environmental factors such as beta-carboline alkaloids and lead.[34]

The severity may vary from a modest, low-amplitude tremor with little disability, partially responsive to alcohol, beta blockers or primidone, to a severe, high-amplitude tremor causing significant handicap and resistant to drug therapy. The tremor is generally greatest on sustained posture but may increase at the termination of a movement. Spillage of cups of tea is a common complaint. Apparent rest tremor of the hands can occur in ET, causing confusion with IPD.[35] ET is usually a vertical up-and-down tremor rather than pill rolling. Other clues to the presence of ET include concurrent vocal, head (titubation) or neck tremor (no–no or yes–yes movements), all of which are uncommon in IPD. In contrast, jaw or leg tremor is highly suggestive of IPD. Cog wheeling may be found in ET but not lead-pipe rigidity or akinesia. Gait ataxia and difficulty in tandem walking may occur.[34]

A postural or kinetic tremor may be seen in association with dystonia and may be misdiagnosed as ET.[36] This type of tremor is often asymmetric or unilateral, and may be task- or position-sensitive, affecting forearms, hands, neck and voice.[29]

In elderly patients the distinction between ET, dystonic tremor and IPD can be very difficult. Some patients who meet the criteria of ET may manifest other mild extrapyramidal signs of uncertain significance, such as modest reduction in facial expression or decreased arm swing. It is suggested that these patients are categorised as having indeterminate tremor syndrome.[29] Ongoing clinical review and functional imaging studies may be necessary to clarify the diagnosis.

Other causes of tremor, such as drugs (e.g. neuroleptics and antiemetics), metabolic disorders (e.g. hyperthyroidism), various cerebral disorders including vascular disease, and peripheral neuropathies[29] should not be overlooked in differential diagnosis.

The recently described Fragile X associated tremor ataxia syndrome (FXTAS) is caused by a trinucleotide repeat expansion in the Fragile X mental retardation gene (FMR1) The syndrome comprises a progressive action tremor, cerebellar dysfunction, parkinsonism and cognitive decline. It occurs typically in middle-aged and elderly men. MRI shows generalised atrophy and distinctive T2 hyperintensities in the middle cerebellar peduncles (the MCP sign). It may be confused with ET and multiple system atrophy.[37]

Other features of IPD
Cognitive dysfunction
Prodromal symptoms of IPD include changes in mood and behaviour but mental status remains relatively normal in early IPD. Signs of significant cognitive impairment at disease onset should suggest other disorders (*see* Table 4.2). Cognitive problems in IPD are discussed elsewhere in this volume.

Ocular dysfunction
Higher-order oculomotor functions are mildly perturbed in IPD[38] but clinically most systems are preserved in contrast to the atypical parkinsonian syndromes.[39] Some IPD patients do complain of blurred vision or difficulty reading caused by weak convergence or tracking problems. In a normal elderly population, broken pursuit movements and mild impairment of upward gaze and defective convergence are common.[39] Prominent visual symptoms or gaze paresis should suggest progressive supranuclear palsy (PSP).

Spontaneous eye blinking is reduced in IPD but less severely than in PSP. Blepharospasm is usually a pointer to another disorder,[13] often PSP, but it may be found in advanced PD.[40] Failure to habituate (continual blinking) when the forehead is tapped is a positive glabellar reflex or Meyerson's sign. This primitive reflex is seen characteristically in IPD, with and without cognitive impairment, but is not specific for IPD.[3] Pertinent neuro-ophthamological examination in parkinsonism is well described by Hardie.[41]

Speech and swallowing, and autonomic dysfunction
The speech of IPD is hypokinetic, typically monotonal, hypophonic and muffled, and lacks prosody. Early or prominent dysarthria or dysphagia suggest other forms of parkinsonism (*see* Table 4.2).

Orthostatic hypotension is common in IPD, particularly in the later stages.[42] Commanding or early autonomic dysfunction or bladder symptoms should bring to mind MSA. Concurrent morbidity or drug therapy (including anti-parkinsonian drugs) may exacerbate or provoke postural hypotension or sphincter disturbance in IPD patients.

Clinical sub-types of IPD

The broad clinical expression of IPD has led to the concept of sub-types of IPD. Age has emerged as one potential determinant of disease course. More rapidly progressive disease is recognised in the elderly[19,20,43] and may be associated with the early postural instability and gait difficulty (PIGD) sub-type. Such axial impairment may result from both disease and ageing effects on non-dopaminergic subcortical structures.[44] Other levodopa-unresponsive features may coexist, such as freezing, dysarthria and dementia.[27] Periventricular hyperintensities on MRI imaging, which increase with age, are reported to be more widespread in patients with more rapid disease progression[45] and dementia. Atypical parkinsonian syndromes should be considered[46] in the differential diagnosis in these cases as well as overlap with common disorders such as stroke and Alzheimer's disease. In contrast to PIGD, tremor-dominant IPD is generally reported to be less aggressive and associated with preserved mental status and younger age at onset.[27,47] There is increasing awareness that the phenotype of IPD may have variable genetic causes although these are more common in younger cases (*see* Chapter 2). The variance which exists in the literature on clinical sub-types of IPD may reflect methodological differences in diagnostic criteria as well as bias in study populations. Recent cluster analyses have refined the methodology and confirm the heterogeneity of Parkinson's disease.[48,49] The latter study confirms a subgroup of older-onset patients with more rapid progression and less motor fluctuations and dyskinesia.

Diagnostic criteria for IPD

A number of diagnostic criteria for IPD have been formulated[28,50,51] which usually require the presence of cardinal signs in association with exclusionary and supportive features. Because of the clinical variability in pathologically confirmed IPD, no criteria are ideal, i.e. 100% sensitivity and 100% specificity. Atypical features were present in 12 out of 100 pathologically confirmed cases of IPD.[52] Early autonomic failure occurred in 2% of these cases, which would usually suggest an alternative diagnosis of multiple system atrophy. A recent study with a high false negative diagnostic rate also highlights the wide phenotypic expression of PD. Atypical features reported included poor levodopa response, early autonomic impairment, early falls and disproportionate antecollis.[11]

Levodopa responsiveness and dyskinesia are supportive features for IPD in most criteria yet 2% of autopsy-proven cases show a poor or absent response to levodopa.[52] Conversely, a positive response is not specific to IPD. Patients with both progressive supranuclear palsy and multiple system atrophy (MSA) may show an initial response to levodopa. Although this response is usually poorly sustained, some cases of MSA derive benefit from levodopa until death.[53]

TABLE 4.5 UK Parkinson's Disease Society Brain Bank clinical diagnostic criteria

STEP 1: Diagnosis of Parkinsonian syndrome

Bradykinesia (slowness of initiation of voluntary movement with progressive reduction in speed and amplitude of repetitive actions) and at least one of the following:

(a) muscular rigidity

(b) 4–6 Hz rest tremor

(c) postural instability not caused by primary visual, vestibular, cerebellar or proprioceptive dysfunction

STEP 2: Exclusion criteria for Parkinson's disease

- History of repeated strokes with stepwise progression of Parkinsonian features
- History of repeated head injury
- History of definite encephalitis
- Oculogyric crisis
- Neuroleptic treatment at onset of symptoms
- More than one affected relative
- Sustained remission
- Strictly unilateral features after three years
- Supranuclear gaze palsy
- Cerebellar signs
- Early severe autonomic involvement
- Early severe dementia with disturbances of memory, language and praxis
- Babinski sign
- Presence of a cerebral tumour or communicating hydrocephalus on CT scan
- Negative response to large doses of levodopa (if malabsorption excluded)
- MPTP exposure

STEP 3: Supportive prospective positive criteria for Parkinson's disease; three or more required for diagnosis of definite Parkinson's disease

- Unilateral onset
- Rest tremor present
- Progressive disorder
- Persistent asymmetry affecting the side of onset most
- Excellent response (70–100%) to levodopa
- Severe levodopa-induced chorea
- Levodopa response for five years or more
- Clinical course of ten years or more

Unilateral onset and persistent asymmetry of signs is considered characteristic of IPD with symmetrical parkinsonism pointing to PSP or MSA. However, symmetrical disease may be commoner in older patients with IPD (>70 years of age) compared with those of younger onset.[19] To add to the diagnostic difficulty, symptoms may begin asymmetrically in PSP[54] and may be unilateral in onset in MSA.[55]

Neuropathological brain examination in conjunction with the clinical history is the gold standard for diagnosis of IPD although there are no universally agreed neuropathological criteria. The United Kingdom Parkinson's Disease Society Brain Bank clinical diagnostic criteria[50] were established on brain-bank experience and are now widely accepted in the UK (*see* Table 4.5). The retrospective application of these criteria in a pathological series[9] produced improvement in diagnostic accuracy from 76% to 82%, but clearly still left 18% of cases misdiagnosed. Using a logistic regression model, selected criteria (asymmetrical onset, no atypical features and no alternative aetiology for parkinsonism) reduced the false positive rate to 7% but excluded 32% of genuine cases.[24] A more recent brain-bank study reports an improvement in diagnostic accuracy although 10% of cases still required revision of diagnosis at post mortem.[56] The recently published UK NICE guidelines recommend the use of UK PD Brain Bank criteria in routine clinical practice.

Different operational circumstances dictate the degree of stringency for diagnostic criteria. Therapeutic research demands high specificity, whereas epidemiological and clinical practice generally requires more sensitive criteria. This is recognised in using probable and possible categories in some criteria that were developed based on literature review.[28] These await prospective validation with neuropathology.

Pharmacological challenge tests

The response to an acute oral dose of levodopa or apomorphine injection is considered positive when there is an improvement of 20% or better on the UPDRS rating scale (Part 3, motor examination). These pharmacological challenge tests help to determine dopaminergic responsiveness in the short term with reasonable precision,[57] but their use as a diagnostic tool is not recommended, mainly because of low sensitivity in de novo patients.[58] Challenge tests may be helpful in the later stages of disease if diagnostic and therapeutic uncertainties persist. A positive challenge test may be useful in demonstrating dopaminergic response objectively, if the therapeutic benefit is uncertain. Determining the response to chronic dopaminergic therapy in older patients may be difficult if they are unable to tolerate adequate dose titration because of postural hypotension or neuropsychiatric symptoms.

Olfactory testing

Significant olfactory dysfunction is an early clinical sign in 90% of patients with PD but not in young-onset parkin patients.[59] Olfaction is generally preserved in patients with vascular parkinsonism.[60] Smell is less commonly affected in MSA and PSP, but may also be diminished in Alzheimer's disease. At present, objective smell testing lacks sufficient discrimination to be utilised in routine clinical practice but this may change with further research.

Neuroimaging

Imaging of the brain is generally unnecessary in patients with features consistent with IPD and a good response to levodopa. However, in the presence of atypical features neuroimaging techniques may be helpful in supporting alternative diagnosis.

Structural imaging

Computerised tomography (CT) of the brain may identify patients with normal pressure hydrocephalus, subcortical vascular disease and rarer causes of parkinsonism such as tumours.

Magnetic resonance imaging (MRI) may demonstrate characteristic findings in atypical disorders. In multiple system atrophy (MSA), infratentorial abnormalities include atrophy and signal change in the pons ('hot cross bun sign') and cerebellar atrophy. Striatal abnormalities include putaminal atrophy and a hyperintense putaminal rim. In PSP, atrophy of the mid-brain, thinning of the quadrigeminal plate and dilatation of the third ventricle may be found. Asymmetrical atrophy of the parietal cortex on MRI is suggestive of corticobasal degeneration. Unfortunately, these MRI changes in the atypical parkinsonian syndromes are often absent in the early stages of disease when diagnosis is most difficult.[61] Other imaging methods which have been used in research settings to aid the distinction of IPD from other atypical syndromes include diffusion-weighted MRI, MRI volumetry and magnetic resonance spectroscopy (MRS).[59]

Functional imaging

Functional imaging techniques such as single-photon emission tomography (SPECT) and positron emission tomography (PET) provide data on dopaminergic system integrity in vivo.[62] In IPD, there is degeneration of the presynaptic dopaminergic neurones but preservation of postsynaptic neurones. Non-idiopathic parkinsonian syndromes such as PSP or MSA demonstrate both pre- and post-synaptic degeneration. PET scanning is a sensitive functional imaging technique but is expensive and is not widely available. For a recent review, see Piccini and Whone.[62] SPECT is more accessible and less costly.

Assessment of presynaptic dopaminergic terminal function in vivo may be performed using SPECT scanning. Using a number of tracers which monitor dopamine transporter function (DAT) including ^{123}I-beta-carbomethoxy-3-beta (4-iodophenyl)-tropane [beta CIT], TRODAT and ^{123}I-FP-CIT. Beta CIT requires 24 hours of equilibration before scanning, which is inconvenient for patient and laboratory; FP CIT scans can be achieved three to six hours after injection. DAT imaging using simple visual assessment discriminates between essential tremor (normal dopamine transporter function) and pre-synaptic parkinsonism such as IPD with high sensitivity and specificity[63] and may detect pre-symptomatic dopamine deficiency.[64] This technique may be a useful tool in difficult cases in determining whether upper-limb tremor is due to essential tremor or dopaminergic deficit. It cannot discriminate accurately between IPD and other forms of presynaptic parkinsonism such as MSA, PSP and dementia with Lewy bodies. As well as in ET, a normal scan is found in drug-induced parkinsonism, psychogenic parkinsonism, Alzheimer's disease and vascular parkinsonism (except with focal basal ganglia infarction). Consequently, the utility of DAT functional imaging in improving the accuracy of clinical diagnosis in clinically uncertain parkinsonian disorders (CUPS) is a burgeoning area of interest. Scans without evidence of dopamine deficiency (SWEDDs) have been reported in around 10% of de novo clinically diagnosed PD in recent trials with SPECT and PET[62] but the significance of this is controversial[59] Prolonged clinical follow-up supports increasing congruence over time between the current working diagnosis and baseline DAT imaging results.[65,66]

SPECT also permits the investigation of striatal post-synaptic D2 receptor status using tracers such as ^{123}I-iodobenzamide, a dopamine D2 receptor ligand. This provides a semiquantitative evaluation of receptor status, which calculates the ratio of uptake in specific (striatal) to non-specific (e.g. occipital) areas.

Concomitant assessment of dopamine terminal and striatal function with PET (or SPECT) is a burgeoning area of interest and may help to discriminate atypical syndromes from IPD but is costly and of limited availability.[61,62] Transcranial sonography is a new diagnostic tool which is currently being investigated for utility in the diagnosis of IPD.

Parkinsonism plus or atypical parkinsonian syndromes
Progressive supranuclear palsy

Progressive supranuclear palsy (PSP) or Steele Richardson Olszewski Syndrome is the commonest atypical parkinsonian syndrome after IPD in old age.[67] It is characterised by a vertical supranuclear gaze palsy and early postural instability.

Subcortical – frontal pathways mediating volitional motor activity, saccadic eye movements, executive function, motivation and social behaviour are perturbed in PSP. Major neurotransmitter systems affected include dopaminergic striatonigral pathways, gaba-ergic, and cholinergic and noradrenergic pathways.[68,69]

The incidence is estimated to be 5.3 new cases per 100 000 person years for ages 50 to 99.[67] The prevalence for persons over 55 years is reported as 5–6 per 100 000.[70,71] These figures are conservative since half the disease course usually elapses before diagnosis[72] and many cases are misdiagnosed.[73]

The incidence of PSP rises steeply with age: 1.7 per 100 000 at 50–59 years, increasing to 14.7 per 100 000 at 80–99 years.[67] Median survival time from symptom onset is around 6–7 (range 2–16) years.[68,74] An older age of onset and classification as probable PSP is associated with poorer survival.[70] Early falls, problems with speech and swallowing, diplopia and early insertion of a gastrostomy also predict reduced survival. The pertinence of a presymptomatic history of hypertension in many cases is uncertain.[74]

The neuropathology of PSP demonstrates neurofibrillary tangles consisting of tau protein in the striatum, pallidum, subthalamic nucleus, substantia nigra, oculomotor complex, peri-aqueductal grey matter, superior colliculi, basis pontis, dentate nuclei and medulla with variable neuronal loss and gliosis.[72] Other neurodegenerative disorders such as corticobasal degeneration, post-encephalitic parkinsonism and the parkinsonism-dementia complex of Guam are also characterised by tau deposition in different forms. PSP and these disorders have been classified as 'tauopathies'.

The aetiology of PSP is unknown but toxic and infectious aetiologies are postulated based on similarities to post-encephalitic parkinsonism and Guam complex. While usually considered a sporadic disease, familial cases are reported.[75] Hereditary PSP may be more common than previously thought.[76] There may also be a genetic predisposition to 'sporadic' PSP. There is an over-representation of the A0 allele of a polymorphic marker of the tau gene in patients with PSP.[77,78] PSP patients display several polymorphisms in tau, representing an extended tau haplotype (H1) which is more common than in the general population.[79] The same association has been reported in patients with corticobasal degeneration and is described as an extended tau haplotype, HapA, which is also found in 33% of controls.[80] Non-genetic factors may trigger or accentuate neuronal degeneration in predisposed patients.[68]

Clinical features (see Table 4.6)

The onset of disease in PSP is insidious and symptoms may evolve in variable order. Mobility problems are the commonest early feature.[70] Typically, patients present with early postural instability and falls. The gait is ataxic, usually wide based and upright with more preservation of arm swing than in IPD. Pseudo-bulbar palsy with dysphagia is often an early feature, unlike IPD, and may be misdiagnosed as motor neurone disease. Dysarthria is characterised by spasticity and ataxia rather than hypophonia as in IPD. The voice may have a growling quality with involuntary groaning. Perseveration, palilalia (repetition of words) and echolalia may intrude in speech.

Parkinsonism in PSP is characterised by symmetrical bradykinesia and axial more than limb rigidity. Distal limb rigidity and bradykinesia are milder than in IPD while nuchal rigidity and dystonia are prominent. Levodopa treatment produces a poor or transient response. The rigid neck may become hyperextended and a hyperlordotic erect posture coupled with impairment of righting reflexes leads to backward falls. The facial appearance in PSP differs from the classic hypomimia of IPD and is described as 'worried or astonished'. The eyebrows are often raised due to frontalis overactivity.

Neurobehavioural changes occur commonly in early disease; primarily apathy, but also disinhibition, dysphoria, anxiety, depression and emotional lability.[81] Emotional lability is very common in PSP, common in MSA and less common in IPD.[82] Patients may be misdiagnosed as having a dementia or psychosis. Mental and physical slowing and social withdrawal may be misinterpreted as normal ageing. Instability and disinhibition lead to impulsive, often dangerous behaviour at home and in traffic. Sitting is often achieved 'en bloc' by toppling into a chair. Frontal lobe behaviours such as automatic imitation of gestures, motor perseveration, forced grasping and a tendency to grab objects placed nearby may be commanding as disease progresses.

Visual disturbances such as diplopia, blurred vision, burning eyes and light sensitivity may antedate the appearance of supranuclear gaze palsy.[83] Some patients complain bitterly of unsuitable glasses despite repeated attendance at opticians.

TABLE 4.6 Clinical features of IPD (Idiopathic Parkinson's disease), PSP (Progressive supranuclear palsy), CBD (Corticobasal degeneration) and MSA (Multiple system atrophy)

	IPD	PSP	CBD	MSA
Median age of onset	~ 60 y	~ 70 yrs	Not known	~ 50 yrs
Median survival	~ Normal	~ 6 yrs	~ 6 yrs	~ 10 yrs
Pill rolling tremor	Common	Rare	Absent	Uncommon
Bradykinesia	Asymmetrical	Symmetrical	Strongly asymmetrical at onset	Symmetrical (but asymmetry well recognised)
Rigidity	Asymmetrical	Axial prominent May be extended neck	Strongly asymmetrical at onset	Symmetrical
Falls	Late	Early ~ 1st year Backwards	Late ~ 3+ yrs (unless leg affected early)	Early ~ 2nd to 3rd yr
Gait	Narrow base, stooped, flexed knees	Wide base, erect, extended knees	Variable base Apraxic Freezing	Narrow base, stooped, shuffling, may be ataxic
Autonomic dysfunction	Late, usually mild (may be drug induced)	Rare	Rare	Common, early and severe
Dysarthria and dysphagia	Late	Early	Early	Early
Facial expression	Hypomimia	Worried or astonished	Hypomimia	Hypomimia
Cognitive impairment	Late	Early	Usually later	Rare
Cortical signs	Absent	Absent	Present +/– 'alien limb'	Absent
Supranuclear palsy	Absent	Vertical > horizontal	Horizontal = vertical	Horizontal > vertical
Blink rate	Low	Very low	Low	Low
Frontal behaviour	Absent	Severe	Moderate	Absent or mild
Cerebellar signs	Absent	Rare	Rare	Common
Levodopa response	Good, sustained	Absent, poor or unsustained	No response	Absent, poor or unsustained (~ 30% may respond initially)

Supranuclear gaze palsy

The hallmark of PSP is a paresis of downward vertical gaze, but this does not begin until a median of four years after disease onset.[84] Gaze restriction can be overcome by the oculocephalic or 'doll's head' manoeuvre, indicating a supranuclear origin. Assessment of reflex movements can be hampered by cervical rigidity. Limitation of upward gaze may antedate or exceed downward gaze problems but this occurs in other neurodegenerative diseases and mild restriction is seen in normal ageing. Limitation of downward gaze is therefore more specific for PSP. Supranuclear gaze palsies are also reported in patients with dementia with Lewy bodies, multiple system atrophy, cerebrovascular disease, Creutzfeld-Jacob disease and Huntington's disease.[72] Horizontal rather than vertical gaze is usually more affected in these disorders.

The earliest ocular sign of PSP is generally slowing of vertical saccades[85] This is tested by asking the patient to make voluntary saccades on command to stationary targets directly ahead and down. Quinn's 'round the houses' sign is seen when vertical excursion shows slight curvature.[86] Breakdown of optokinetic nystagmus in the vertical plane is also an early sensitive indicator of PSP.[87]

Vertical eye movements are characteristically more affected than horizontal movements in PSP, although in the later stages gaze may be affected in all directions. Pursuit movements are usually preserved initially but become saccadic as disease progresses. In the terminal stages the patient may lose all eye movements, including those to reflex manoeuvres.

Eyelid abnormalities are common in PSP. Blink rate is often reduced to less than five per minute and artificial tears may be required to prevent exposure keratitis. Involuntary eye closure may be noted. Difficulty opening the eyes may be caused by true blepharospasm or levator inhibition due to apraxia. In late disease, the combination of eyelid abnormalities, facial dystonia and gaze abnormalities gives rise to a peculiar staring non-blinking facies.[83]

Cognitive syndrome

The cognitive syndrome of PSP generally conforms to a specific pattern comprising cognitive slowing, impairment of executive function and forgetfulness.[88] The cognitive impairment may be severe enough to be considered dementia as disease progresses although the deficits remain specific. PSP is considered the prototype of subcortical – frontal dementia. Cortical functions such as language, praxis and gnosis are generally unaffected except for a reduction in spontaneous speech and mild word-finding difficulty.[72] Executive dysfunction and slow information processing is demonstrable with difficulties in initiation and fluency, concept formation and problem solving. Memory function improves in cued recall situations. Bedside and neuropsychological tests useful in defining cognitive abnormalities in PSP are given in Litvan *et al.*[85] In contrast to PSP, frontal-lobe features in IPD and MSA are usually mild and may be evident only on detailed neuropsychological testing.[89] The Frontal Assessment Battery (FAB) and the Addenbrokes cognitive examination (ACE) may be useful bedside tests for discriminating these akinetic rigid syndromes.[90,91]

Other clinical features of PSP include pyramidal tract signs, cerebellar ataxia, major depression, myoclonus,[83] focal dystonia,[92] sleep disturbances,[93] and urinary frequency. Autonomic failure is not part of PSP but urinary and faecal incontinence[94] as well as orthostatic hypotension can occur in advanced disease. Resting tremor is rare and usually modest.[83]

Clinical phenotypes and variants

The classical picture of PSP is unmistakable but the spectrum of clinical expression is extremely wide.[73] Ophthalmoplegia never occurs in some cases.[95] Multiple lacunar infarcts in old age may mimic the clinical syndrome of PSP.[96] Some patients with an isolated cognitive syndrome without prominent motor signs may be misdiagnosed as dementia with Lewy bodies, Pick's disease, Creutzfeld–Jacob disease or even Alzheimer's disease despite the lack of 'cortical' dementia.[73] Asymmetry of signs and limb apraxia, while uncommon and generally mild, may cause diagnostic confusion with corticobasal degeneration.[54]

Two distinct phenotypes of PSP have been described using factor analysis in a brain-bank series of 103 consecutive cases.[97] The first phenotype, occurring in around two-thirds of cases, broadly conforms to classical PSP (early falls, supranuclear palsy and cognitive dysfunction) and has been named Richardson's syndrome (RS). A second group (PSP-P) with longer survival and older age at death was characterised by asymmetric onset, tremor and initial response to levodopa. These patients were often misdiagnosed as IPD. Differences in tau-tangle composition between the groups may contribute to the clinical differences. The syndrome of primary progressive freezing gait (PPFG) may be a smaller third sub-type of PSP.[97]

Pure akinesia is a syndrome first reported in Japan, characterised by progressive akinesia of gait, speech and handwriting without tremor, rigidity or dementia. It is suggested this is a clinical variant of PSP and may occur before ocular abnormalities.[98]

Diagnostic criteria

Different sets of criteria have been proposed for the diagnosis of PSP.[83,54,73,99] An international workshop sponsored by NINDS and the Society for Progressive Supranuclear Palsy[85] has published a set of diagnostic criteria based on literature review and expert consensus which aims to improve diagnostic accuracy specifying levels of diagnostic certainty. When tested in a detailed autopsy-confirmed set of cases, the criteria for probable PSP were highly specific (100%) but not very sensitive (50%). The possible PSP criteria achieved 83% sensitivity and 93% specificity. The latter possible criteria are more suitable for clinical care but show similar positive predictive value (around 80%) to earlier criteria which are less rigid.[83] None of the existing operational criteria improves accuracy of the final specialist clinical diagnosis.[100]

Corticobasal degeneration (CBD)

CBD is a rare sporadic progressive neurodegenerative disorder with onset in the sixth decade or later.[101] Very rare familial cases are described. Emerging evidence suggests that PSP and CBD are closely related neurodegenerative disorders with similar clinical, pathological and genetic features. Recently CBD and PSP phenotypes have been described in a single family.[102] Neurochemical findings common to both disorders include aggregations of isoforms of 'four repeat tau protein' due to splicing of exon 10. CBD and PSP are both homozygous for the 'H1-tau' haplotype. However, molecular pathology and biochemistry demonstrate some differences between the disorders.[86]

Neuropathological features in CBD may overlap not only with PSP, but also with Alzheimer's disease and focal or asymmetric cortical degenerations such as Pick's disease, frontotemporal dementia linked to chromosome 17 and amyotrophic lateral sclerosis with frontal dementia.[103] Neuropathology shows neuronal loss and formation of ballooned achromatic neurons in the cortex and degeneration of substantia nigra. Tau immunoreactive astrocytic plaques are characteristic for CBD.[104]

Other heterogeneous substrates including Pick's disease, Alzheimer's disease, PSP and cerebrovascular disease may produce a clinical syndrome of CBD if the lesions correspond to the classical topography of the disorder.[105]

No data are available on prevalence or incidence, but CBD is probably under-diagnosed.[106] The median survival is six to eight years.[107,108]

Clinical features of corticobasal degeneration[108] (see Table 4.6)
CBD usually includes a combination of:
1. movement disorders (asymmetric akinesia and rigidity not responsive to levodopa, limb dystonia, focal stimulus sensitive myoclonus, action tremor, postural instability) and
2. higher cortical dysfunction (ideomotor or ideational apraxia, alien limb, cortical sensory loss, dementia, aphasia, frontal release reflexes) and
3. other manifestations (supranuclear gaze palsy, pyramidal tract signs, pseudobulbar palsy, cerebellar signs, pain).

The commonest presenting complaint is clumsiness of one hand and arm.[109] Classically, patients develop a unilateral jerky, tremulous, akinetic rigid and apraxic extremity, usually the arm, with accompanying dystonia. The posture is often of a flexed hand and forearm with adduction of the arm. Cortical sensory signs develop concurrently in the form of agraphesthesia, astereognosis and tactile sensory extinction. Ideomotor apraxia[110] (difficulty initiating voluntary movements, making fine finger movements and copying hand postures) is a key finding in CBD.[106] Apraxia can be masked by concurrent rigidity and immobility as the limb progresses to functional uselessness with a dystonic clenched fist. Examining the opposite limb may reveal an abnormality even if asymptomatic, indicating early involvement of the contralateral cortex.

The 'alien limb phenomenon' (ALP) is very suggestive of CBD but is variably present[109] and not specific.[111] Such an 'alien limb' has 'a mind of its own', drifting uncontrollably into space or crossing the midline and interfering with the contralateral limb or the examiner. Complex behaviour (groping and manipulation) should be present for true ALP rather than simple levitation with non-purposeful behaviour.

Over a number of years, symptoms and signs in CBD usually spread to the ipsilateral or to the corresponding contralateral limb but remain distinctly asymmetric. Rigid immobility ensues in the terminal phase with hypostatic complications. For a review of clinical diagnostic criteria see Mahapatra *et al.* (2004).[104]

Diagnostic problems in corticobasal degeneration

The clinical features of CBD show considerable heterogeneity and are recognised as including cognitive decline, dementia and altered behaviour (depression, apathy, irritability, anxiety, agitation and obsessive-compulsive disorders) with mild, delayed or entirely absent motor symptoms.[107,112,104] Non-fluent aphasia is a common feature of CBD. CBD overlaps clinically with other causes of frontal dementia.[104]

CBD can be confused with PSP but cognitive problems and difficulty in walking usually occur rather later in classical CBD (unless the leg is affected first).[72] Limb dystonia may be an early feature in some cases of PSP which are misdiagnosed initially as CBD.[92] In contrast to PSP, the supranuclear gaze palsy in CBD affects equally both horizontal and vertical gaze. The gaze abnormality in early disease is apraxic with patients struggling to generate saccades to command.[38,72] Prominent eye blinks or head thrusts may be used to initiate saccade generation. Once achieved, gaze may be unrestricted. Such difficulties are most prominent in the direction of the more affected side of the body. These findings, combined with jerky pursuit-movements maximal in the opposite direction, strongly suggest CBD as the cause of the gaze palsy.[39]

In early disease, an asymmetrical rigid syndrome may be mistaken for IPD. Helpful distinguishing features include lack of response to levodopa, and cortical signs. The eye movement abnormalities exceed those of comparable IPD patients.[38] Myoclonus of the fingers and jerky action tremor are distinct from classical IPD rest tremor.[109]

Multiple system atrophy

Multiple system atrophy (MSA) is a sporadic, progressive neurodegenerative disorder of unknown aetiology, characterised by any combination of parkinsonism, cerebellar, autonomic, urinary and pyramidal dysfunction.[113] Neuropathology demonstrates neuronal loss and gliosis in some or all of the following: inferior olives, pons, cerebellum, substantia nigra, locus coeruleus, striatum and interomedial lateral columns of the spinal cord. Lewy bodies are usually absent.

MSA median survival is around 8 to 10 years,[53,67] with substantial individual variation.[113] Older age at onset is associated with shorter survival.[53]

Clinical features (see Table 4.6)

Autonomic dysfunction

Autonomic dysfunction (AuD) (orthostatic hypotension, urinary and male erectile dysfunction, constipation and decreased sweating) is invariable during the disease course,[53] but may be absent at disease onset. Orthostatic hypotension (OH) may be symptomatic or asymptomatic. Postural faintness is reported more commonly than recurrent syncope[53] but this may represent selection bias of more prominent parkinsonism from movement-disorder clinics. Since patients with IPD also develop AuD, distinction from MSA can be difficult. AuD in MSA tends to affect more than one autonomic domain, is generally more severe, and may antedate parkinsonism.[119] The older patient with parkinsonism may have other concurrent causes for OH such as drug treatment, diabetes mellitus and cerebrovascular disease. Neurovascular instability and OH may be prominent in dementia with Lewy bodies and Alzheimer's disease.[120] Diagnosis of MSA should be circumspect if AuD is limited to one domain.

Bladder dysfunction is an important indicator of possible MSA.[121] Atrophy of the brainstem leads to detrusor hyperreflexia, while loss of anterior horn cells in Onuf's nucleus produces sphincter weakness. Cell loss in the interomediolateral columns impairs parasympathetic innervation of the bladder and causes atonia with retention and overflow incontinence. Detrusor instability may be an early feature with progression to failure of bladder emptying and high residual volume.[121] In the elderly, other potential causes of urinary dysfunction, such as abnormal detrusor behaviour, concomitant cerebral and urological pathology including prostatic outflow obstruction in men, should be considered before attributing symptoms to MSA.

Impotence is the commonest early sign of AuD in males with MSA, but is a non-specific feature in older men. Sleep apnoea, new or increased snoring and stridor are suggestive of MSA.[118,122]

Parkinsonism and motor signs in MSA

Parkinsonism is the most common initial motor disorder in MSA, even allowing for ascertainment bias.[123,82] Severe and early dysphagia and dysarthria as well as pseudobulbar crying or laughing are characteristic of MSA. Speech is typically slurred with hypophonic monotony, sometimes with a scanning quality where cerebellar dysfunction is prominent, followed in later disease by a quivering strained quality of voice. Tremor in MSA tends to be jerky and irregular. Pill-rolling tremor is uncommon.

Cerebellar dysfunction in MSA

A pure cerebellar syndrome is uncommon in MSA[116] but cerebellar features often coexist with parkinsonism.[55] Cerebellar signs seen in MSA include gait ataxia, finger nose or heel shin dysmetria, intention tremor and nystagmus. Various other eye signs are described with disproportionate impairment of slow–phase eye movements.[39] Smooth pursuit movements commonly become saccadic. Mild supranuclear palsy may occur in any direction of gaze in MSA. Marked supranuclear downgaze palsy with significant slowing of saccades suggests PSP. Cerebellar signs may be difficult to discern in late disease, when parkinsonism is pronounced.

Pyramidal dysfunction in MSA

Pyramidal tract signs (extensor plantar responses and hyperreflexia) are common in MSA, but weakness and spastic gait are not. Pyramidal tract signs in older patients with parkinsonism may be due to comorbid cerebrovascular disease or cervical myelopathy.

Other clinical pointers to MSA

Disproportionate antecollis, Pisa syndrome (lateral deviation of the spine) contracted or dusky violaceous extremities, involuntary inspiratory sighs and wheelchair dependence are other pointers to MSA.[13,82] REM sleep behaviour disorder occurs in several synucleinopathies including IPD, but is very common in MSA and may antedate other CNS symptoms by years.[124] Episodes of intense sleep-related vocalisations or extreme motor activity occur during REM sleep without loss of muscle tone and are accompanied by subsequent recall of vivid dreaming. Dementia is not part of MSA but a dysexecutive syndrome similar to IPD may occur.[89] A mild peripheral neuropathy is reported in some cases.[118]

Levodopa response in MSA

Absent, poor or waning response to levodopa is a hallmark of MSA; however, approximately 30% of patients may have a good initial response to levodopa, falling to around 10% in late disease.[53,118] Dyskinesias due to levodopa may be atypical and are often unilateral or dystonic affecting the head, face and neck[118] and may mimic a 'risus sardonicus'.[113]

Diagnostic problems in MSA

There is a low clinical sensitivity for the diagnosis of MSA.[123] Neurologists with expertise in movement disorders correctly identified only 25% and 50% of patients with MSA at the first and last clinic visit, on average six years after symptom onset.[125] Early severe autonomic failure, absence of cognitive impairment, early cerebellar symptoms and early gait disturbance were identified as the best predictive features for MSA.[125] However, gait disturbance and instability within the first year of disease onset suggests PSP.[94] Gait abnormality in MSA usually emerges two to three years after symptom onset.

MSA presenting as pure parkinsonism causes most diagnostic confusion with IPD.[126] Rapid progression, symmetrical onset, absence of tremor at onset and no response to levodopa were reported to be more positively associated with MSA than with IPD in 16 consecutive autopsy-confirmed cases of MSA.[127] However, parkinsonism was asymmetric in 74% of 100 patients in a clinical series,[53] and unilateral in onset in 49% of 203 literature cases.[55]

Diagnostic criteria for MSA

Diagnostic criteria for MSA have been formulated by Quinn[118] and by a consensus committee of the American Autonomic Society and the American Academy of Neurology.[128,114]

Patients are classified as MSA-P if parkinsonian features predominate or MSA-C if cerebellar features predominate.[114] These terms are intended to replace the SND and sporadic OPCA types of MSA.

Urogenital criteria which favour a diagnosis of MSA include urinary symptoms preceding or presenting with parkinsonism, urinary incontinence, post-micturition residual volume >100 ml, worsening bladder control after urological surgery.[121]

In elderly patients, a high prevalence of concurrent pathology may simulate features of MSA and impair the specificity of diagnostic criteria. Characteristically, autonomic, urinary and corticospinal dysfunction should not be explained by drug therapy or other pathology.[128]

Laboratory tests including autonomic function tests, sphincter electromyography, neuroimaging, functional cardiac imaging[113] and neuroendocrine testing[129] may support the diagnosis of MSA but lack sensitivity in early disease.[114] Quinn emphasises that 'The (relatively cheap) skills of an informed clinician remain more important than specialised investigations in the diagnosis of MSA'.[82]

Other neurodegenerative disorders associated with parkinsonism

Dementia with Lewy bodies

Dementia with Lewy bodies (DLB) is characterised by a progressive dementia with a fluctuating course, extrapyramidal signs (EPS), visual hallucinations and increased sensitivity to neuroleptic drugs. Patients may present with cognitive impairment or with EPS. It is uncertain whether DLB is a distinct nosological entity or more likely representative of one part of the spectrum of Lewy body diseases that includes IPD. DLB should be diagnosed when dementia occurs before or concurrently with parkinsonism (if present). Dementia occurring one year after the onset of IPD has hitherto been classified as Parkinson's disease with dementia (PDD) but the revised clinical criteria for DLB recognise difficulties in the strict application of this rule in clinical practice.[130] There is, as yet, no clear agreement in the literature regarding a difference, if any, in the profile of the parkinsonian syndrome in DLB as compared with IPD; this may reflect bias in retrospective retrieval of data in autopsy studies as well as differing 'sampling' times during disease progression. The parkinsonian syndrome in DLB is more commonly a modest akinetic rigid syndrome without classical rest tremor. As well as PDD, the main differential is Alzheimer's disease.

Alzheimer's disease (AD)

Extrapyramidal signs (EPS) are common in patients with Alzheimer's disease.[131] Rigidity and bradykinesia are most prevalent with resting tremor and abnormalities of gait are less frequent.[131,132] EPS can be detected at any stage of the dementing process, although are commoner in the later stages of illness.[132] AD patients with EPS have greater cognitive and functional impairment than those without EPS.[133]

Secondary causes of parkinsonism

Drug-induced parkinsonism

Drug-induced parkinsonism (DIP) is a common cause of parkinsonism in elderly patients[8] and may affect up to 40% of exposed individuals.[134] In a US Medicaid programme, elderly patients taking neuroleptics were 5.4 times more likely to begin antiparkinsonian drugs than non-users.[135]

Neuroleptic drugs (dopamine receptor blocking compounds such as phenothiazines, butyrephenones, thioxanthenes and benzamides, or dopamine-depleting drugs such as reserpine and tetrabenazine) are most often involved as precipitants. Substituted benzamides such as metoclopramide, or prochlorperazine – a phenothiazine derivative – are often prescribed for non-psychiatric conditions such as nausea or 'dizziness' in elderly patients and these drugs are commonly implicated in DIP.

Apart from advancing age, reported risk factors for DIP include female gender[8] and high drug dosage,[135] but a clear dose-response curve has not been established.[134] Neuroleptic-induced parkinsonism generally starts within three months, usually 10 to 30 days after beginning treatment, but immediate onset within hours of exposure or more delayed emergence is reported.[134]

Newer 'atypical neuroleptics' such as clozapine, olanzapine, or quetiapine may still produce significant extrapyramidal effects in elderly subjects. Calcium channel blocking drugs may possess anti-dopaminergic effects[134] and are recognised as a cause of DIP. Most substantiated are reports implicating the piperazine derivatives, flunarizine and cinnarizine.[136]

A number of other agents are reported to provoke DIP but the putative mechanism and role of these agents in causation is unclear. Amiodarone and sodium valproate cause postural tremor[29] but cases of DIP are well described with the latter.[134,136] Isolated case reports of DIP exist for sundry drugs including lithium, sulindac, phenelzine, procaine, meperidine, amphotericin, captopril, cephaloridine and various cytotoxic agents.[134] Selective serotonin re-uptake inhibitor antidepressant drugs such as fluoxetine have been implicated as rare causes of DIP.[1,136]

Clinical features of DIP

Drug-induced parkinsonism is classically a symmetrical akinetic rigid syndrome. Some cases may be indistinguishable from IPD with asymmetric onset and resting tremor. Supporting features for the diagnosis of DIP include concurrent high-frequency (7 to 8 Hz) postural or action tremor, perioral tremor (rabbit syndrome), superimposed tardive dyskinesia and akathisia. Resolution of DIP usually occurs within three months following drug withdrawal but some patients may have signs for up to one year before remission.[134] In a proportion of affected individuals, parkinsonism may persist or recur with progression to IPD. Drug-induced parkinsonism appears a risk factor for subsequent development of IPD.[137] These patients may have a subclinical dopamine deficiency which has been unmasked by dopaminergic blockade or depletion. PET studies support this proposal. While reduced fluorodopa uptake on PET scanning does not invariably predict worsening parkinsonism in DIP, a normal PET scan correlates well with recovery.[138] FP CIT SPECT (DAT) may also aid in diagnosis of drug-induced parkinsonism.[139]

Normal-pressure hydrocephalus

At all ages, an akinetic rigid syndrome may complicate non-communicating hydrocephalus.[140] In older patients, normal-pressure hydrocephalus (NPH) has received most attention as a cause of parkinsonism.[141]

The clinical syndrome of NPH includes the gradual onset of gait disturbance, incontinence and dementia, but all three components may not always be present. The gait abnormalities may comprise elements of magnetic gait, start hesitation, apraxia and ataxia with a lurching quality. Characteristic features include a wide base, normal leg function when recumbent, poor tandem gait, brisk leg tendon jerks and spasticity. In addition to gait disturbance, other typical features of parkinsonism have been described in NPH, including rest tremor, hypomimia, hypophonia, decreased arm swing, akinesia and rigidity.[140] Parkinsonism may or may not improve with levodopa.[140]

Vascular parkinsonism

Macdonald Critchley introduced the term *arteriosclerotic parkinsonism* in 1929, reporting that a flexed posture, slowness of movement and a shuffling gait might be produced by 'cerebral arteriosclerosis'. Criticism of this concept followed and Critchley redefined the syndrome in 1981 as arteriosclerotic pseudoparkinsonism,[142] as distinct from Parkinson's disease. He recognised that the disorder occurred mainly in elderly hypertensive patients and that it was associated with a stepwise progression. Other clinical features included pyramidal and pseudobulbar signs, emotional lability and dementia. Since then a number of different terms, such as *lower-body parkinsonism*,[143] *lower-half parkinsonism*,[144] *vascular pseudoparkinsonism*[145] or simply *vascular parkinsonism*[146] have been employed in the literature to describe a similar syndrome occurring in association with neuroimaging evidence of subcortical ischaemia or lacunar infarcts. Although the relevance of these vascular lesions as a cause of the clinical features remains controversial,[147] increasing evidence supports a causal relationship.[148] Intrinsic vascular lesions of the basal ganglia or disruption of fronto-striatal pathways are suggested as plausible mechanisms.[146] However, the expression of the syndrome in individual patients appears unpredictable in relation to the extent of vascular lesion load and site of lesion.[148]

In MRI studies, subcortical white-matter lesions appear more prevalent in patients with 'suspected vascular parkinsonism' (lower-half parkinsonism with frontal gait disorder) than in those with IPD or hypertension.[149] Two different types of vascular parkinsonism have been postulated.[149] First, an acute onset is reported with lesions predominantly affecting the subcortical grey nuclei (striatum, globus pallidus and thalamus); second, a more insidious onset is seen with diffuse subcortical white-matter lesions. Territorial stroke is less commonly associated with parkinsonian signs than are lacunar events.[150] Resting tremor of non-pill-rolling type was reported in nearly 20% of stroke patients with one or more parkinsonian signs.[150] Less commonly, basal ganglia lacunar states may produce a clinical syndrome indistinguishable from IPD, including levodopa responsiveness.[151,152]

Most reports highlight the abnormality of gait,[143,145,146,153] while noting a relative absence of parkinsonian features above the waist. These cases may be more correctly described as vascular pseudoparkinsonism.

Clinicopathological studies are of interest. Binswanger's disease (BD) or subcortical arteriosclerotic encephalopathy generally occurs in patients with vascular risk factors and may present with a gait disorder with elements of parkinsonism and ataxia. Reports of levodopa-responsive parkinsonism (with no concurrent Lewy body pathology) and a progressive supranuclear palsy-like syndrome have extended the clinical spectrum of BD.[154]

Predominantly symmetrical axial parkinsonism occurring in two men in their ninth decade has been reported in association with dilatation of the perivascular spaces (etat crible) of the striatum confirmed with neuropathology.[155] One case also had typical pathology of IPD.

Because of the heterogeneity of clinical expression and course in previous studies, a precise definition of vascular parkinsonism (VP) is elusive. Typically, core features comprise predominant lower-body parkinsonism, pyramidal tract and pseudobulbar signs, associated risk factors for stroke, absence of tremor or postural tremor with an overall poorer response to levodopa than in IPD.[143,153,156] However, a recent clinicopathological study suggests a significant response to levodopa in VP in a substantial number of patients, particularly where lesions occur in or nearby the nigrostriatal pathway.[157] Confusingly, levodopa-induced dyskinesia may occur in some VP patients.[158] The concept of VP remains under debate[148] but different phenotypes of parkinsonism, associated with cerebrovascular disease are recognised (*see* Table 4.7). IPD and cerebrovascular disease are both common disorders of the elderly: coexistent pathology may produce an 'overlap syndrome' with some degree of slowing, rigidity or gait disturbance attributable to vascular disease. This should be considered as a cause of disproportionate motor disability and disappointing levodopa response in older patients with IPD. Characteristic dopaminergic deficit on presynaptic SPECT scanning may suggest concurrent IPD[159] and may predict a good therapeutic response.[160] Combined DAT/D2 receptor studies may be of further diagnostic value.[161]

TABLE 4.7 Cerebrovascular disease and associated parkinsonian syndromes

- Lower-body parkinsonism (prominent gait disturbance, absent or atypical resting tremor, poor L-Dopa response)
- Progressive supranuclear-palsy-like syndrome
- Unilateral parkinsonism
- Parkinsonism indistinguishable from IPD
- Overlap syndromes associated with co-morbid Lewy body and cerebrovascular pathology

Conclusion

Idiopathic Parkinson's disease and other parkinsonian syndromes are clinical diagnoses, and ongoing review of atypical features for IPD will increase the diagnostic accuracy. In the older patient, the astute clinician will weigh up potential confounders to accurate diagnosis, such as centrally acting drugs or common concurrent morbidity like cerebral arteriopathy, diabetes or arthritis. The possibility of overlap syndromes or more than one diagnosis should always be considered. A summary of a practical clinical approach for diagnosis is shown in Figure 4.1. Where available, plain and

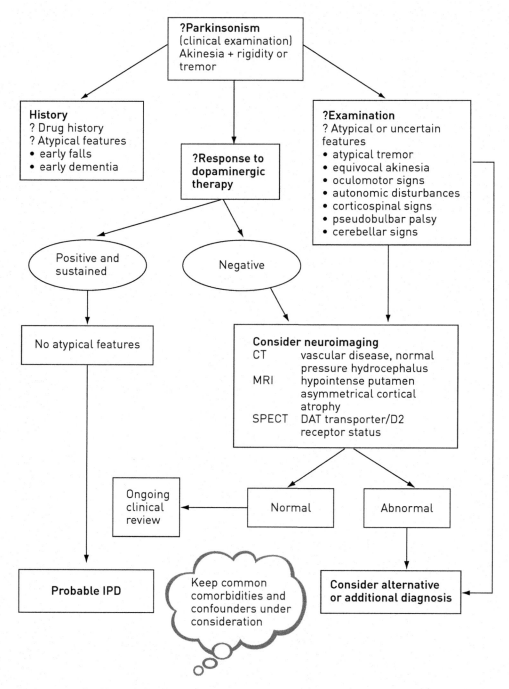

FIGURE 4.1 Outline of diagnostic approach for IPD in the older patient.

functional neuroimaging may be used as an adjunct to clinical diagnosis in the presence of atypical features or a poor or unsustained response to dopaminergic therapy. Finally, it should be remembered that even in expert hands, some cases of parkinsonism will be unclassifiable.[162] The emergence of genetic factors and molecular biology will increasingly challenge our traditional clinicopathological diagnostic approach to parkinsonian disorders.

REFERENCES

1 Riley DE, Lang AE. Non Parkinson akinetic rigid syndromes. *Cur Opin Neurol.* 1996; **9**: 321–6.
2 Louis ED, Marder K, Cote L, *et al.* Prevalence of a history of shaking in persons 65 years of age and older: diagnostic and functional correlates. *Mov Disord.* 1996; **11**: 63–9.
3 Waite LM, Broe GA, Creasey H, *et al.* Neurological signs, aging, and the neurodegenerative syndromes. *Arch Neurol.* 1996; **53**: 498–502.
4 Bennet DA, Beckett LA, Murray AM, *et al.* Prevalence of parkinsonian signs and associated mortality in a community population of older people. *N Eng J Med.* 1996; **334**: 71–6.
5 Moghal S, Rajput AH, D'Arcy C, *et al.* Prevalence of movement disorders in elderly community residents. *Neuroepidemiology.* 1994; **13**: 175–8.
6 Boyle P, Wilson R, Aggarwal N, *et al.* Parkinsonian signs in subjects with mild cognitive impairment. *Neurology.* 2005; **65**: 1901–6.
7 Louis ED, Tang M-X, Mayeux R. Parkinsonian signs in older people in a community based study. *Arch Neurol.* 2004; **61**: 1273–6.
8 Bower JH, Maraganore DM, McDonnell SK, *et al.* Incidence and distribution of parkinsonism in Olmstead County, Minnesota, 1976–1990. *Neurology.* 1999; **52**: 1214–20.
9 Hughes AJ, Daniel SE, Kilford L, *et al.* Accuracy of clinical diagnosis of idiopathic Parkinson's disease: a clinico-pathological study of 100 cases. *J Neurol Neurosurg Psychiatry.* 1992; **55**: 181–4.
10 Rajput AH, Rozdilsky R, Rajput A. Accuracy of clinical diagnosis in parkinsonism: a prospective study. *Can J Neurol Sci.* 1991; **18**: 275–8.
11 Hughes AJ, Daniel SE, Ben-Shlomo Y, *et al.* The accuracy of diagnosis of parkinsonian syndromes in a specialist movement disorder service. *Brain.* 2002; **125**: 861–70.
12 Jankovic J, Rajput AH, McDermott M, *et al.* The evolution of diagnosis in early Parkinson disease. *Arch Neurol.* 2000; 369–72.
13 Quinn N. Parkinsonism: recognition and differential diagnosis. *BMJ.* 1995; **310**: 447–52.
14 Meara J, Bhowmick BK, Hobson P. Accuracy of diagnosis in patients with presumed Parkinson's disease. *Age Ageing.* 1999; **28**: 99–103.
15 Schrag A, Ben-Shlomo Y, Quinn NP. How valid is the clinical diagnosis of Parkinson's disease in the community? *J Neurol Neurosurg Psychiatry.* 2002; **73**: 529–34.
16 Espay A, Li J-Y, Johnston L, *et al.* Mirror movements in parkinsonism: evaluation of a new clinical sign. *J Neurol Neurosurg Psychiatry.* 2005; **76**: 1355–9.
17 Rajput AH. Movement disorders and aging. In: Watts RL, Koller WC, editors. *Movement Disorders: neurological principles and practice.* New York: McGraw Hill; 1997: 673–86.
18 van Hilten JJ, Braat AM, van der Velde EA, *et al.* Hypokinesia in Parkinson's disease: influence of age, disease severity, and disease duration. *Mov Disord.* 1995; **10**: 424–32.
19 Hely MA, Morris JGL, Reid WGJ, *et al.* Age at onset: the major determinant of outcome in Parkinson's disease. *Acta Neurol Scand.* 1995; **92**: 455–63.
20 Diamond SG, Markham CH, Hoehn MM, *et al.* Effect of age at onset on progression and mortality in Parkinson's disease. *Neurology.* 1989; **39**: 1190.
21 Munhoz R, Li J-Y, Kurtinecz M, *et al.* Evaluation of the pull test technique in assessing postural instability in Parkinson's disease. *Neurology.* 2004; **62**: 125–7.

22 Charlett A, Weller C, Purkiss AG, *et al.* Breadth of base whilst walking: effect of ageing and parkinsonism. *Age Ageing.* 1998; **27**: 49–54.

23 Calne D. A definition of Parkinson's disease. *Parkinsonism and Related Disorders.* 2005; **11**: S39–S40.

24 Hughes AJ, Ben-Shlomo Y, Daniel SE, *et al.* What features improve the accuracy of clinical diagnosis in Parkinson's disease: A clinicopathologic study. *Neurology.* 1992; **42**: 1142–6.

25 Toth C, Rajput M, Rajput AH. Anomalies of asymmetry of clinical signs in parkinsonism. *Mov Disord.* 2004; **19**: 151–7.

26 Calne D, Snow BJ, Lee C. Criteria for diagnosing Parkinson's disease. *Ann Neurol.* 1992; **32**: 125–7.

27 Poewe WH, Wenning GK. The natural history of Parkinson's disease. *Ann Neurol.* 1998; **44**: S1–S9.

28 Gelb DJ, Oliver E, Gilman S. Diagnostic criteria for Parkinson Disease. *Arch Neurol.* 1999; **56**: 33–9.

29 Deuschl G, Bain P, Brin M, Ad Hoc Scientific Committee. Consensus Statement of the Movement Disorder Society on Tremor. *Mov Disord.* 1998; **13**: 2–23.

30 Quinn NP. Parkinson's disease: clinical features. In: Quinn NP, editor. *Bailliere's Clinical Neurology: parkinsonism.* London: Bailliere Tindall; 1997: 1–13.

31 Brooks DJ, Playford ED, Ibantz V, *et al.* Isolated tremor and disruption of the nigrostriatal pathway. *Neurology.* 1992; **42**: 1554–60.

32 Louis ED, Ottman R, Hauser WA. How common is the most common adult movement disorder? Estimates of the prevalence of essential tremor throughout the world. *Mov Disord.* 1998; **13**: 5–10.

33 Bain P, Findley LJ, Thompson PD, *et al.* A study of hereditary essential tremor. *Brain.* 1994; **117**: 805–24.

34 Louis ED. Essential tremor. *Lancet Neurol.* 2005; **4**: 100–10.

35 Cohen O, Pullman S, Jurewicz E, *et al.* Rest tremor in patients with essential tremor. *Arch Neurol.* 2003; **60**: 405–10.

36 Schrag A, Muenchau A, Bhatia K, *et al.* Overdiagnosis of essential tremor. *Lancet.* 1999; **353**: 1498–9.

37 Hall D, Berry-Kravis E, Jaquemont S, *et al.* Initial diagnosis given to persons with the fragile X associated tremor/ataxia syndrome (FXTAS). *Neurology.* 2005; **65**: 299–301.

38 Vidailhet M, Rivaud S, Goulder-Khouja N, *et al.* Eye movements in parkinsonian syndromes. *Ann Neurol.* 1994; **35**: 420–6.

39 Stell R, Bronstein AM. Eye movement abnormalities in extrapyramidal disease. In: Marsden CD, Fahn S, editors. *Movement Disorders 3.* Oxford: Butterworth Heinemann; 1994: 88–116.

40 Biousse V, Skibell B, Watts RL, *et al.* Ophthalmological features of Parkinson's disease. *Neurology.* 2004; **62**: 177–88.

41 Hardie R. The differential diagnosis of Parkinson's disease. *Reviews in Clinical Gerontology.* 1995; **5**: 155–63.

42 Pogarell O, Oertel WH. Parkinsonian syndromes and Parkinson's disease. In: Le Witt P, Oertel WH, editors. *Parkinson's Disease: the treatment options.* London: Martin Dunitz; 1999: 1–10.

43 Diederich NJ, Moore C, Leurgans S, *et al.* Parkinson disease with old age onset: a comparative study with subjects with middle age onset. *Arch Neurol.* 2006; **60**: 529–33.

44 Levy G, Louis ED, Cote L, *et al.* Contribution of aging to the severity of different motor signs in Parkinson disease. *Arch Neurol.* 2005; **62**: 467–72.

45 Piccini P, Pavese N, Canapicchi R, *et al.* White matter hyperintensities in Parkinson's disease. *Arch Neurol.* 1995; **52**: 191–4.

46 Rajput AH, Pahwa R, Pahwa P, *et al.* Prognostic significance of the onset mode in parkinsonism. *Neurology.* 1993; **43**: 829–30.

47 Roos RAC, Jongen JCF, van der Velde EA. Clinical course of patients with idiopathic Parkinson's disease. *Mov Disord.* 1996; **11**: 236–42.

48 Lewis S, Foltynie T, Blackwell A, *et al.* Heterogeneity of Parkinson's disease in the early clinical stages using a data driven approach. *J Neurol Neurosurg Psychiatry.* 2005; **76**: 343–8.

49 Schrag A, Quinn NP, Ben-Shlomo Y. Heterogeneity of Parkinson's disease. *J Neurol Neurosurg Psychiatry.* 2006; **77**: 275–6.

50 Gibb WR, Lees AJ. The relevance of the Lewy body to the pathogenesis of idiopathic Parkinson's disease. *J Neurol Neurosurg Psychiatry.* 1988; **51**: 752.

51 Ward CD, Gibb WR. Research diagnostic criteria for Parkinson's disease. *Adv Neurology.* 1990; **53**: 245–9.

52 Hughes AJ, Daniel SE, Blankson S, *et al.* A clinicopathologic study of 100 cases of Parkinson's disease. *Arch Neurol.* 1993; **50**: 140–8.

53 Wenning GK, Ben-Shlomo Y, Magalhaes M, *et al.* Clinical features and natural history of multiple system atrophy: An analysis of 100 cases. *Brain.* 1994; **117**: 835–45.

54 Collins SJ, Ahlskog JE, Parisi JE, *et al.* Progressive supranuclear palsy: neuropathologically based diagnostic clinical criteria. *J Neurol Neurosurg Psychiatry.* 1995; **58**: 167–73.

55 Wenning GK, Tison F, Ben-Shlomo Y, *et al.* Multiple system atrophy: a review of 203 pathologically proven cases. *Mov Disord.* 1997; **12**: 133–47.

56 Hughes AJ, Daniel SE, Lees AJ. Improved accuracy of clinical diagnosis of Lewy body Parkinson's disease. *Neurology.* 2001; **57**: 1497–9.

57 Hughes AJ, Lees AJ, Stern GM. Apomorphine test to predict dopaminergic responsiveness in parkinsonian syndromes. *Lancet.* 1990; **336**: 32–4.

58 Bhatia K, Brooks DJ, Burn DJ, *et al.* Guidelines for the management of Parkinson's disease. *Hospital Medicine.* 1998; **59**: 469–79.

59 Tolosa E, Wenning GK, Poewe WH. The diagnosis of Parkinson's disease. *Lancet Neurol.* 2006; **5**: 75–86.

60 Katzenschlager R, Zijlmans JCM, Evans A, *et al.* Olfactory function distinguishes vascular parkinsonism from Parkinson's disease. *J Neurol Neurosurg Psychiatry.* 2004; **75**: 1749–52.

61 Brooks DJ. Diagnosis and management of atypical parkinsonian syndromes. *Neurology in Practice.* 2002; **72**: i10–i16.

62 Piccini P, Whone A. Functional brain imaging in the differential diagnosis of Parkinson's disease. *Lancet Neurol.* 2004; **3**: 284–90.

63 Benamer HTS, Patterson J, Grosset DG. Accurate differentiation of parkinsonism and essential tremor using visual assessment of [123I] FP-CIT SPECT imaging: the FP CIT study group. *Mov Disord.* 2000; **15**: 503–10.

64 Marshall V, Grosset DG. Role of dopamine transporter imaging in routine clinical practice. *Mov Disord.* 2003; **18**: 1415–23.

65 Catafau A, Tolosa E. Clinically uncertain parkinsonian syndrome group: impact of dopamine transporter spect using 123i ioflupane on diagnosis and management of patients with clinically uncertain parkinsonian syndromes. *Mov Disord.* 2004; **19**: 1175–82.

66 Booij J, Speelman JD, Horstink MIM, *et al.* The clinical benefit of imaging striatal dopamine transporters with [I 123] FP-CIT SPET in differentiating patients with presynaptic parkinsonism from those with other forms of parkinsonism. *Eur J Nucl Med.* 2001; **28**: 266–72.

67 Bower JH, Maraganore DM, McDonnell SK, *et al.* Incidence of progressive supranuclear palsy and multiple system atrophy in Olmsted County, Minnesota, 1976 to 1990. *Neurology.* 1997; **49**: 1284–8.

68 Litvan I. Progressive supranuclear palsy revisited. *Acta Neurol Scand.* 1998; **98**: 73–84.

69 Rampello L, Butta V, Raffaele R, *et al.* Progressive supranuclear palsy: a systematic review. *Neurobiol Dis.* 2005; **20**: 179–86.

70 Nath U, Ben-Shlomo Y, Thomson R, *et al.* Clinical features and natural history of progressive supranuclear palsy. *Neurology.* 2003; **60**: 910–6.

71 Schrag A, Ben-Shlomo Y, Quinn NP. Prevalence of progressive supranuclear palsy and multiple system atrophy: a cross sectional study. *Lancet.* 1999; **354**: 1771–5.

72 Litvan I. Progressive supranuclear palsy and corticobasal degeneration. In: Quinn NP, editor. *Bailliere's Clinical Neurology: parkinsonism.* London: Bailliere Tindall; 1997: 167–85.

73 Valldeoriola F, Tolosa E, Valls-Sole J. Differential diagnosis and clinical diagnostic criteria of

progressive supranuclear palsy. In: Battistin L, Scarlato G, Caraceni T, Ruggieri S, editors. *Advances in Neurology*. Philadelphia: Lippincott-Raven; 1996: 405–11.

74 Burn DJ. The natural history of PSP. *Mov Disord*. 2006; **21**: 434.

75 Tetrud JW, Golbe LI, Forno LS, *et al*. Autopsy proven progressive supranuclear palsy in two siblings. *Neurology*. 1996; **46**: 931–4.

76 Rojo A, Pernaute RS, Fontan A, *et al*. Clinical genetics of familial progressive supranuclear palsy. *Brain*. 1999; **122**: 1233–45.

77 Higgins J, Litvan I, Pho L, *et al*. Progressive supranuclear palsy is in linkage dysequilibrium with the tau and not the alpha synuclein gene. *Neurology*. 1998; **50**: 270–3.

78 Morris HM, Janssen JC, Bandemann O, *et al*. The tau gene A0 polymorphism in progressive supranuclear palsy and related neurodegenerative diseases. *J Neurol Neurosurg Psychiatry*. 1999; **66**: 663–7.

79 Baker M, Litvan I, Houlden H, *et al*. Association of an extended haplotype in the tau gene with progressive supranuclear palsy. *Hum Mol Genet*. 1999; **8**: 711–5.

80 Houden H, Baker M, Morris H. Corticobasal degeneration and progressive supranuclear palsy share a common tau haplotype. *Neurology*. 2001; **56**: 1702–6.

81 Litvan I, Mega MS, Cummings JL, *et al*. Neuropsychiatric aspects of progressive supranuclear palsy. *Neurology*. 1996; **47**: 1184–9.

82 Quinn NP. How to diagnose multiple system atrophy. *Mov Disord*. 2005; **20** Suppl 12: S5–S10.

83 Lees AJ. The Steele Richardson Olszewski syndrome (progressive supranuclear palsy). In: Marsden CD, Fahn S, editors. *Movement Disorders 2*. Oxford: Butterworth Heinemann; 1987: 272–87.

84 Golbe LI, David PH, Schoenberg BS, *et al*. Prevalence and natural history of progressive supranuclear palsy. *Neurology*. 1988; **38**: 1031–4.

85 Litvan I, Agid Y, Calne D, *et al*. Clinical research criteria for the diagnosis of progressive supranuclear palsy (Steel-Richardson-Olszewski syndrome): Report of the NINDS-SPSP International Workshop. *Neurology*. 1996; **47**: 1–9.

86 Scaravilli T, Tolosa E, Ferrer I. Progressive supranuclear palsy and corticobasal degeneration: lumping versus splitting. *Mov Disord*. 2005; **20** Suppl 12: S21–S28.

87 Golbe LI. Progressive supranuclear palsy. In: Watts RL, Koller WC, editors. *Movement Disorders: neurologic principles and practice*. New York: McGraw Hill; 1997: 279–95.

88 Dubois B, Deweer B, Pillon B. The cognitive syndrome of progressive supranuclear palsy. In: Battistin L, Scarlato G, Caraceni T, Ruggieri S, editors. *Advances in Neurology*. Philadelphia: Lippincott-Raven; 1996: 398–9.

89 Pillon B, Goulder-Khouja N, Deweer B, *et al*. Neuropsychological pattern of striatonigral degeneration: comparison with Parkinson's disease and progressive supranuclear palsy. *J Neurol Neurosurg Psychiatry*. 1995; **58**: 174–9.

90 Paviour D, Winterburn D, Simmonds S, *et al*. Can the frontal asssessment battery (FAB) differentiate bradykinetic rigid syndromes? Relation of the FAB to formal neuropsychological testing. *Neurocase*. 2005; **11**: 274–82.

91 Bak T, Rogers T, Crawford L, *et al*. Cognitive bedside assessment in atypical parkinsonian syndromes. *J Neurol Neurosurg Psychiatry*. 2005; **76**: 420–2.

92 Barclay CL, Lang AE. Dystonia in progressive supranuclear palsy. *J Neurol Neurosurg Psychiatry*. 1997; **62**: 352–6.

93 De Bruin VS, Machado C, Howard RS, *et al*. Nocturnal and respiratory disturbances in Steele-Richardson-Olszewski syndrome (progressive supranuclear palsy). *Postgrad Med J*. 1996; **72**: 293–6.

94 Litvan I, Campbell G, Mangone CA, *et al*. Which clinical features differentiate progressive supranuclear palsy (Steele-Richardson-Olszewski syndrome) from related disorders? A clinicopathological study. *Brain*. 1997; **120**: 65–74.

95 Daniel SE, De Bruin VMS, Lees AJ. The clinical and pathological spectrum of Steele-Richardson-Olszewski syndrome (progressive supranuclear palsy): a reappraisal. *Brain*. 1995; **118**: 759–70.

96 Ghika J, Bougousslavsky J. Presymptomatic hypertension is a major feature in the diagnosis of progressive supranuclear palsy. *Arch Neurol.* 1997; **54**: 1104–8.

97 Williams D, de Silva R, Paviour D, *et al.* Characteristics of two distinct clinical phenotypes in pathologically proven progressive supranuclear palsy: Richardson's syndrome and PSP – parkinsonism. *Brain.* 2005; **128**: 1247–58.

98 Riley DE, Fogt N, Leigh RJ. The syndrome of 'pure akinesia' and its relationship to progressive supranuclear palsy. *Neurology.* 1994; **44**: 1025–9.

99 Litvan I, Bhatia K, Burn DJ, *et al.* SIC Task Force appraisal of clinical diagnostic criteria for parkinsonian disorders. *Mov Disord.* 2003; **18**: 467–86.

100 Osaki Y, Ben-Shlomo Y, Lees AJ, *et al.* Accuracy of clinical diagnosis of progressive supranuclear palsy. *Mov Disord.* 2004; **19**: 181–9.

101 Bhatia KP, Brooks DJ, Burn DJ, *et al.* Updated guidelines for the management of Parkinson's disease. *Hospital Medicine.* 2001; **62**: 456–70.

102 Tuite P, Clark H, Bergeron C, *et al.* Clinical and pathological evidence of corticobasal degeneration and progressive supra nuclear palsy in familial tauopathy. *Arch Neurol.* 2005; **62**: 1453–7.

103 Schneider JA, Watts RL, Gearing M, *et al.* Corticobasal degeneration: neuropathologic and clinical heterogeneity. *Neurology.* 1997; **48**: 959–69.

104 Mahapatra R, Edwards M, Schott J, *et al.* Corticobasal degeneration. *Lancet Neurol.* 2004; **3**: 736–43.

105 Maraganore DM, Boeve BF, Parisi JE. Disorders mimicking the 'classical' clinical syndrome of corticobasal degeneration. *Mov Disord.* 1996; **11**: 347.

106 Litvan I, Agid Y, Goetz CG, *et al.* Accuracy of the clinical diagnosis of corticobasal degeneration: a clinicopathologic study. *Neurology.* 1997; **48**: 119–25.

107 Wenning GK, Litvan I, Jankovic J, *et al.* Natural history and survival of 14 patients with corticobasal degeneration confirmed at postmortem examination. *J Neurol Neurosurg Psychiatry.* 1998; **64**: 184–9.

108 Kompoliti K, Goetz CG, Boeve BF, *et al.* Clinical presentation and pharmacological therapy in corticobasal degeneration. *Arch Neurol.* 1998; **55**: 957–61.

109 Rinne JO, Lee MS, Thompson PD, *et al.* Corticobasal degeneration: a clinical study of 36 cases. *Brain.* 1994; **117**: 1183–96.

110 Leiguarda R, Lees AJ, Merello M, *et al.* The nature of apraxia in corticobasal degeneration. *J Neurol Neurosurg Psychiatry.* 1994; **57**: 455–9.

111 Ball JA, Lantos P, Jackson M, *et al.* Alien hand sign in association with Alzheimer's pathology. *J Neurol Neurosurg Psychiatry.* 1993; **56**: 1020–3.

112 Bergeron C, Pollanen MS, Weyer L, *et al.* Unusual clinical presentations of corticobasal ganglionic degeneration. *Ann Neurol.* 1996; **40**: 893–900.

113 Wenning GK, Colosimo C, Geser F, *et al.* Multiple system atrophy. *Lancet Neurol.* 2004; **3**: 93–103.

114 Gilman S, Low P, Quinn N, *et al.* Consensus statement on the diagnosis of multiple system atrophy. *Clinical Autonomic Research.* 1998; **8**: 359–62.

115 Lantos PL. The cellular and molecular pathology of multiple system atrophy. *Mov Disord.* 1997; **12**: 822.

116 Kaufmann H. Multiple system atrophy. *Cur Opin Neurol.* 1998; **11**: 351–5.

117 Jellinger KA. The neuropathologic diagnosis of secondary parkinsonian syndromes. In: Battistin L, Scarlato G, Caraceni T, Ruggieri S, editors. *Advances in Neurology.* Philadelphia: Lippincott-Raven; 1996: 293–303.

118 Quinn NP, Wenning GK. Multiple system atrophy. In: Battistin L, Scarlato G, Caraceni T, Ruggieri S, editors. *Advances in Neurology.* Philadelphia: Lippincott-Raven; 1996: 413–19.

119 Magalhaes M, Wenning GK, Daniel SE, *et al.* Autonomic dysfunction in pathologically confirmed multiple system atrophy and idiopathic Parkinson's disease: a retrospective comparison. *Acta Neurol Scand.* 1995; **91**: 98–102.

120 Ballard C, Shaw F, McKeith I, *et al*. High prevalence of neurovascular instability in neurodegenerative dementias. *Neurology*. 1998; **51**: 1760–2.
121 Fowler C. Neurological disorders of micturition and their treatment. *Brain*. 1999; **122**: 1213–31.
122 Quinn NP. How to diagnose multiple system atrophy. *Mov Disord*. 2005; **20** Suppl 12: S5–S10.
123 Wenning GK, Quinn NP. Multiple system atrophy. In: Quinn NP, editor. *Bailliere's Clinical Neurology: parkinsonism*. London: Bailliere Tindall; 1997: 187–204.
124 Plazzi G, Cortelli P, Montagna P, *et al*. REM sleep behaviour disorder differentiates pure autonomic failure from multiple system atrophy with autonomic failure. *J Neurol Neurosurg Psychiatry*. 1998; **64**: 683–5.
125 Litvan I, Goetz CG, Jankovic J, *et al*. What is the accuracy of the clinical diagnosis of multiple system atrophy? A clinicopathologic study. *Arch Neurol*. 1997; **54**: 937–44.
126 Albanese A, Colosimo C, Lees AJ, *et al*. The clinical diagnosis of multiple system atrophy presenting as pure parkinsonism. In: Battistin L, Scarlato G, Caraceni T, Ruggieri S, editors. *Advances in Neurology*. Philadelphia: Lippincott-Raven; 1996: 393–7.
127 Colosimo C, Albanese A, Hughes AJ, *et al*. Some specific clinical features differentiate multiple system atrophy (striatonigral variety) from Parkinson's disease. *Arch Neurol*. 1995; **52**: 294–8.
128 Consensus Committee of the American Autonomic Society and the American Academy of Neurology. Consensus statement on the definition of orthostatic hypotension, pure autonomic failure and multiple system atrophy. *Neurology*. 1996; **46**: 1470.
129 Kimber JR, Watson L, Mathias C. Distinction of idiopathic Parkinson's disease from multiple system atrophy by stimulation of growth hormone release with clonidine. *Lancet*. 1997; **349**: 1877–81.
130 McKeith I, Dickson D, Lowe J, *et al*. Diagnosis and management of dementia with Lewy bodies. Third report of the DLB consortium. *Neurology*. 2005; **65**: 1863–72.
131 Perl DP, Olanow CW, Calne D. Alzheimer's disease and Parkinson's disease: distinct entities or extremes of a spectrum of neurodegeneration? *Ann Neurol*. 1998; **44**: S19–S31.
132 Mitchell SL. Extrapyramidal features in Alzheimer's disease. *Age Ageing*. 1999; **28**: 401–9.
133 Clark CM, Ewbank D, Lerner A, *et al*. The relationship between extrapyramidal signs and cognitive performance in patients with Alzheimer's disease enrolled in the CERAD study. *Neurology*. 1997; **49**: 70–5.
134 Montastruc JL, Llau ME, Rascol O, *et al*. Drug-induced Parkinsonism. *Fundam Clin Pharmacol*. 1994; **8**: 293–306.
135 Avorn J, Bohn RL, Mogun H, *et al*. Neuroleptic drug exposure and treatment of parkinsonism in the elderly: a case-control study. *Am J Med*. 1995; **99**: 48–54.
136 Hubble JP. Drug-induced parkinsonism. In: Watts RL, Koller WC, editors. *Movement Disorders: neurological principles and practice*. New York: McGraw Hill; 1997: 325–30.
137 Chabolla DR, Maraganore DM, Ahlskog JE, *et al*. Drug-induced parkinsonism as a risk factor for Parkinson's disease: a historical cohort study in Olmstead County, Minnesota. *Mayo Clinic Proceedings*. 1998; **73**: 724–7.
138 Burn DJ, Brooks DJ. Nigral dysfunction in drug-induced parkinsonsim: an 18F-dopa PET study. *Neurology*. 1993; **43**: 552–6.
139 Macphee GJA. Valproate induced parkinsonism. *J R Coll Physicians Edinb*. 2005; **35**: 214–6.
140 Curran T, Lang AE. Parkinsonian syndromes associated with hydrocephalus: case reports, a review of the literature, and pathophysiological hypotheses. *Mov Disord*. 1994; **9**: 508–20.
141 Graff-Radford NR. Normal pressure hydrocephalus. *The Neurologist*. 1999; **5**: 194–204.
142 Critchley M. Arteriosclerotic pseudoparkinsonism. In: Rose FC, Capildeo R, editors. *Research Progress in Parkinson's Disease*. London: Pitman; 1981: 745–52.
143 Fitzgerald PM, Jankovic J. Lower body parkinsonism: evidence for vascular etiology. *Mov Disord*. 1989; **4**: 249–60.
144 Thompson PD, Marsden CD. Gait disorder of subcortical arteriosclerotic encephalopathy: Binswanger's disease. *Mov Disord*. 1987; **4**: 1–8.

145 Chang CM, Yu YL, Ng HK, *et al.* Vascular pseudoparkinsonism. *Acta Neurol Scand.* 1992; **86**: 588–592.

146 Winikates J, Jankovic J. Clinical correlates of vascular parkinsonism. *Arch Neurol.* 1999; **56**: 98–102.

147 Fenelon G, Houeto JL. Vascular parkinsonism: a controversial concept. *Revue Neurologique.* 1998; **154**: 291–302.

148 Sibon I, Tison F. Vascular parkinsonism. *Cur Opin Neurol.* 2004; **17**: 49–54.

149 Zijlmans JCM, Thijssen HOM, Vogels JM, *et al.* MRI in patients with suspected vascular parkinsonism. *Neurology.* 1995; **45**: 2183–8.

150 van Zagten M, Lodder J, Kessels F. Gait disorder and parkinsonian signs in patients with stroke related to small deep infarcts and white matter lesions. *Mov Disord.* 1998; **13**: 89–95.

151 Murrow RW, Schweiger GD, Kepes JJ, *et al.* Parkinsonism due to a basal ganglia lacunar state: clinicopathological correlation. *Neurology.* 1990; **40**: 897–900.

152 Inzelberg R, Bornstein NM, Reider I, *et al.* Basal ganglia lacunes and parkinsonism. *Neuroepidemiology.* 1994; **13**: 108–12.

153 Zijlmans JCM, Poels PJE, van der Straaten J, *et al.* Quantitative gait analysis in patients with vascular parkinsonism. *Mov Disord.* 1996; **11**: 501–8.

154 Mark MH, Sage JI, Walters AS, *et al.* Binswanger's disease presenting as levodopa-responsive parkinsonism: clinicopathologic study of three cases. *Mov Disord.* 1995; **10**: 450–4.

155 Fenelon G, Gray F, Wallays C, *et al.* Parkinsonism and dilatation of the perivascular spaces (etat crible) of the striatum: a clinical, magnetic resonance imaging, and pathological study. *Mov Disord.* 1995; **10**: 754–60.

156 Yamanouchi H, Nagura H. Neurological signs and frontal white matter lesions in vascular parkinsonism: a clinicopathologic study. *Stroke.* 1997; **28**: 965–9.

157 Zijlmans JCM, Daniel SE, Hughes AJ, *et al.* Clinicopathological investigation of vascular parkinsonism, including clinical criteria for diagnosis. *Mov Disord.* 2004; **19**: 630–40.

158 Zijlmans JCM, Katzenschlager R, Daniel SE, *et al.* The l dopa response in vascular parkinsonism. *J Neurol Neurosurg Psychiatry.* 2004; **75**: 545–7.

159 Katzenschlager R, Zijlmans JCM, Evans A, *et al.* [123]I beta CIT distinguishes vascular parkinsonism from parkinson's disease. *J Neurol Neurosurg Psychiatry.* 2004; **75**: 1749–52.

160 Lorberboym M, Djaldetti R, Melamed E, *et al.* [123]I FP CIT SPECT imaging of dopamine transporters in patients with cerebrovascular disease and clinical diagnosis of vascular parkinsonism. *J Nucl Med.* 2004; **45**: 1688–93.

161 Plotkin M, Amthauer H, Quill S, *et al.* Imaging of dopamine transporters and D2 receptors in vascular parkinsonism: a report of four cases. *J Neural Transm.* 2005; **112**: 1355–61.

162 Katzenschlager R, Cardozo A, Cobo M, *et al.* Unclassifiable parkinsonism in two European tertiary referral centres for movement disorders. *Mov Disord.* 2003; **18**: 1123–31.

5

Assessment and quality of life

DUNCAN FORSYTH AND JOLYON MEARA

Introduction

Assessment is the process of careful measurement and evaluation leading to an informed decision about possible interventions designed to improve functional ability and maximise independence – it should include re-evaluation to determine outcome.[1] Assessment is therefore key to any purposeful health or welfare activity, and is particularly important in the rehabilitative approach to the long-term management of conditions such as Parkinson's disease (PD).[2] Without appropriate assessment, diagnoses can be missed; treatment opportunities overlooked; remediable handicap can increase; and the effectiveness of interventions can never be established. Timely and appropriate assessment should lead to interventions that improve the quality of life for patients and carers.

Key aspects to consider in the assessment process include the following.

- ➤ The need for and purpose of the assessment must be clear to both the individual being assessed and the assessor.
- ➤ Who is most appropriate to undertake a given assessment (nurse, doctor, therapist, social worker) and where should this take place?
- ➤ How competent is the assessor in their knowledge and understanding of Parkinson's?
- ➤ Functional capacity can vary enormously in response to drug treatment, hence the timing of the assessment in relation to drug therapy is important.
- ➤ The assessment will inevitably comprise both subjective and objective components, incorporating history, examination and observation. This may require the use of standardised and validated assessment tools. It will require a carer's perspective.
- ➤ Assessment is a dynamic process that should involve the patient and carer(s) as active partners in the assessment process. The assessment should identify the impact of PD on the lives of both sufferer and carer(s).
- ➤ The results of the assessment will inform further discussion between the subject being assessed, their carer(s) and the multidisciplinary team, in the formulation of an appropriate management strategy individualised to the individual concerned.
- ➤ Inevitably, as PD progresses, new problems will arise and it will be necessary to reassess and redefine potentially effective interventions.

Comprehensive assessment is time consuming but essential if we are to provide the best possible care to the person with PD. This should cover physical, psychological, social, environmental and quality-of-life domains.[3] No single health or social care professional has the expertise to perform such an assessment in isolation, and so PD needs to be managed by a multiprofessional health and social care team. Unnecessary duplication should be avoided by common shared records (e.g. a single assessment process), or at the very least accurate and timely communication between different health and social care professionals. Each re-assessment should build upon information already gathered and seek to define changes in health and social status that will influence further management strategies. It will not be necessary to reassess everything all the time, yet everything will need re-assessing in time! The complexity of PD and, therefore, of its assessment can present considerable challenges.

Adequate assessment will not only serve to guide the treatment regime for each Parkinson's patient, but can also influence the provision of healthcare resources for Parkinson's services.

Challenges in the assessment of PD

Parkinson's disease is a progressive neurological disorder with a long clinical evolution. Although the primary lesion involves the nigrostriatal tract, causing a disorder of motor control (bradykinesia, rigidity and tremor), primary and secondary changes can involve many areas of the nervous system, from the mesenteric plexus in the gut to the retina. This can result in a complex picture of neurological damage and diverse symptoms such as poor memory, anxiety, depression, apathy, constipation, urinary incontinence, dizziness, impotence and sleep disorder. Consequently, assessment of motor function alone can rarely describe the full impact of PD on an individual's disadvantage and quality of life.

Psychological dysfunction can occur directly as the result of the dopaminergic deficiency in PD and indirectly as a consequence of rapidly changing motor disability and physical handicap. Concerns over other people's perception of the PD sufferer, or the carer, reduce the opportunities to socialise (*see* Table 5.1). Anxiety exacerbates tremor and dysphonia, heightening self-awareness, embarrassment and risk of depression; this frequently results in further social isolation for both sufferer and carer.

Mobility problems make travelling difficult (including attendance at clinic appointments), and nocturnal symptoms disturb both partners. The assessment process may also be hindered by the effect PD commonly has on language, communication and cognitive function (dysphonia, dysarthria, bradyphrenia, dysexecutive or frontotemporal dementia). Other external factors (emotional and/or psychological) may also hinder the individual's ability to buffer the symptoms of PD and need to be enquired about.

TABLE 5.1 Social impact of Parkinson's disease

Stigma	% suffering
Complain of poor social functioning	29
No longer participate in social activities	40
Feel rejected by family (sometime/all the time)	38/14
Feel miserable and depressed	78
Plan life around medication	75
Experience side effects of medication	64
Experience 'wearing-off'	45
Sleep disturbance	75
Balance problems	72
Difficulties with walking	75
Complain of poor memory	75

Parkinson's disease shows a strong age-associated risk, with most people with PD being over the age of 70 years. This presents further difficulties in the assessment process as the effects of other disease states (co-morbidities) interact in complex ways with the impairments, disabilities and handicaps of PD. Determining whether co-existent cardiac, respiratory or joint disease contribute more to frailty, handicap and disadvantage than PD can be difficult. Interpreting the physical assessment may be hindered by the presence of co-morbid conditions, e.g. the presence of arthritis or joint replacements may render assessment of tone impossible. Furthermore, declining physical function may be mis-attributed to PD as new diagnoses are overlooked (e.g. the gradual development of anaemia secondary to underlying colonic cancer being the cause of fatigue rather than progression of PD). Finally, clinicopathological studies have shown that several neuropathological processes coexist in older patients with PD[4,5], including vascular damage, Alzheimer's disease and Alzheimer-type pathology. Put simply, there are more types of Parkinson's in older age.

Why and when assessment is important in PD

To establish the presence and type of parkinsonism

Accurate diagnosis is essential for appropriate management and prognosis. The diagnosis of parkinsonism and what type of parkinsonism is present can present considerable difficulties in elderly subjects. Even in expert hands, clinical diagnosis is far from secure,[4,5] and this is even more evident in community studies of PD and parkinsonism.[6] Obtaining a good history, careful observation and neurological examination can often establish the diagnosis without much difficulty. The use of formal clinical diagnostic assessment criteria can improve the accuracy of diagnosis of PD[7] and similar use of criteria for essential tremor[8] and other disorders commonly mistaken for PD should also help to reduce diagnostic errors (*see* Box 5.1). However, the diagnosis should always be under review to ensure that the progression of disease and response to treatments is compatible with a diagnosis of PD.[7] Occasionally, it will be necessary to resort to neuro-imaging,[9] e.g. where clinical diagnostic accuracy is hindered by co-morbidities, such as osteoarthrits, limiting assessment of gait and rigidity.

BOX 5.1 Common conditions misdiagnosed as Parkinson's disease

Essential tremor
Multiple system atrophy (MSA)
Progressive supranuclear palsy
Frontal gait apraxia
Other tremulous conditions
- Adverse drug effects
  - Lithium
  - Amiodarone
  - SSRIs
- Thyrotoxicosis
- Anxiety

To monitor the response to treatment and disease progression

Early stages of PD may not require drug treatment; the decision to implement any therapeutic intervention will be determined by assessing the impact of PD on the individual (the 'nuisance value' of their symptoms to them). Assessing response to any therapeutic intervention in PD (physiotherapy or pharmacotherapy) requires both objective and subjective analysis, for the impact of treatment may not always be readily discernible on questioning alone. Assessment of the response to drug treatment can help to confirm the diagnosis of PD and direct further treatment.

➤ How well have motor symptoms responded?
➤ Do motor symptoms remain responsive to drug treatment as the disease progresses?
➤ Is therapeutic response limited by early onset of drug toxicity (side effects)?

A good response can often be determined simply from the way the individual walks into the room and through their own reports and those of their family as to how they have been managing. However, the subjective response to drug treatment can be less clear-cut in elderly patients and should always be accompanied by an objective assessment of the motor response using measures of bradykinesia, tremor and rigidity and comparing these with pre-treatment levels. Each assessment must also enquire about 'gaps' in therapeutic efficacy, e.g. 'wearing-off' and nocturnal symptoms (fragmented sleep, cramps, nightmares, parasomnias, difficulty moving in bed, nocturia, etc). This approach will help to determine the best symptomatic individual response that can be achieved with drug treatment; that is, it will make tailoring of treatment to the individual possible, rather than a 'one-size-fits-all' approach. Assessment of side effects from drug treatment is also important at every encounter, particularly looking for dyskinesias, postural hypotension, sleep disturbance, drowsiness, cognitive impairment and psychosis. The early development of such problems indicates a poor prognosis, suggests a parkinsonism rather than PD, limits therapeutic options, and will influence caregiver strain.

Where there is diagnostic uncertainty, formal brief challenge tests to indicate responsiveness to dopaminergic stimulation (using single large doses of levodopa or subcutaneous apomorphine) have been developed to predict the diagnosis and the likely response to longer-term treatment.[10,11] However, these challenge tests are not recommended since they have poor specificity and sensitivity and are no real substitute for a therapeutic trial of levodopa treatment of several weeks' duration.[12] Acute 'therapeutic trials' in cases of difficult tremor or possible drug-induced parkinsonism should not be necessary these days with the increasing availability of functional imaging (DAT scans) to aid the diagnosis.[13]

Regular assessment of motor, autonomic and cognitive function can help to monitor disease progression, the continuing response of signs and symptoms to drug treatment, and the advent of complications/drug side effects. This approach will also demonstrate the development of non-motor, disabling symptoms such as drooling, dysarthria, dysphagia, freezing and falls, which respond poorly to drug treatment and hence need other management strategies. The frequency of review will be determined by a complex interplay between:

➤ stage of disease
➤ how fast the disease is moving (its trajectory) – itself a function of the stage and type of disease

➤ expected time to see the impact of the last therapeutic intervention (e.g. the effect of introducing a COMT-inhibitor will be evident within 2–4 weeks)
➤ expected time to see resolution of drug side effects
➤ clinical staff workload (necessary or appropriate frequency of review).

When assessing response to any therapeutic intervention, a limited number of questions need to be addressed:
➤ Have symptoms and signs improved with treatment?
➤ Is the response 'good enough' as far as the patient is concerned (assuming realistic expectations)?
➤ Are there any unresolved issues?
➤ Have there been any adverse effects of medication?

The more detailed assessments[14] that are required in the work-up for neurosurgery are dealt with in Chapter 17.

To manage advanced disease with complex problems

Comprehensive assessment becomes increasingly important with disease progression and the frequent interplay of other co-morbidities. The symptoms of late-stage disease often do not respond to dopaminergic drugs and increasing side effects limit treatment. Cognitive impairment becomes more prevalent, either due to PD or to co-existent Alzheimer's or vascular dementia, and increases vulnerability to neuropsychiatric side effects of dopaminergic therapy. Assessment can help to define the major problems and determine how these can be ameliorated. Very often, decisions need to be made about reducing dopaminergic drug treatment. Formal assessment of mood and anxiety with self-rating scales can help detect underlying depression and stress in both patient and carer. This stage imperceptibly merges with the assessment needs of palliative care, where the emphasis of assessment/management veers more towards the needs of carers, in order to sustain them in their caring role (*see also* Chapters 6 and 20).

To assess the impact of PD on the patient

Whilst there is no doubt that physician and patient alike seek to optimise the control of PD symptoms, we cannot hope to improve the quality of our patients' lives if we do not understand how their PD affects them as individuals. Nocturnal problems are common in PD, including early and frequent wakening, cramps, pains and nightmares.[15] These have an important impact upon the quality of life (QoL) of both sufferer and spouse. Just as PD is protean in its manifestations, so we must be diverse in our efforts to improve the QoL of the PD sufferers and their carers. A functional-status approach alone is not appreciated and only leads to dissatisfaction among sufferers and carers.

The Global Parkinson's Disease Survey (GPDS) (*see* Table 5.2) was the first in-depth international survey of QoL in PD.[16] The GPDS demonstrated that QoL in PD is affected by factors other than disease severity and medication usage. Only 17.3%

of the variation in QoL was explained by the disease stage (Hoehn and Yahr) and medication usage. Almost 60% of the variation in QoL can be explained by knowing the disease stage, medication usage, presence of depressive symptoms, the patient's level of satisfaction with the explanation of the diagnosis and their current level of optimism. Thus, the GPDS has helped to identify those factors which might be important in improving the QoL of PD sufferers.

Subsequent research has identified that depression, disability, postural instability, and cognitive impairment have the greatest influence on QoL in PD.[17] The improvement of these features should therefore become an important target in the treatment of the disease.

TABLE 5.2 Profile of Parkinson's patients and carers from six countries participating in the Global Parkinson's Disease Survey

	Patient profile	Carer profile
Males (%)	60	23
Age 60–74 years (%)	52	43
Access to carer (%)	74	–
Retired (%)	–	45
Median caregiving (h/day)	–	17
Median time as carer (years)	–	6.5
Levodopa treatment (%)	88	–
Dopamine agonist treatment (%)	60	–

Source: Findley (1999)[16]

Depressive symptoms may be present in around two-thirds of PD sufferers and one-third of carers.[18] Carers are more likely to suffer depression when the PD sufferer is depressed. In community-living PD sufferers, depressive symptoms, presence of sleep disturbance, and low degree of independence are associated with higher stress levels and reduced QOL.[19] Thus, it is important to screen for depression, for it is common; potentially treatable; significantly affects the QOL of PD sufferers, and adds to the distress of caregivers. The Geriatric Depression Scale (GDS-15)[20,21] is a self-reported screening instrument, which has been validated in elderly community-dwelling Parkinson's sufferers and their carers.[18] (*see also* Chapter 6).

To assess the impact of PD on the patient's family

Caring in chronic disease is largely informal family care,[22] thus PD does not just affect the sufferer, it also impacts upon their family and friends. The assessment of the needs of families and carers is therefore an important part in the management of PD and becomes increasingly so as PD progresses and the burden of care increases. Carer spouses of PD sufferers are more likely than non-carer controls to fare worse from the perspective of social functioning, psychological well-being and physical health.[23] They are less likely to get out of the house at least once per week, or to have had a holiday in the last year. Depression and anxiety are common in carers of people with PD,[18,24] with an almost fivefold increase in psychiatric morbidity in the carers, who are also more likely to suffer chronic illness.[23] The physical, social and psychological strain on carers increases in proportion to the level of care they are having to provide.[25]

Carers' needs fall broadly into the following areas:
> information
> reduction in physical and psychological burden
> a good night's sleep
> knowledge of and access to benefits, e.g. Attendance Allowance
> respite care.

Identification of such needs should lead to a reduction in carer distress by providing appropriate resources that support and do not undermine the carer's role. This may include the provision of physical care support, respite care, social support and financial aid. On occasions, the perceived needs of carers may be in conflict with the needs of the person for whom they are caring.

The Caregiver Strain Index (CSI) is a 13-item (brief), easily administered questionnaire that assesses the physical, social and emotional impact of dependency and caring upon the carer. The CSI has been shown to be valid across generations.[26] As PD progresses, carer strain accumulates; their lives become less predictable; the positive quality of the relationship declines; and carers are more likely to become depressed. Carer stress also shows a strong correlation with levels of depression in the PD sufferer.[24]

Specific assessment tools such as the Geriatric Depression Scale[20] and Carer Strain Index[26] can be useful in detecting depression and strain in carers. Standardised assessments of health-related quality of life, cognitive function and anxiety might also prove to be useful in carers.

To address problems with medication regime

At each assessment it is important to determine whether there are any problems associated with the medication regimen. Difficulties in getting washed and dressed in the morning may result from adhering rigidly to these tasks before going downstairs for breakfast when the first dose of medication is then taken. Blister packs may be difficult to open due to problems with manual dexterity, either due directly to PD or to co-existent arthritis. Tremor or dyskinesias may render liquid preparations and dosette boxes impossible to manage. Cognitive impairment may necessitate supervised medicating, as even alarming pill dispensers may be inaudible to those with profound deafness. Side effects of individual drug classes will be dealt with in Chapter 16. Ensuring that hospital and care home staff understand the importance of adhering to the PD sufferer's unique dosing schedule will minimise the risk of unnecessary problems arising such as: loss of motor control; delirium; falls; postural hypotension; immobility leading to pressure sores, hypostatic pneumonia, deep vein thrombosis and pulmonary embolism; problems with communication and swallowing.

To support research in PD

Basic medical research, pharmaceutical company-sponsored drug research and health service research into PD can all require specialised assessment techniques. The level and intensity of assessment in research is necessarily greater than that normally possible in everyday clinical practice. The observation that patients in clinical trials do better than those given normal clinical care may partly reflect this fact.

Assessment domains in PD

Disease-specific clinical rating scales

The advent of drug treatments for PD necessitated the development of more formal assessment of impairments in PD.[27] The assessment of the motor impairments of rigidity, tremor and bradykinesia should be an integral part of any neurological examination, and assigned a subjective value, e.g. at the very least, graded 'mild', 'moderate' or 'severe'. The sensitivity of this approach is likely to be fairly crude and the discriminative power very limited. However, it has the benefit of being quick and easy to do and may be sufficient if there is continuity of care for the individual patient (e.g. they are seen by the same assessor at each clinic visit).

More formalised clinical rating scales have been developed based on sign-and-symptom test items and/or the effect of PD on activities of daily living (ADL). Examples of the first include items such as walking pattern, finger movements, standing up from a chair, or amplitude of resting tremor. Examples of the second include the effect of PD on washing, dressing, feeding and household chores. Well-recognised clinical rating scales include the Hoehn and Yahr scale,[28] the Columbian Rating Scale,[29] the Northwestern University Disability Scale,[30] the Webster Scale[31] and the Unified Parkinson's Disease Rating Scale (UPDRS)[32]. Existing clinical rating scales cover many domains of assessment in PD and also tend to blur the distinction between impairments, disabilities and handicaps or disadvantages.[33] Sections of clinical rating scales can either be scored independently or can be summated to reach a grand total. The lack of any weighting of scores on test items makes the clinical interpretation of overall global scores and changes in scores difficult.[33] Clinical rating scales are often used as outcome measures in drug studies in PD, though the manipulation of such numerical 'results' are difficult to interpret given the subjective nature of the rating scales.[34] Many of these scales also have the disadvantage that they are too time consuming for use in routine clinical practice.

As the most popular clinical rating scale in present use, the US-derived UPDRS deserves further comment.[32] The UPDRS is a very large scale, largely derived from several other scales. As the UPDRS takes around 20–40 minutes to administer, it is rarely used in clinical practice in its entirety outside of research studies. Although an attempt at a comprehensive assessment of PD, the UPDRS fails to cover adequately important non-motor features of PD, such as sleep disturbance, cognitive function, bladder and bowel symptoms, and axial and balance problems. The reliability and validity of the UPDRS have also been questioned.[35,36,37] However, despite its limitations, it has become the 'gold standard' clinical rating scale, supplanting the hopelessly inadequate and flawed Hoehn and Yahr scale.

The reliability of sign-and-symptom tests has been investigated by showing video recordings of patient performances to a group of neurologists and non-medical undergraduates. This demonstrated that reliability was unsatisfactory in both groups, largely due to the inherent peculiarities and ambiguities of particular patient performances and contextual factors.[38] This same study also investigated the convergent validity of five clinical rating scales, both ADL and sign-and-symptom based, in 49 patients with PD.[38] There was good evidence of convergent validity between the scales studied, but considerable redundancy in the number of test items was apparent. The investigators concluded that the sensitivity of rating scales to clinical interventions was limited by the raters' capacity for absolute categorical judgement and that valid objective measures needed to be developed.

Physical
Motor
Simply stating whether or not the individual has tremor, extrapyramidal-type rigidity or problems walking is insufficient. Site, side and severity of tremor, rigidity or dyskinesia should be defined (e.g. jaw, orofacial, truncal, whole body and which limbs). Is tremor or dyskinesia constant or intermittent? What proportion of the waking day do dyskinesias occupy and what is the relationship to timing of drug doses. Enquire about wearing-off symptoms and dystonia. Describe standing posture, gait pattern and walking speed (measured over 5 m or 10 m), ability to stand from sitting and to negotiate doorways or other obstacles. The motor section of the UPDRS, a timed and observed 10-metre walk along with a simple measure of hand bradykinesia such as finger tapping on a counter device or touching each armrest of a chair with each hand in turn over a period of 30 seconds for each hand (two-touch test), can all be completed in around 10–15 minutes and so should be part of the routine assessment of every PD patient. Detailing the motor abnormalities will also aid in assessing the impact of therapy (physical and pharmacological). All motor abnormalities will be worse when the individual is stressed (physically or emotionally).

Normative values for these tests do not exist in elderly subjects. More detailed tests of motor function involving reaction and movement times and mechanically estimated measures of limb rigidity have been described, but are still largely confined to use in movement-disorder laboratories. [39,40]

Sensory
Painful symptoms are common in PD and must be asked about. No specialised assessment scales have been developed for these symptoms, though painful symptoms are represented, albeit poorly, in one item of the UPDRS. They either result from the primary disease process or arise secondarily from rigidity. Painful symptoms may occur:
- as part of nocturnal sleep disturbance
- when drugs 'wear off' (e.g. early morning dystonic cramps), or
- as part of an acute 'off' response when drug treatment temporarily fails to work.

Autonomic function

Autonomic dysfunction is common in PD either due to direct involvement of the autonomic system or as a side effect of dopaminergic medication. Early severe autonomic dysfunction raises the possibility of diagnoses other than PD (e.g. MSA). Impairment of autonomic function may also arise from co-morbidity (e.g. diabetes) as well as from concurrent drug therapy, such as thiazide diuretics to treat hypertension.

Postural hypotension can be extremely disabling and potentially very hazardous, leading to falls and injury. Assessment of PD must include lying (after five minutes' rest) and standing (immediate and after two minutes) blood pressure and pulse.[41] This assessment must be undertaken:

> if the individual has postural symptoms (e.g. dizziness, lightheadiness on standing)
> new onset of falls
> after any change in dopaminergic therapy (dosing or class of drug). The most appropriate time to assess for drug related side effects, in the absence of new symptoms suggestive of postural hypotension, will largely be determined by the time to maximum effect of the drug.

Other symptoms of autonomic impairment such as frequency of micturition, constipation, impotence and abnormal sweating also need to be elicited. An autonomic symptom checklist has been developed for use in PD.[42] Symptoms of autonomic dysfunction correlate poorly with objective tests of autonomic function. Older patients with PD rarely complete details of any sexual problem on the checklist (personal observations).

Activities of daily living

Stiffness and poverty of movement will impact on personal (PADL), domestic (DADL) and extended (EADL) activities of daily living, so no assessment is complete without enquiring about the individual's ability (or problems they encounter trying) to undertake basic activities:

> washing
> dressing
> grooming
> toileting
> feeding
> cooking
> cleaning
> gardening
> getting out of the house
> driving a car or riding a bicycle.

Self-reported disability in PD patients compares well with assessments made by relatives and observers.[43] A brief self-report ADL scale has been found to correlate well with measures of disease severity and quality of life in PD.[44]

The impact of PD on functional capacity is easily captured by the use of existing generic ADL scales. An instrumental ADL scale such as the Nottingham Extended ADL Index[45] can be used in this situation, combined with the Barthel ADL scale.[46] The UPDRS contains a subsection of ADL elements that could also be used.

Mental health

Mood

Depression is common in PD, and may respond well to antidepressant medication. Discussion of mood with the patient and recognition of the part that mood disorders play in the clinical expression of PD can in itself be a therapeutic exercise. It is difficult to determine which came first, mood disturbance causing deterioration in motor function or declining motor function ± poor response to medication leading to secondary anxiety and/or depression.

Several self-rated mood questionnaires exist to detect depression and anxiety, such as the Geriatric Depression Scale,[47] the Beck Depression Inventory[48] and the Hospital Anxiety and Depression Scale.[49] At appropriate cut-off scores, these scales show acceptable sensitivity and specificity for syndromic depression when compared with formal psychiatric diagnosis.[21] Depression can pre-date the motor onset of PD, and the risk of depression seems particularly high around the time of diagnosis and when major changes in disability occur. These findings reflect both the biological and reactive elements of depression in PD.

A busy outpatient clinic is not an ideal place to administer such instruments unless a quiet room that affords privacy can be provided. Although designed as self-rated instruments, in reality the nurse or relative often helps patients to fill in the responses. This can directly affect the results – as can the sight of the scoring sheet or any suggestion that the questionnaire is designed to detect 'depression'.

In older age it has been suggested by some that the simple question 'Are you depressed?' may be all one needs to ask.[50] (*See also* Chapter 6.)

Cognitive function

Cognitive impairment is also common in PD, ranging from mild evidence of frontal lobe dysfunction to frank dementia. Many elderly patients and their carers complain of problems with apathy, passivity, poor concentration and impaired short-term memory. A considerable proportion of elderly patients with late-onset PD will progress to dementia. Screening tests of cognitive function are important to define groups of patients at risk of dementia and to identify patients who will be poorly tolerant of dopaminergic therapy, especially dopamine agonist and anticholinergic drug therapy. The rate of cognitive decline in the individual patient can help in determining future treatment strategy and in providing a prognosis for the patient and carer. The trajectory for dementia is often steeper than that for motor symptoms. Better knowledge of the risk factors for dementia in PD may in the future permit early interventions that are designed to slow the development of dementia in at-risk groups. Early detection of cognitive impairment and/or psychosis will help direct carers to other support systems, e.g. community mental health teams; respite care.[51]

Three useful tests of cognitive function are the Folstein Mini Mental State Examination (MMSE),[52] the CAMCOG assessment,[53] and the Addenbrooke's Cognitive Examination (ACE-R).[54] The revised CAMCOG (CAMCOG-R) has the addition of more specific tests of executive function.[55] The MMSE is a brief global test of cognitive function, but suffers from lack of specificity and ceiling effects. Age, language and past educational achievement influence performance on the MMSE and so must be taken into account when interpreting the scores ascertained. In community-dwelling individuals, with clinically probable PD, CAMCOG assessment was more sensitive to early cognitive decline than the MMSE.[56] Since the CAMCOG takes 30 minutes to administer, a useful strategy might be to use the MMSE as a screening tool and to reserve the CAMCOG assessment for patients with borderline scores on the MMSE and for patients with evident cognitive impairment that requires further definition. Alternatively, the ACE-R takes approximately 15 minutes to complete, has the MMSE and clock drawing embedded in it, and includes assessment of frontal executive function.

The paired associates learning (CANTAB-PAL) test usefully discriminates between dementia and depression,[57] can be downloaded to a palm-held computer but has not been validated in a Parkinson's population and may not be appropriate for tremulous patients. (*See also* Chapter 6.)

Sleep and nocturnal problems

Nocturnal problems affecting sleep occur in up to 98% of PD sufferers.[15] Not surprisingly, improvements in sleep quality produce improvements in motor symptoms of PD.[15,58,59] Sleep problems may be grouped into four broad categories: insomnia, motor, urinary and neuropsychiatric.[60] Excessive day-time somnolence (EDS) may be caused by or cause nocturnal sleep disturbance.[61]

Enquiry about sleep-related problems should be a routine part of the assessment of all PD patients. As the UPDRS [32] contains only one sleep-related question, there has been a need to develop specific scales for assessing sleep disturbance in PD. The Pittsburgh Sleep Quality Index, Stanford Sleepiness Scale and Karolinska Sleepiness Scales are neither disease-specific nor sufficiently comprehensive to cover the sleep problems associated with PD. The Epworth Sleepiness Scale (ESS) is a self-adminstered questionnaire restricted to assessing EDS in eight day-time situations.[62] Interpretation of the ESS suffers from cross-cultural differences and uncertain test-retest reliability. The SCOPA-SLEEP Scale is a short, two-part scale assessing day-time sleepiness and nocturnal sleep[63] and whilst this has been shown to be both valid and reliable, it does not address some problems specific to PD. The Parkinson's Disease Sleep Scale (PDSS) is a 15-question validated instrument for quantifying sleep problems in PD.[64] The PDSS has robust test-retest reliability and good discriminatory power between PD patients and controls. (*See also* Chapter 9.)

Social and environmental (quality of life)

PD has a major adverse impact on the lives of both sufferer and carer(s), not just in terms of functional impairment, but also through its impact on their emotional and social life. Housing, driving ability and the availability of public transport or access to shopping are likely to be major determinants of quality of life in PD. Driving assessments are considered in Chapter 11. The social support of patients and carers may be an important determinant of access to, and utilisation of, health and social services.[65]

Given the pervasive nature of PD, there is clearly a need for self-rated quality-of-life (QoL) assessment scales in the assessment of any new treatments. This is especially so, as there appears to be poor correlation between the physician's perception of their patient's quality of life and the patient's own perception. QoL instruments measure the impact of PD on general well-being that other rating clinical scales cannot fully appreciate. Neurological assessment scales, e.g. UPDRS, simply describe the signs and symptoms of PD without attending to the many dimensions of the disease, including its emotional and social impact on sufferer and carer. Health-related quality-of-life measures can be used in PD to measure the complex interaction between PD and quality of life. Generic measures such as the Short Form-36 (SF-36) have largely been found to be unsuited to older people. Disease-specific measures such as the PDQ-39 and the PDQL have been developed and validated in PD.[66,67,68]

Carers may be restricted by their anxieties over leaving the PD sufferer unattended; for example, the fear of their falling. Patient well-being has been shown to be proportional to their perception of control over their symptoms. The extent to which the individual feels in control of their disease/life also influences their level of dependency upon others, with more optimistic individuals requiring less assistance.[69] It is therefore not surprising that caregiver strain has also been shown to be inversely proportional to the sufferer's perception of control over their symptoms.[70]

Quality-of-life assessment

In the absence of a cure for PD, therapies are directed at maintenance of function and limitation of symptoms. Thus, whether in the context of clinical trials or routine clinics, it is important that when assessing the impact of any therapy (pharmacological or physical), we consider the whole patient and not just the motor components. QoL is a better indicator of successful management than, for example, the degree of reduction in 'off' time. What matters is how the patient feels, rather than how the doctors think they ought to feel on the basis of motor function. For example, a reduction in 'off' time attests to the physical impact of a treatment, but tells us nothing about the quality of the 'on' time gained or any effect of the treatment on the quality of the remaining 'off' time.

Generic scales

Generic scales, such as the Sickness Impact Scale (SIP), which contains 153 questions, and the Nottingham Health Profile (NHP), which contains 38 questions, assess the impact of disease on quality of life but do not focus on the specific problems of PD. The NHP was developed to measure effects on QoL at the severe end of ill health and thus may not detect small improvements in QoL.[71] The SF-36 consists of 19 items relating to physical, psychological and social function; 11 relating to well-being; and

5 relating to general health perception. The items relating to vigorous activities/work in the SF-36 may not be pertinent to older people, and may lead to an age-related increase in omissions. The SF-36 has also been criticised for its possible floor effects. Although the items relating to physical and social function in the SF-36 appear to correlate with Hoehn and Yahr scores, the SF-36 is unlikely to be a sensitive measure of change in disease after any intervention.[66,72]

Disease-specific scales

Disease-specific scales, such as the PDQL and PDQ-39, can be self-rated and measure the impact of PD upon QoL. The PDQL has 37 items: 14 relate to Parkinson's symptoms; 9 to emotional functioning; 7 to systemic symptoms; and 7 to social functioning. Using the PDQL, older age, depression, cognitive impairment and disease severity are all associated with lower health-related QoL.[68] The PDQL requires longitudinal validation, and thus cannot be recommended for assessing the impact of any therapeutic interventions.[73]

The PDQ-39 has 10 items relating to mobility; 6 to activities of daily living; 6 to emotional well-being; 4 to stigma; 3 to social support; 4 to cognition; 3 to communication; and 3 to bodily discomfort. The PDQ-39 has been shown to have good reliability, validity, responsiveness and reproducibility. The mobility and the activities of daily living (ADL) domains of the PDQ-39 show a correlation with the severity of the disease, as assessed by the Hoehn and Yahr scale. These domains also appear to be responsive to disease progression. This longitudinal validity means that the profile response to the PDQ-39 may be useful in studying the impact of a therapeutic intervention upon different aspects of function and well-being in PD. A summary index (PDSI) can also be used from the responses to the PDQ-39 to summarise the overall impact of disease and the effect of therapeutic interventions upon function and well-being. The PDSI has also been shown to correlate with disease severity assessed by both Hoehn and Yahr, or the Columbia rating scale.[74,75,76] Depression, disability (disease severity), postural instability and cognitive impairment appear to have greatest influence on QoL in PD, as assessed by the PDQ-39.[17]

TABLE 5.3 Clinical features associated with significantly impaired quality-of-life scores

Depression (BDI>17)	<0.001
MMSE<25	<0.001
History of hallucinations	0.026
History of falls	<0.001
Postural instability	<0.001
Gait impairment	<0.001
Akinetic-rigid subtype	0.005

Adapted from: Schrag *et al.*[17]

Specialist assessment in PD

What patients and carers want is:
- information
- to be listened to
- support – both practical and emotional
- access to other professionals as required.

Initial assessment will often indicate the need for more specialist assessments by a wide range of health and welfare professions, including the physiotherapist, occupational therapist, speech and language therapist, dietician, dentist, chiropodist, orthoptist, clinical psychologist, neurosurgeon, ophthalmologist, old-age psychiatrist and urologist. The Parkinson's nurse and the Parkinson's specialist have pivotal roles in co-ordinating these professionals, all of whom must share information with one another so that it is clear who is doing what to whom, when and why.

The QoL of PD sufferers who have contact with a PD nurse is enhanced because they are less likely to fall, suffer fractures, or be institutionalised.[77] These practical benefits of PD nurses are probably attributable to their effects on monitoring and giving advice on drug therapy within primary care.

Team working is essential in providing a quality service to the PD sufferer and their carers.[78] Multidisciplinary clinics, with ready access to physiotherapist, occupational therapist, speech and language therapist, and availability of other disciplines as needed – for example, dietician and clinical psychologist – help to improve the quality of care provided. Consideration must also be given as to how one meets the needs of PD sufferers in nursing homes, who may not be able physically to attend these clinics.

TABLE 5.4 Potential benefits of early involvement of a Parkinson's team

- Making sure diagnosis is correct
- Ensuring access to specialist clinic (follow-up)
- Sharing of knowledge
- Disease control
- Patient support systems
- Impact of current illness on function
- PD pharmacology
- Management of parkinsonian complications
- Reduce complications
- Better understanding of complex drug regimes
- Use of apomorphine if unable to take oral medications
- Reduced length of stay
- Facilitate discharge

At some time in their life, the PD sufferer may require some form of surgery, not necessarily as a direct consequence of their PD. This can be a traumatic experience, with many experiencing post-operative confusion, loss of symptom control, or other complications of the disease, due to failure to receive their medication on time.[79] Such experiences lead to PD sufferers wanting to avoid hospital admission. It is important to improve PD patients' experience of hospitalisation by ensuring that they are seen by a member of the specialist PD team whenever (and for whatever reason) they are hospitalised.

A practical approach to assessment and improving quality of life in PD

Detailed assessments take time and, outside of research programmes, are not feasible – particularly for the practitioner working without the support of a large team. Several of the suggested assessments are self-rated, though elderly patients will often require some help with completion. Non-medical personnel given adequate training can administer the UPDRS, MMSE, ACE-R and CAMCOG assessments. Nursing staff can often fulfil this role, and assessment is seen as an important function of Parkinson Disease Specialist Nurse (*see* Chapter 15).

TABLE 5.5 Suggested minimum assessment guideline for older patients with Parkinson's disease (PD) and minimum (in brackets) frequency of repeat assessment

Body weight (annual)
Supine and standing blood pressure and pulse (after any change in dosing or if postural symptoms of falls develop)
Clinical diagnostic criteria for PD (mental checklist at each consultation)
Motor subsection of UPDRS or four-point tremor, rigidity and dyskinesia scale (each consultation)
MMSE and CLOX or ACE-R (with MMSE embedded in it) (annual or if cognitive problems develop)
Geriatric Depression Scale (GDS-15) (annual or if depressive symptoms occur or if response to treatment is not as expected)
Barthel ADL/Nottingham Extended ADL Index (annual)
Timed 10-metre walk or timed get up and go (each consultation)
Two-touch test of upper-limb bradykinesia (each consultation)
PDQ-39 (annual)
PDSS (annual or if sleep problems arise)

A suggested minimum assessment guideline in PD on first referral is shown in Table 5.5. This can easily be fitted in to a 30-minute follow-up consultation with enough time to discuss management strategies and thereby empower the person with PD. How often such assessments need to be repeated will be determined by the rate of disease progression and how frequently treatment is changed; a possible minimum frequency for re-assessment is also shown in Table 5.5. Assessment of motor function needs to be taken at a standardised time for each patient in relation to drug treatment if significant dose response fluctuations occur. In most cases, this means assessing motor function when the patient is reasonably 'on' in terms of response to drug treatment. In many older patients, response fluctuations are not evident and motor evaluation can be carried out at any time.

A better understanding of those features of PD that have the greatest impact on patient and carer well-being will be important in the development of new and improved management strategies. Current treatment algorithms focus on drug therapy and pay little attention to other aspects of the disease or non-drug therapies. Whilst control of symptoms is important, the PD team must also recognise the strong relationship between depression and QoL in PD, and consider measures to manage this. Attention must also be given to the explanation of the diagnosis and maintaining patient optimism. The importance of the first consultation cannot be overemphasised, as it provides the foundation upon which to build a supportive, patient-focused, disease management strategy.

REFERENCES

1 Barer D. Assessment in rehabilitation. *Rev Clin Gerontol.* 1993; **3**: 169–86.
2 Ward CD. Rehabilitation in Parkinson's disease. *Rev Clin Gerontol.* 1992; **2**: 254–68.
3 Struck AE, Siu AL, Wieland GD, *et al.* Comprehensive geriatric assessment: a meta-analysis of controlled trials. *Lancet.* 1993; **342**: 1032–6.
4 Hughes AJ, Daniel SE, Kilford L, *et al.* The accuracy of clinical diagnosis of idiopathic Parkinson's disease: a clinicopathological study. *J Neurol Neurosurg Psychiatry.* 1992; **55**: 181–4.
5 Rajput AH, Rozdilsky B, Rajput A. Accuracy of diagnosis in Parkinsonism: a prospective study. *Can J Neurol Sci.* 1991; **18**: 275–8.
6 Meara RJ, Bhowmick BK, Hobson JP. Accuracy of diagnosis in patients with presumed Parkinson's disease in a community based register. *Age Ageing.* 1999; **28**: 99–102.
7 Gibb WRG, Lees AJ. The relevance of the Lewy body to the pathogenesis of idiopathic Parkinson's disease. *J Neurol Neurosurg Psychiatry.* 1988; **51**: 745–52.
8 Findley LJ, Koller WC. Definitions and behavioural classifications. In: Findley LJ, Koller WC, editors. *Handbook of Tremor Disorders.* Neurological Disease and Therapy, Vol. 30. New York: Marcel-Dekker Inc.; 1995: 1–5.
9 Catafau A, Tolosa E. Impact of dopamine transporter SPECT using ^{123}I-Ioflupane on diagnosis and management of patients with clinically uncertain parkinsonian syndromes (CUPS Study). DaTSCAN Clinically Uncertain Parkinsonian Syndromes Study Group. *Mov Disord.* 2004; **19/10**: 1175–82.
10 D'Costa DF, Sheehan LJ, Phillips PA, *et al.* The levodopa test in Parkinson's disease. *Age Ageing.* 1995; **24**: 210–12.
11 Hughes AJ, Lees AJ, Stern GM. Apomorphine test to predict dopaminergic responsiveness in parkinsonian patients. *Lancet.* 1990; **336**: 32–4.
12 Hughes AJ, Lees AJ, Stern GM. Challenge tests to predict the dopaminergic response in untreated Parkinson's disease. *Neurology.* 1991; **41**: 1723–5.
13 Benamer HTS, Patterson J, Grosset DG, *et al.* Accurate differentiation of parkinsonism and essential tremor using visual assessment of [I-123]-FP-CIT SPECT imaging: the [I-123]-FP-CIT study group. *Mov Disord.* 2000; **15/3**: 503–10.
14 Langston JW, Widner H, Goetz CG. Core assessment programme for intracerebral transplantation (CAPIT). *Mov Disord.* 1992; **7**: 2–13.

15 Lees AJ, Blackburn NA, Campell VL. The night time problems of Parkinson's disease. *Clin Neuropharmacol.* 1988; **6**: 512–19.

16 Findley L. *Investigating factors which may influence quality of life in Parkinson's disease.* Proceedings of 13th International Congress on Parkinson's Disease; 1999 July 24–28; Vancouver, Canada. (Abstract.)

17 Schrag A, Jahanshahi M, Quinn N. What contributes to quality of life in patients with Parkinson's disease? *J Neurol Neurosurg Psychiatry.* 2000; **69**: 308–12.

18 Meara RJ, Mitchelmore E, Hobson JP. Use of the GDS-15 as a screening instrument for depressive symptomatology in patients with Parkinson's disease and their carers in the community. *Age Ageing.* 1999; **28**: 35–8.

19 Karlsen KH, Larsen JP, Tandberg E, *et al.* Influence of clinical and demographic variables on quality of life in patients with Parkinson's disease. *J Neurol Neurosurg Psychiatry.* 1999; **66**: 431–5.

20 Yesavage JA, Brink TL. Development and validation of a geriatric depression screening scale: a preliminary report. *J Psychiatr Res.* 1983; **17**: 37–49.

21 Jackson R, Baldwin B. Detecting depression in elderly medically ill patients: the use of the Geriatric Depression Scale compared with medical and nursing observations. *Age Ageing.* 1993; **22**: 349–43.

22 Nolan M, Grant G, Keady J, editors. *Understanding Family Care.* Buckingham: Open University Press; 1996.

23 O'Reilly F, Finnan F, Allwright S, *et al.* The effects of caring for a spouse with Parkinson's disease on social, psychological and physical well-being. *Br J Gen Pract.* 1996; **46**: 507–12.

24 Miller E, Berrios GE, Politynska BE. Caring for someone with Parkinson's disease: factors that contribute to distress. *Int J Geriatr Psychiatry.* 1996; **11**: 263–8.

25 Carter JH, Stewart BJ, Archbold PG, *et al.* (Parkinson's Study Group). Living with a person who has Parkinson's disease: the spouse's perspective by stage of disease. *Mov Disord.* 1998; **13**: 20–8.

26 Robinson BC. Validation of a caregiver strain index. *J Gerontol.* 1983; **38**: 344–8.

27 Marsden CD, Schachter M. Assessment of extrapyramidal disorders. *Br J Clin Pharmacol.* 1981; **11**: 129–51.

28 Hoehn MM, Yahr MD. Parkinsonism: onset, progression and mortality. *Neurology.* 1967; **17**: 427–42.

29 Lang AET, Fahn S. Assessment of Parkinson's disease. In: Munsat TL, editor. *Quantification of Neurologic Deficit.* Stoneham, MA: Butterworths; 1989: 285–309.

30 Canter CD, de la Torre A, Mier M. A method for evaluating disability in patients with Parkinson's disease. *J Nerv Ment Dis.* 1961; **133**: 143–7.

31 Webster DD. Clinical analysis of the disability in Parkinson's disease. *Mod Treat.* 1968; **5**: 257–82.

32 Fahn S, Elton RL. Members of the UPDRS Committee. Unified Parkinson's Disease Rating Scale. In: Fahn S, Marsden CD, Calne DB, Goldstein M, editors. *Recent Developments in Parkinson's Disease.* Florham Park, NJ: Macmillan Health Care Information; 1987: 153–64.

33 Wade DT, editor. *Measurement in Neurological Rehabilitation.* Oxford: Oxford University Press; 1992.

34 Martinez-Martin P. Rating scales in Parkinson's disease. In: Jankovic J, Tolosa E, editors. *Parkinson's Disease and Movement Disorders.* Baltimore: Williams and Wilkins; 1993: 281–92.

35 Martinez-Martin P, Gil-Nagel A, Morlan Gracia L, *et al.* and The Co-operative Multicentric Group. Unified Parkinson's Disease Rating Scale Characteristics and Structure. *Mov Disord.* 1994; **9**: 76–83.

36 van Hiltern JJ, van der Zwan AD, Zwinderman AH, *et al.* Rating impairment and disability in Parkinson's disease: evaluation of the Unified Parkinson's Disease Rating Scale. *Mov Disord.* 1994; **9**: 84–8.

37 Stebbins GT, Goetz CG, Lang AE, *et al.* Factor analysis of the motor section of the Unified Parkinson's Disease Rating Scale during the off-state. *Mov Disord.* 1999; **14**: 585–9.

38 Henderson L, Kennard C, Crawford TJ, *et al.* Scales for rating motor impairment in Parkinson's disease: studies of reliability and convergent validity. *J Neurol Neurosurg Psychiatry.* 1991; **54**: 18–24.

39 Teravainen H, Calne D. Quantitative assessment of Parkinsonian deficits. In: Rinne UK, Klinger M, Stamm G, editors. *Parkinson's Disease: current progress, problems and management.* Holland: Elsevier/North Holland Biomedical Press; 1980: 145–64.

40 Ward CD, Sanes JN, Dambrosia JM, *et al.* Methods for evaluating treatment in Parkinson's Disease. In: Fahn S, Calne DB, Shoulson I, editors. *Advances in Neurology, vol. 37: Experimental Therapeutics of Movement Disorders.* New York; Raven Press: 1983: 1–7.

41 Mathias CJ, Bannister R. Investigation of autonomic disorders. In: Bannister R., Mathias CJ, editors. *Autonomic Failure.* Oxford: Oxford University Press; 1992: 255–90.

42 Berrios GE, Campbell C, Politynska BE. Autonomic failure, depression and anxiety in Parkinson's disease. *Br J Psychiatry.* 1995; **166**: 789–92.

43 Brown RG, MacCarthy B, Jahanshahi M, *et al.* Accuracy of self-reported disability in patients with parkinsonism. *Arch Neurol.* 1989; **46**: 955–9.

44 Edwards NI, Meara RJ, Hobson JP. The Parkinson's disease Activities of Daily Living scale: a new simple and brief subjective measure of disability in Parkinson's disease. *Age Ageing.* 1999; **28** (suppl. 2): 107.

45 Nouri FM, Lincoln NB. An extended activities of daily living scale for stroke patients. *Clin Rehab.* 1987; **1**: 301–5.

46 Collin C, Wade DT, Davis S, *et al.* The Barthel ADL index: a reliability study. *Int Disability Stud.* 1988; **10**: 61–3.

47 D'Ath P, Katona P, Mullan E, *et al.* Screening, detection and management of depression in elderly primary care attenders. I: The acceptability and performance of the 15 item Geriatric Depression Scale (GDS15) and the development of short versions. *Family Practice.* 1994; **11**: 260–6.

48 Beck AT, Ward CH, Mendelson M, *et al.* An inventory for measuring depression. *Arch Gen Psychiatry.* 1961; **4**: 53–63.

49 Zigmond AS, Snaith RP. The Hospital Anxiety and Depression Scale. *Acta Psychiatr Scand.* 1983; **17**: 361–70.

50 Almeida OP, Almeida SA. Short versions of the geriatric depression scale: a study of their validity for the diagnosis of a major depressive episode according to ICD-10 and DSM-IV. *Int J Geriatr Psychiatry.* 1999; **14**(10): 858–65.

51 Delirious about dementia: towards better services for patients with cognitive impairment by geriatricians. www.bgs.org.uk/Publications/Publications%20Downloads/Delirious-about-dementia.pdf (accessed April 2006).

52 Folstein MF, Folstein SE, McHugh PR. 'Mini-Mental State': a practical method for grading the cognitive state of patients for the clinician. *J Psychiatr Res.* 1975; **12**: 189–98.

53 Huppert FA, Brayne C, Gill C. CAMCOG: a concise neuropsychological test to assist dementia diagnosis: socio-demographic determinants in an elderly population sample. *Br J Clin Psychol.* 1995; **34**: 529–41.

54 Mathuranath PS, Nestor PJ, Berrios GE, *et al.* A brief cognitive test battery to differentiate Alzheimer's disease and frontotemporal dementia. *Neurology.* 2000; **55**(11): 1613–20.

55 Leeds L, Meara RJ, Woods RT, *et al.* A validation of the new executive functioning sub-tests of the revised CAMCOG with the Ravens Coloured Progressive Matrices and the Weigl–Grewel Neuropsychological tests in elderly stroke survivors. *Age Ageing.* 1999; **28** (suppl. 2): 62.

56 Hobson JP, Meara RJ. The detection of dementia and cognitive impairment in a community population of elderly Parkinson's disease subjects by use of the CAMCOG neuropsychological test. *Age Ageing.* 1999; **2**: 39–43.

57 Swainson R, Hodges JR, Galton CJ, *et al.* Early detection and differential diagnosis of Alzheimer's disease and depression with neuropsychological tasks. *Dement Geriatr Cogn Disord.* 2001; **12**(4): 265–80.

58 Tandberg E, Larsen JP, Karlsen K. Excessive daytime sleepiness and sleep benefit in Parkinson's disease: a community-based study. *Mov Disord.* 1999; **14**: 922–7.

59 Karlsen K, Larsen JP, Tandberg E, *et al.* Fatigue in patients with Parkinson's disease. *Mov Disord.* 1999; **14**: 237–41.

60 Chaudhuri KR. Nocturnal symptom complex in PD and its management. *Neurology.* 2003; **61** (suppl. 3): S17–23.

61 MacMahon D. Why excessive daytime sleepiness is an important issue in Parkinson's disease. *Adv Clin Neurol Rehabil.* 2005; **5**: 46–9.

62 Johns MW. A new method for measuring daytime sleepiness: the Epworth Sleepiness Scale. *Sleep.* 1991; **14**: 540–5.

63 Marinus J, Visser M, van Hilten JJ, *et al.* Assessment of sleep and sleepiness in Parkinson's disease. *Sleep.* 2003; **26**: 1049–54.

64 Chaudhuri KR, Pal S, Di Marco A, *et al.* The Parkinson's disease sleep scale: a new instrument for assessing sleep and nocturnal disability in Parkinson's disease. *J Neurol Neurosurg Psychiatry.* 2002; **73**: 629–35.

65 Hobson JP, Meara RJ. Coping and support networks for people with Parkinson's disease. In: Percival R, Hobson JP, editors. *Parkinson's Disease: studies in psychological and social care.* Leicester: BPS Books (The British Psychological Society); 1999: 217–28.

66 Jenkinson C, Peto V, Fitzpatrick R, *et al.* Self-reported functioning and well-being in patients with Parkinson's disease: comparison of the Short-form Health Survey (SF-36) and the Parkinson's Disease Questionnaire (PDQ-39). *Age Ageing.* 1995; **24**: 505–9.

67 de Boer AGEM, Wijker W, Speelman JD, *et al.* Quality of life in patients with Parkinson's disease: development of a questionnaire. *J Neurol Neurosurg Psychiatry.* 1996; **61**: 70–4.

68 Hobson JP, Holden A, Meara RJ. Measuring the impact of Parkinson's disease with the Parkinson's Disease Quality of Life questionnaire (PDQL). *Age Ageing.* 1999; **28**: 341–6.

69 Shifren K. Individual differences in the perception of optimism and disease severity: a study among individuals with Parkinson's disease. *J Behav Med.* 1996; **19**: 241–71.

70 Wallhagen MI, Brod M. Perceived control and well-being in Parkinson's disease. *West J Nurs Res.* 1997; **19**: 11–31.

71 Jenkinson C, Fitzpatrick R, Argyle M. The Nottingham Health Profile: an analysis of its sensitivity in differentiating illness groups. *Soc Sci Med.* 1988; **27**: 1411–14.

72 Hayes V, Morris J, Wolfe C, *et al.* The SF-36 health survey questionnaire: is it suitable for use in older adults? *Age Ageing.* 1995; **24**: 120–5.

73 de Boer AG, Wijker W, Speelman JD, *et al.* Quality of life in patients with Parkinson's disease: development of a questionnaire. *J Neurol Neurosurg Psychiatry.* 1996; **61**: 70–4.

74 Fitzpatrick R, Peto V, Jenkinson C, *et al.* Health-related quality of life in Parkinson's disease: a study of outpatient clinic attenders. *Mov Disord.* 1997; **12**: 916–22.

75 Harrison JE, Preston S, Blunt SB. Measuring symptom change in patients with Parkinson's disease. *Age Ageing.* 2000; **29**: 41–5.

76 Jenkinson C, Fitzpatrick R, Peto V, *et al.* The Parkinson's Disease Questionnaire (PDQ-39): development and validation of a Parkinson's disease summary index score. *Age Ageing.* 1997; **26**: 353–7.

77 Jarman B. The Imperial College School of Medicine Parkinson's disease nurse specialist project. Presented at: 'The science and practice of multidisciplinary care in Parkinson's disease'; 1998, 12 June. The Royal College of Physicians, London.

78 Firth-Cozens J. Celebrating teamwork. *Qual Healthcare.* 1998; **7** (suppl. I): S3–S7.

79 Barber M, Stewart D, Scott S, *et al.* Patient and carer perception of the management of Parkinson's disease in the peri-operative period. *Age Ageing.* 1999; **28** (suppl. 2): 99 (Abstract 149).

PART 3

Non-motor dysfunction

Neuropsychiatry

JOHN HINDLE

Introduction

Parkinson's disease (PD) is a complex disorder with neurological and psychiatric components. The older term for the condition was *paralysis agitans*, with paralysis at that time meaning 'abolition of movement and sensation'. Dr James Parkinson, in his essay on the shaking palsy, famously described the senses and intellect as being uninjured.[1] Parkinson was open to the possibility of psychiatric disturbance in the condition, and quoted one case of a patient who became melancholy and dejected, mute, then spitting.[1] An historical re-reading of the 'senses and intellect uninjured' suggests the true interpretation to be that sensory modalities remain uninjured (distinguishing it from other causes of paralysis) and that intelligence is normal.[2] Although psychiatric abnormalities were recognised in the nineteenth century by Charcot in Paris and Gowers in London, they were only judged to be an intrinsic part of the condition in the early twentieth century. Benjamin Ball, the first professor of psychiatry in Paris, was an exception and, in 1881, quite correctly stated that 'a large number of parkinsonian patients present psychological disorders extending from simple irritability to psychosis; I would say that a slight degree of cognitive impairment is the rule'.[2] We now recognise that psychiatric problems in PD can include cognitive impairment, dementia, depression, psychosis, anxiety, mania and impulse control disorders including hypersexuality and gambling. There are complex interactions between motor function, emotions, cognition, and the effects of treatment and chronic disability. Today, the most problematic psychiatric disorders are often secondary to the combined effects of the disease and treatment.

The importance of mental state

The maintenance of mental health in PD may be more important than the physical state. Depression and cognition may affect the quality of life of patients and stress their carers more than physical disability.[3,4] Psychosis is disruptive to normal life, and often involves a substantial increase in demands on the primary healthcare team. The development of psychosis may predict institutionalisation and early death.[5] The development of depression and dementia is also associated with increased mortality.[6] Cognitive impairment may limit performance of complex psychomotor tasks such as driving.[7] Mild cognitive impairment can be detected even early in the disease.[8] An understanding of the psychiatry of PD is therefore important.

Heterogeneity in the psychiatry of PD

The complexity of the psychiatry of PD is a manifestation of the heterogeneity of PD itself. This heterogeneity has no simple explanation. The psychiatric symptoms are a manifestation of the system failure brought about by the underlying disease processes. In older patients, the variation in psychiatric manifestations may be greater due the effects of ageing and the effects of co-morbid conditions such as cerebrovascular disease. An interaction between genes, the environment, the biology of the brain and ageing may bring an increased liability to develop protein deposition, leading to cell loss and neurodegeneration. The hallmark of this neurodegenerative process in PD is the intracellular inclusion body known as the Lewy body. Variations in the distribution of this pathology may lead to a spectrum of conditions with varying motor and psychiatric features, including idiopathic PD, Parkinson's disease dementia (PDD) and dementia with Lewy bodies (DLB).

It is useful to attempt to distinguish primary psychiatric phenomena, which are due to the disease itself, from secondary phenomena which may be due to the effects of treatment, other superimposed conditions or the effects of the psychosocial stress of chronic disability. The primary psychiatric abnormalities were well described prior to the use of levodopa and surgery by Mjones in 1949, who summarised these as abnormalities of personality, memory, depression and anxiety.[9] In considering these, it is important not to include those patients suffering from parkinsonism secondary to the encephalitis lethargica pandemic in 1917–21, which caused more florid psychiatric phenomena including severe personality change and psychosis.

Parkinsonian 'personality'

Early in the twentieth century, there was increasing interest in descriptive psychopathology. The influence of Freud and his pupils produced a fascination with the power of the mind and personality. Theories of the effects of suppressed emotion and psychogenesis of disease increased interest in the effects of personality as a cause of PD. Preceding the motor syndrome, patients were said to be industrious, introverted, punctual, inflexible, reliable, exacting, morally rigid and to exhibit reduced novelty-seeking behaviour.[10] It now seems most likely that these traits are in fact a manifestation of mild affective and cognitive changes very early in the disease, since it is recognised that anxiety and depression may be presenting features of PD reflecting early pathology in the brain stem and limbic connections.[11] Abnormalities of neurotransmitters preceding the motor symptoms may manifest in psychological changes. For example, it is possible that deficiency of serotonin may contribute to pre-morbid shyness. A study of personality, depression and pre-morbid lifestyle in twin pairs discordant for PD gives some support for the existence of a genetically determined non-motor syndrome of PD prior to the onset of motor symptoms.[12] In a systematic review of the literature, the general descriptions of PD patients included being nervous, cautious, rigid and conventional. The studies were all retrospective. To confirm that 'pre-morbid' personality traits precede PD onset, prospective research correlating personality characteristics to activities or changes in the brain is required. The term *pre-morbid* is difficult to define due to the unknown latent period before onset of PD.[13]

Psychogenic parkinsonism has been described in patients with normal positron emission tomography (PET) scans, some of whom had spontaneous remission. This condition is extremely rare and is a diagnosis of exclusion.[14] More commonly, psychogenic symptoms can complicate the presentation of PD.

Measurement in neuropsychiatry

Psychometric testing, electrical measurement and imaging techniques can be used in the assessment of cognitive and psychiatric processes in PD. A range of psychometric tests and rating scales is required to examine the spectrum of cognitive and psychological abnormalities in PD (*see* Table 6.1). Clinical assessment of the mental state is also covered in Chapter 5, on the assessment of PD.

TABLE 6.1 Examples of neuropsychological tests in Parkinson's disease

Function	Examples of tests
Global cognition	Mini Mental State Examination (MMSE)
	Cambridge Cognitive Examination (CAMCOG)
	Rivermead Behavioural Memory Test (RBMT)
	Mattis Dementia Rating Scale (DRS)
	Addenbrookes Cognitive Examination (ACE-R)
Episodic memory	Three-word recall from MMSE
Executive function	CAMCOG-R (extra subsection for executive function)
	Wisconsin Card Sorting Test
	STROOP test
	Digit recall
	Verbal fluency
	Trail making
Frontal lobe	Frontal assessment battery
	Verbal fluency 'F,A,S' test
	Proverbs/Similarities
	Go-no-go tests
	Cognitive estimates
Working memory	Digit span
Behaviour	Apathy scale
Visuospatial	Picture completion – Weschler Adult Intelligence Scale (WAIS)
	Clock drawing

The standard electroencephalogram (EEG) is not very helpful in PD and should be normal, except in PD dementia (PDD) in which there may be some background slowing. Specific EEG responses to a single stimulus, known as event-related potentials (ERP), have been studied extensively. The time to a positive deflection on the ERP is called the latency. The peak at 200 millisecond (P_{200}) is due to activation of association areas, and the peak at 300 milliseconds (P_{300}) is due to thinking time and reflects uncertainty. The latency of these peak responses is delayed in PD, and also in Alzheimer's and Huntington's diseases, reflecting abnormal central processing.[15] In addition, the ERP can be studied in relation to preparation for movement – the movement-related potential (MRP). A negative deflection (*bereitschaftspotential*) prior to a movement reflects the ability to anticipate and prepare for an action and is also impaired in PD.[16] Brain electrical activity mapping (BEAM), which gives a contoured map of the intensity of electrical activity in response to a stimulus, has been studied.[15] Structural imaging using computed tomography (CT) and magnetic resonance imaging (MRI) is used to measure the size of subcortical areas. Functional imaging is much more useful in the study of cognition since areas of increased cerebral blood flow and metabolism can be demonstrated during the performance of specific tasks. Scans are performed at rest and during activation, then subtracted to demonstrate specific areas of activation. Positron emission tomography (PET) is performed in specialist centres using a cyclotron to manufacture the short-lived isotopes. Single photon emission tomography (SPECT) utilises CT techniques to enhance isotope brain scans produced from improved radiotracer biochemicals that emit gamma rays. The technique is not as quantifiable as PET and the resolution is poorer, but it is more accessible and has been used in the differential diagnosis of PD.[17] PET, and to a lesser extent SPECT studies, have demonstrated neurochemical changes in depression, attentional deficits, cognitive dysfunction and dementia in PD.[16] A more rapid change in cerebral blood flow can be detected using functional magnetic resonance scanning (FMRI). This technique uses MRI technology to monitor the change in resonance which occurs when oxyhaemoglobin changes to deoxyhaemoglobin, thus measuring blood flow and metabolism. FMRI has, for example, demonstrated altered cortical visual processing in PD patients with recurrent visual hallucinations.[18] Proton magnetic resonance spectroscopy, which measures metabolite signals from neurones, has been used to study small changes in cortical metabolism in early non-demented PD patients.[19] Transcranial sonography has also been used as a tool for the early preclinical diagnosis of PD in those at risk and as a tool in the study of depression in PD.

Cognitive functions in PD

Cognition is the process by which knowledge is acquired, and this includes perception, intuition and reasoning.[20] Modern studies of cognition in PD began with Aubrin in 1937, who, supervised by Guillain-Barré, performed one of the earliest experiments to use psychometric instruments for the measurement of cognition in PD.[2]

In order to understand the effects of PD on cognition, it is important to have a basic understanding of the functional anatomy of the basal ganglia connections. In a very simplified model it is useful to consider the basal ganglia connections as a series of parallel functionally segregated motor, occulomotor and complex circuits. The motor circuits, which are involved in automatic motor function and automatic (implicit) learning, are under-active in PD. Implicit processes, which are not available to conscious thought, include conditioning, priming and automatic motor skills. The complex circuits include dorsolateral, pre-frontal and anterior cingulate loops, which mediate the cognitive processes involved in explicit learning, problem solving and attention, are also under-active in PD.[21,22] Explicit processes are available to conscious thought, and include short- and long-term memory. Short-term or working memory can either be verbal or visuo-spatial. Long-term memory can be either be episodic (recalled in a specific time frame) or semantic (recalled outside a time frame, e.g. grass is green).[20] The reduction in number of neurones in the lateral part of the substantia nigra compacta correlates with the motor severity of PD, whereas the number of neurones in the medial substantia nigra compacta correlates with abnormalities of cognition.[23] Limbic dopaminergic pathways linked through the medial substantia nigra modulate these circuits. There are also other interconnecting loops within the striatum and linking thalamocortical circuits modulated by other neurotransmitters. Malfunction of these interconnections may contribute to cognitive dysfunction in PD. Compensatory over-activity of the cerebellar motor pathways occurs in PD and these pathways involve more conscious processes such as attention and cueing.[24]

Cognitive processes can be distributed or localised in the brain (*see* Table 6.2),[20] and the fact that many of these functions are impaired in PD reflects the extensive connections of the basal ganglia with other brain areas. Higher animals are able to produce adaptive behaviour through connections between the basal ganglia and the prefrontal cortex. The basal ganglia tend to select routine, over-learned or safe behaviours. In normal circumstances these behaviours are suppressed through connections with the prefrontal cortex, which interacts more with the environment to produce adaptive behaviour appropriate to the situation. Interruption of this system in the prefrontal cortex tends to produce perseveration and disinhibition, whereas a basal ganglia lesion tends to produce a difficulty in acquiring new behaviours and a predominance of over-learned behaviour.[25]

TABLE 6.2 Structure of cognition and memory

Cognition – Distributed	Cognition – Localised
Attention – Reticular activating system and association areas	**Dominant hemisphere** – Language, calculation, praxis
Memory – Limbic, hippocampus, diencephalon	**Non-dominant** – Spatial attention, visuoperceptual skills, construction, language prosody, vigilance
Higher functions – Frontal	
Memory – Explicit	**Memory – Implicit**
Short term (working memory) – Verbal, spatial	Conditioning
	Priming
	Motor skills
Long term – Episodic, semantic	

The basal ganglia are involved in the generation, maintenance, switching and blending of motor, cognitive and behavioural patterns or sets. A basal ganglia lesion leads to difficulties with procedural mobilisation due to problems selecting, activating and maintaining behaviours, with difficulty formulating strategies and preparing for action.[21,25]

Mild cognitive impairment in PD

Patients with PD demonstrate slowing of movement (bradykinesia), and in addition show variable degrees of slowing of thought and speech. This was thought to be similar to the psychomotor retardation seen in depression by the French psychiatrist Ball in 1881 and was defined as bradyphrenia by Naville in 1922.[2] Bradyphrenia is most severe in progressive supranuclear palsy (PSP), in which patients may take minutes to respond. Although bradyphrenia represents some slowing of central processing, it is important to distinguish this from other forms of cognitive deterioration seen in PD.

In the non-demented PD patient with mild cognitive impairment, the core deficit is of planning abilities sometimes called the dysexecutive syndrome.[26] This produces abnormalities of the executive functions of abstract reasoning, planning, set shifting, working memory, semantic memory, temporal sequencing, and abnormal procedural learning evidenced by slowing of serial reaction times.[26] These abnormalities of frontal lobe function may be associated with apathy.

There is a debate as to whether there is a primary memory storage deficit in PD or whether deficits of memory are due mainly to a deficit of retrieval. Most studies show a combination of deficits of encoding, recognition and retrieval of memories rather than a primary storage deficit.[27] Most PD patients with mild cognitive impairment have a characteristic frontostriatal executive pattern of deficits but a smaller number have a more significant primary memory deficit of temporal lobe amnestic pattern similar to, and possibly due to, early Alzheimer's disease.

There is evidence of visuospatial dysfunction in PD with reduction in central processing speed and reduced useful visual field.[28] These visual abnormalities may predict poor performance in complex psychomotor tasks. Studies have shown that slowing of the processing of visual information may be a predictor of poor driving ability in PD[7] and of accident risk in older adults.[29] Other studies have shown no clear relationship between cognition and safe driving in PD.[30] Specific tests have been developed which measure the limitations of useful visual field as a predictor of poor driving performance.

Under-activation of the prefrontal and supplementary motor areas with compensatory increased activation of lateral prefrontal, cerebellar and hippocampal areas have been shown on PET scans. These abnormalities occur not only when a task is actually performed but also when subjects imagine performing the task. This evidence supports the use of compensatory cueing strategies, which utilise the activated brain areas in therapy.

Some evidence of mild cognitive impairment may be present in patients even at diagnosis, with more global impairment in older age.[8] Age of disease onset is a critical determinant of cognitive deterioration in PD. Older age of disease onset predicts consistently cognitive decline above and beyond normal ageing and disease duration, with specific deterioration in visuospatial ability, immediate and delayed verbal memory and executive functions.[31] It is important to recognise that impairments can be demonstrated even in young-onset patients.[32]

There has been a debate as to whether mild cognitive impairment increases the risk of developing dementia. Mild cognitive impairment with early abnormalities on tests of verbal fluency, the picture completion section of the Wechsler Adult Intelligence Scale and the interference section of the STROOP test (a test of divided attention) may predict the development of dementia.[33] A recent study has shown that mild cognitive impairment may lead to dementia in 60% cases over four years with an odds ratio of more than five[34] with the time to onset of dementia being a median of 10.5 years. Mild cognitive impairment is associated with more severe motor symptoms, may have a predictive effect on prognosis and may predict the development of dementia.[35] The motor subtype of postural instability and gait disorder may be associated with faster cognitive decline and a risk of dementia.[36]

The effects of treatment on cognition

The effects of treatment on cognition are confusing. Levodopa would be expected to improve function mediated by dopaminergic pathways, but the effects are difficult to separate from the effects of disease severity and motor performance. Many cognitive abnormalities are dependent on dopaminergic frontostriatal dysfunction. The effects of dopaminergic treatments can be seen by improvement in some cognitive functions in fluctuating patients who are in an 'on' period.[37] This dopaminergic deficit may be due to alteration of the outflow of the caudate nuclei to the frontal lobes or due to diminished dopaminergic activity in the frontal lobes themselves, caused by degeneration of mesocortical projections. Functional imaging studies using fMRI and PET have shown under-activation and reduced dopaminergic levels in the caudate and dorsolateralprefrontal cortex to be associated with executive dysfunction[38] but the model is complicated by other evidence of differential effects of dopamine on cognition. Paradoxically, high dopamine activity in the dorsolateralprefrontal cortex in early disease may impair working memory, with this effect reducing with disease progression. Genetic abnormalities leading to higher prefrontal dopamine associated with cognitive impairment also demonstrate this effect.[39] Some components of recognition memory and enforcement learning are more impaired on levodopa.[40] These differential effects on enforced learning may lead to poor gambling decisions in medicated patients. There is an inverted 'U'-shaped curve for dopaminergic regulation of prefrontal function which is responsible for this confusing picture. Executive function may improve initially on therapy to a suboptimal level[41] with further impairment at higher levels of dopaminergic stimulation and wearing off.[42]

There is conflicting evidence regarding any specific cognitive deficit associated with modern stereotactic surgery in PD. Subgroup analysis shows that post-operative cognitive decline may be more common in older patients and patients taking higher doses of levodopa undergoing pallidal stimulation.[43] There are some reports of altered attention, verbal fluency and executive function following deep-brain stimulation but most long-term studies show either no change from baseline or some changes in verbal fluency alone.[44]

In summary, mild cognitive impairment in PD mainly affects the domains of executive function, working memory, visuospatial function and retrieval of information in the absence of any significant storage deficit and can be described as a dysexecutive visuospatial or subcorticofrontal pattern. The deficits in PD tend to lead patients to be more reactive rather than predictive in relation to the environment in cognitive, behavioural and motor activities, and this deficit increases with older age of disease onset.

Parkinson's disease dementia (PDD)

The term *dementia* has been used for centuries, but it first acquired a medical connotation in the eighteenth century. In the *Encyclopédie* of 1765, Diderot and D'Alembert described people with dementia as having weakening of understanding and memory, inability to remember anything, having no judgement and being sluggish and retarded.[2] This may have been the first description of dementia with parkinsonism. The syndrome of dementia is a more global decline of intellect, memory and personality than the cognitive deficits of PD described above, and interferes with everyday activities through changes in emotional control, motivation or social behaviour. There may be behavioural changes including apathy, personality changes, sleep disorder and day-time sleepiness. Recurrent visual hallucinations are often present, together with secondary delusions.

Epidemiology of Parkinson's disease dementia

The age-specific prevalence of dementia (from all causes) in the normal population increases with increasing age. The relative risk of developing dementia in PD at all ages is higher than that of age-matched controls, but also increases with increasing age. In clinical practice, therefore, dementia is common in the older PD patient but relatively less common in the young. Overall, a review of the literature suggests that between 24 and 31% of Parkinson's disease patients have dementia and 3–4% of the dementia population would have Parkinson's disease dementia. The most accurate prevalence figures for PDD are derived from community studies. A community study of PD patients using the CAMCOG (cognitive section of the Cambridge examination for mental disorders) as a screening tool showed a total of 44% to meet DSM-IV criteria for dementia. This study also confirmed the high false-positive rate of the commonly used mini mental state examination (MMSE) for detecting dementia in PD.[45] PD patients have a five times greater risk of developing dementia than the normal population with 10% of PD patients developing dementia each year. The later age of the onset of Parkinson's; the longer duration of symptoms; the presence of hallucinations, impaired memory and language function, all predict the development of dementia. Dementia itself is a significant predictor for institutional placement.[45] Other studies have shown that PDD is more common with an age of onset of PD greater than 60 years and in late-stage disease with more severe extrapyramidal syndrome, particularly in patients who develop psychosis and confusion on levodopa.[33]

Cognitive deficits in Parkinson's disease dementia

The pattern of deficits in PDD is a more severe version of that seen in mild cognitive impairment in PD affecting the domains of executive function, working memory, visuospatial function and retrieval of information in the absence of any significant storage deficit which can be described as a dysexecutive visuospatial dementia. Patients may develop a severe disturbance of planning (dysexecutive syndrome), slowing of thought (bradyphrenia) and a recall memory deficit which responds to external cues or reminders which is described as subcortical dementia. Since this deficit of recall is not primarily due to memory disruption, there is debate about the use of the term *dementia* in these patients. The term *subcortical dementia* was first used in 1974, and there is still some debate as to the clinical usefulness of distinguishing subcortical from cortical dementia.[22] Since patients demonstrate frontal lobe dysfunction, including impaired verbal fluency, the condition can be termed a subcorticofrontal dementia. An even better descriptive term for this form of dementia is a dysexecutive visuospatial dementia.

Parkinson's disease dementia and dementia with Lewy bodies (DLB)

The main differential diagnosis of PDD is dementia with Lewy bodies which may represent 15–20% of all causes of dementia in general. Studies have shown that attentional deficits and fluctuation occur in both DLB and PDD suggesting that the distinction is arbitrary.[46] In reality, these conditions are part of a clinico–pathological syndrome forming a spectrum of disease rather than distinct entities. DLB patients have early onset of cognitive deficit with fluctuation, early hallucinosis, visuospatial dysfunction, disturbances of consciousness and severe motor problems.[47] DLB has a male preponderance. When comparing DLB with PDD, both have visuospatial disturbances, which fit with hypo-activity in the cortical areas involved in visual processing.[48] There is no difference in the characteristics of recurrent visual hallucinations between PDD and DLB.[49] In comparing DLB with Alzheimer's disease (AD), the DLB patients suffered more visual hallucinations, disturbances of consciousness and parkinsonism than the AD patients. Patients with AD have difficulty drawing clocks but improve on copying clocks when compared with PD patients.[50] A small proportion of patients with AD (6.7%) may develop parkinsonism, but this is usually late in the disease.

Aetiology: pathology of Parkinson's disease dementia

The development of PDD is associated with subcortical loss of ascending projections from brainstem nuclei and disconnection of prefrontal connections to the caudate nuclei. This can be caused by intrinsic cortical pathology with the formation of Lewy bodies, dystrophic Lewy neurites, Alzheimer-like changes with plaques and vascular disease. Ageing itself can be associated with some incidental Lewy body formation and Alzheimer-like changes which complicate the picture. In a pathological study of dementia in general, 85% had Alzheimer pathology, 29% infarcts and 15% Lewy bodies. The most significant finding was the high prevalence of mixed pathology (38.8%).[51] Although this study was not specifically concerned with PDD, it does confirm the heterogeneity of dementia and the fact that clinical diagnostic criteria may not be good at picking up this mixed pathology.

Lewy bodies

In post-mortem studies, dementia may be associated with increasing density of cortical intracellular inclusion bodies (Lewy bodies) which, in its most advanced form, is called dementia with Lewy bodies (DLB). In some studies there was a direct correlation between the density of acortical Lewy bodies and the severity of dementia, with a high sensitivity (91%) and high specificity (90%) of these markers for dementia in PD.[52] Some cortical Lewy bodies are present in PD but occur in larger numbers in PDD and DLB. It is the presence of parahippocampal Lewy bodies which is the main predictor of dementia being present in both PDD and DLB.[53]

The greater severity of executive impairment in DLB than PDD may relate to the greater loss of frontohippocampal projections in DLB. The differing pattern of pathology in the striatum may account for the differences in parkinsonism. In some patients with PDD, frontosubcortical changes are the main contributing factor to dementia, whereas in other patients, cortical and hippocampal changes are more important.[54] Cortical Lewy bodies, especially in the amygdala and ventral visual pathways, are associated with visual hallucinations.

Extrapyramidal signs are much more common in AD than in age-matched controls, are more common in older patients, and tend to predict a worse prognosis, with increased mortality. The pathological basis for extrapyramidal signs in AD is heterogeneous, but is most probably associated with the presence of subcortical Lewy bodies.[55]

Alzheimer pathology

There is continued debate about the relationship of Alzheimer pathology and PDD/DLB. In one post-mortem pathological study of hospitalised PD, patients with dementia had a higher degree of cortical Alzheimer pathology, but the correlation of neurofibrillary changes, cortical Lewy bodies and dementia was poor.[56] The Lewy-body neurofilaments and Alzheimer tangles share common characteristics, and these two pathologies appear more frequently together than expected by chance, suggesting some relationship between them. There is more Alzheimer-like amyloid deposition in DLB than in PD or normals, with studies suggesting a possible interaction between the amyloid-producing protein (abeta peptide) and the protein deposited in PD (alpha synuclein).[57] There is also evidence that deposition of beta-amyloid protein is more marked and more closely related to cognitive impairment in DLB than in PDD, possibly contributing to early dementia. The percentage of patients with high plaque counts is greater in DLB than in PDD, which in turn is much greater than in PD with no dementia.[53] Superimposed Alzheimer pathology may alter the presentation of PDD and DLB with an increased likelihood of misdiagnosis.[58]

Cell loss

One consistently reported pathological difference between PDD and DLB is the greater neuronal loss in the substantia nigra in PDD and greater cell loss in the hippocampus in DLB.[59] Cell loss also occurs in the basal forebrain cholinergic system and relates to both the duration and severity of dementia in PDD and DLB. This cell loss occurs before the onset of dementia and may relate to mild cognitive impairment. Cell loss is mainly cortical in AD.

Extrapyramidal signs occur early in DLB and late in AD. In both AD and DLB, rigidity and bradykinesia are symmetrical and rest tremor is uncommon. The latter may be due to the different pattern of striatal cell loss in the putamen in these conditions, compared with PD.

Vascular disease

The role of white matter vascular lesions in PDD is unclear. Vascular mixed pathology in dementia without PD is more common than pure vascular dementia, and it may be the case in PD that vascular lesions add to the burden of pathology causing dementia. White matter hyper-intensities on MRI scans progress regardless of the type of dementia and largely reflect the vascular burden at onset.[60]

Summary of pathology of dementia

The pathological causes of dementia and cognitive impairment in PD are likely to be a mixture of Lewy body, Alzheimer and vascular pathological changes, which increase the probability of dementia (*see* Figure 6.1). The development of cortical Lewy bodies and/or Alzheimer pathology is most associated with the onset of dementia.[56] Dual

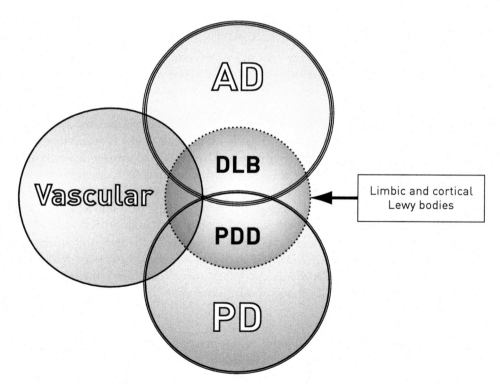

Limbic and cortical Lewy bodies

FIGURE 6.1 Schematic representation of possible relationships of PD/PDD/DLB/AD.

plaque and Lewy body pathologies are associated with DLB, whereas the development of limbic para-hippocampal and cortical Lewy bodies is associated particularly with PDD.[53] This combination of pathologies is related to interacting abnormal metabolism of proteins which underpins the cognitive impairment in PDD and DLB.[61] The clinical presentation of dementia may be altered by the relative burden of Alzheimer's pathology or superimposed vascular pathology.

Aetiology: neurochemistry of Parkinson's disease dementia

Cholinergic deficiency, dopaminergic hypo- and hyper-activation and noradrenergic mechanisms have been postulated for the cognitive changes in PD. Methyl-phenyl-tetrahydropyridine (MPTP) selectively destroys nigrostriatal dopaminergic neurones, and people exposed to this develop parkinsonism, with deficits in planning and internal control. We have seen that dopaminergic stimulation has a 'U'-shaped response with only a weak positive effect on cognition in early disease and a deleterious effect in later disease in PD. This dopamine deficiency is compounded by loss of inputs from the cholinergic and noradrenergic systems. Noradrenergic deficiency may produce attention deficits, which potentially may be correctable with noradrenaline precursors or re-uptake inhibitors.[62] The role of serotonin (5HT) in cognition in PD has hardly been studied except for some small experiments using acute tryptophan depletion which demonstrate impaired memory consolidation.[63] The most consistent body of evidence suggests that substantial ascending cholinergic deficits accompany the development of PDD. Atrophy of the nucleus basalis in PD produces a marked cholinergic underactivity. Cognitive deficits increase with reduced cortical cholinergic and particularly nicotinic receptor binding.[64] Nicotine increases the availability of dopamine, improving motor function and some aspects of cognition in normals, AD and possibly PD.[64] Reduced cholineacetyltransferase in the prefrontal cortex correlates with cognitive dysfunction.[65] Tests of executive function and working memory correlate with cortical acetylcholinesterase (AchE) and imaging of cholinergic function using PET shows that, compared with controls, AchE activity was lowest in patients with PDD (–20%), followed by PD without dementia (–13%) and AD patients with similar levels of dementia (–9%).[66] On the basis of these cholinergic deficits, cholinergic enhancement strategies using AchE inhibitors may be more effective in PDD than in AD.

Diagnosis of Parkinson's disease dementia

The difficulty of diagnosing dementia in PD is compounded by fluctuation in the condition; the presence of the motor deficit; the effects of treatment and the presence of vascular disease, acute confusion and depression. PDD occurs in the presence of well-established PD. There is a slow onset of impairment in more than one cognitive domain which impairs daily life or social function. Sometimes the timing of the development of motor and cognitive symptoms is unclear, leading to difficulties distinguishing from DLB. The consensus criteria for the clinical diagnosis of DLB (see Table 6.3) have been revised recently.[47] DLB should be diagnosed when dementia occurs before or concurrently with parkinsonism. PDD should be used to describe dementia that occurs in the context of well-established Parkinson's disease. For research purposes, the existing one-year rule between the onset of dementia and parkinsonism for DLB is still to be recommended.

TABLE 6.3 A summary of the revised international consensus criteria for the diagnosis of dementia with Lewy bodies (DLB)

1	**Central feature**
	Progressive cognitive decline interfering with normal social and occupational function. Memory impairment not necessarily present in early stages but evident with progression
	Prominent subcorticofrontal, attentional and visuospatial deficits
2	**Core features**
	Fluctuating cognition
	Recurrent visual hallucinations
	Spontaneous motor features of parkinsonism
3	**Suggestive features**
	REM sleep behaviour disorder
	Severe neuroleptic sensitivity
	Low SPECT (DAT) or PET dopamine transporter uptake
4	**Supportive features** (common but not diagnostic)
	Repeated falls
	Syncope/transient loss of consciousness
	Severe autonomic dysfunction
	Hallucinations in other modalities
	Systematised delusions
	Depression
	Relative preservation of medial temporal lobe structures on CT/MRI
	Abnormal myocardial scinigraphy
	Prominent slow waves on EEG with temporal lobe transient sharp waves
5	**Diagnosis less likely in the presence of:**
	Cerebrovascular disease on clinical examination or imaging
	Any other physical illness or brain disorder sufficient to account for the condition if parkinsonism appears only in the stage of severe dementia
6	**Temporal sequence**
	DLB should be diagnosed when dementia occurs before or concurrently with parkinsonism
	PDD should be used to describe dementia that occurs in the context of well-established Parkinson's disease

Source: McKeith et al.[47]

Assessment of Parkinson's disease dementia

A general medical assessment should include tests of thyroid function and vitamin B_{12} levels. Screening for PDD is important but needs to include a more extensive assessment than the Mini Mental State Examination (MMSE) which does not pick up the executive dysfunction which may be an early sign of PDD. Assessment needs to include tests of intellectual function, episodic memory, frontal and executive functioning, instrumental planning functions, behaviour and activities of daily living. For the assessment of intellectual and memory functions, various screening tools have been used, including the Mattis dementia rating scale and the CAMCOG[67] with more extensive tests of executive function including verbal fluency, digit recall, trail making and the Wisconsin card sorting test (*see* Table 6.1). Instrumental and planning functions can be assessed using clock drawing and apathy by using an apathy scale. It may be useful to combine screening tools with tests of frontal lobe function such as the frontal assessment battery (FAB) which is a 10-minute clinical schedule.[68] In practice, the Addenbrookes Cognitive Examination (ACE-R) includes components of frontal function, clock drawing and MMSE score and this may be a useful, easy-to-use screening tool.[69] Identifying fluctuations by asking four questions about the presence of day-time drowsiness and lethargy; day-time sleep of two or more hours; staring into space for long periods, and episodes of disorganised speech may be useful in distinguishing DLB/PDD from Alzheimer's disease.[70] In assessing response to treatment, it may be useful to focus on clinically relevant outcomes (clinimetric outcomes) by targeting particular functional and symptom domains such as the ability to dress, the ability to hold a conversation or the presence of disturbing hallucinations. This could be done through assessment by an occupational therapist.

Access to detailed and repeated neuropsychological assessment by a clinical psychologist integrated with the interdisciplinary team is helpful in the assessment and management of cognitive changes and dementia in PD. Assessment of the capacity of patients to make decisions can be difficult due to speech problems and the fluctuation of cognition. It is important to understand that patients must be assumed to have capacity unless specific criteria are met, since there is a tendency to try to make decisions for patients without their full participation. Loss of capacity may occur when the abilities to understand, retain and manipulate information are lost, or when/if the patient is unable to communicate choice. Decisions must be free from coercion, and this includes internal coercion from delusions and psychosis. Loss of capacity is not assumed because a diagnosis of PD dementia has been made. Often capacity may vary and may need to be assessed in relation to a specific decision at a specific point in time. An independent assessment from a psychogeriatrician can be helpful in these circumstances.

Management of Parkinson's disease dementia

It is easy for patients to 'fall between two stools' because of the combination of major physical and cognitive symptoms. Therefore, early liaison with psychogeriatric services is important in order to develop a joint management plan, which must involve liaison with social services and provision of appropriate social and respite care. Since the dementia of PD is due to a spectrum of disorders, including AD, the principles of clinical management of patients with dementia in PD are no different to those for patients with other forms of dementia. These principles, which focus on carers, cognition, assessment, liaison and medical treatment can be summarised using the acronym 'CALM' (*see* Table 6.4) and applied through an algorithm for the medical management (*see* Figure 6.2). There needs to be a careful explanation of the diagnosis, particularly to carers. Clear goals need to be set, targeting and prioritising symptoms. Co-morbid psychiatric symptoms such as depression and sleep behaviour disorder need to be assessed and treated. Environmental modifications and cueing should be considered since patients may benefit from external cues for memory and movement. Sedation, especially typical neuroleptics, should be avoided if possible, but where agitation and restlessness are a problem, a small dose of a benzodiazepine can be tried.

TABLE 6.4 The principles of management of PDD 'CALM'

Carer support	Appropriate and timely social and respite care, support groups, advice lines
Cognitive strategies	Use of cueing and attentional strategies for movement and memory
Assessment	Full and regular interdisciplinary assessment – cognition, capacity, mood, psychosis, motor, autonomic, ADL and social function
Liaison	Close liaison between specialist, psychogeriatrician and primary healthcare team. Key role of PD nurse specialist
Medical care	Avoid neuroleptics, consider cholinesterase inhibitors, manage sleep disturbance, manage hallucinosis and psychosis. Avoid hospitalisation and anaesthesia where possible

Management of hallucinations is of major importance, particularly for the relatives. The principles of management of psychosis and hallucinations, where present, should be followed as described in the section on psychosis below, taking into account the following aspects of management of cognition. In optimising anti-parkinsonian medications, the regime needs to balance controlling motor function whilst avoiding deleterious cognitive and behavioural effects of dopamine stimulation. Some interesting early work has suggested a possibility that amantadine may have a role in delaying the onset of dementia, although further work is needed to confirm this.[71] Cholinesterase inhibitors should be considered once anti-parkinsonian medication is optimised. Treatment should be considered where dementia has been diagnosed which is interfering with executive function and daily activities. The presence of hallucinosis or psychosis may justify earlier treatment. There is evidence from randomised placebo–controlled trials for the effectiveness and safety of cholinesterase inhibitors in the treatment of PDD with their use supported by the NICE guidelines and other evidence-based reviews.[72,73] The largest study utilised rivastigmine which, to date, is the only licensed treatment in the UK.[74] An extension of a 24–week study of rivastigmine to 48 weeks showed good long-term safety and efficacy, especially

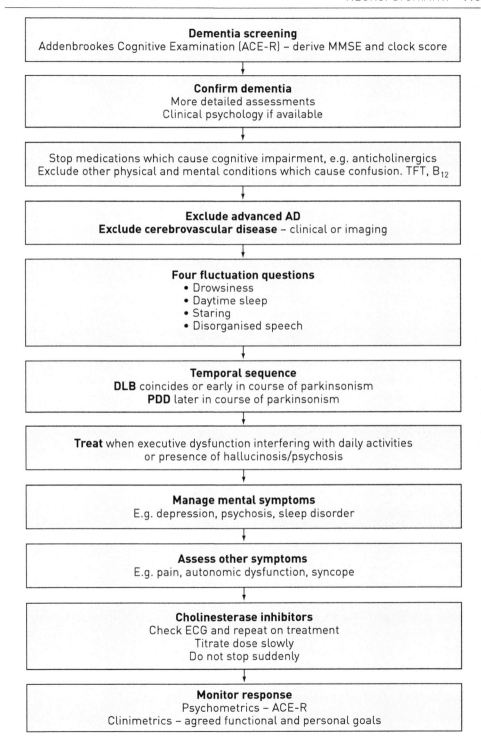

Dementia screening
Addenbrookes Cognitive Examination (ACE-R) – derive MMSE and clock score

Confirm dementia
More detailed assessments
Clinical psychology if available

Stop medications which cause cognitive impairment, e.g. anticholinergics
Exclude other physical and mental conditions which cause confusion. TFT, B_{12}

Exclude advanced AD
Exclude cerebrovascular disease – clinical or imaging

Four fluctuation questions
- Drowsiness
- Daytime sleep
- Staring
- Disorganised speech

Temporal sequence
DLB coincides or early in course of parkinsonism
PDD later in course of parkinsonism

Treat when executive dysfunction interfering with daily activities
or presence of hallucinosis/psychosis

Manage mental symptoms
E.g. depression, psychosis, sleep disorder

Assess other symptoms
E.g. pain, autonomic dysfunction, syncope

Cholinesterase inhibitors
Check ECG and repeat on treatment
Titrate dose slowly
Do not stop suddenly

Monitor response
Psychometrics – ACE-R
Clinimetrics – agreed functional and personal goals

FIGURE 6.2 Suggested medical management of PDD.

in its effects on recurrent visual hallucinations.[75] It is likely that donepezil and galantamine are also effective. Since cholinesterase inhibitors can cause bradycardia rarely, an electrocardiogram (ECG) should be checked before commencement to exclude pre-existing bradycardia or bundle branch block.[76] Rivastigmine should be carefully titrated through recommended increments, at intervals of least 2–3 weeks, while monitoring the patient's mental, physical and cognitive state. Rapid withdrawal can lead to an acute cognitive and behavioural decline and should be avoided.[77] Side effects of cholinesterase inhibitors include nausea and vomiting, anorexia, nightmares, hyper-salivation and breakthrough tremor. It is possible that the development of cognitive impairment in PD may be associated with an alteration in the perception of pain which make the assessment of pain difficult.[78] Depression is common in PDD but easily missed and may require the use of specific assessment scales such as the Cornell validated for depression in dementia.[79]

It is useful for patients and relatives to complete an enduring power of attorney at an early stage which, under new legislation in England and Wales, will include the ability of the attorney to make treatment decisions on behalf of the patient. This process allows an appointed attorney to continue to look after the affairs and interests of the patient if they lose capacity. Where loss of capacity is demonstrated, it is important for the carers to be fully involved in decisions on respite and long-term residential or nursing home care, since they possess vital knowledge of those for whom they care.

In some areas there is provision of respite care for the patient and carer together. PDD patients may worsen in hospital because of the change in environment and accidental alteration of drug timing. Support for carers is vital, since the 24-hour burden of care is stressful and demanding. Ultimately many cases will not be manageable in the home environment and dementia is a common reason for nursing home admission.

Mood disorders in PD

Mood disorders in Parkinson's disease – apathy

Apathy, with or without depression, is common in PD, occurring in over one third-of cases. It seems to be associated more with frontal cognitive impairment than with depression.[80] Apathy may overlap with anhedonia (the lack of ability to enjoy) which in turn overlaps with depression. The presence of apathy can be extremely frustrating and distressing for carers who are trying to help maintain the independence of the sufferer. Apathy can be measured using the Apathy Evaluation Scale or the Starkstein Apathy Rating Scale but these are not often used in daily practice.[81,82] Treatment of apathy is difficult with most anti-parkinsonian drug groups having been tried. Limited evidence favours a trial of cholinesterase inhibitors.

Mood disorders in Parkinson's disease – depression

Depressive symptoms are common in PD, especially in elderly patients.[4] Depression in Parkinson's disease (dPD) is associated with a poor quality of life,[83] excess disability and carer stress[84] and treatment of depression can reduce functional disability.[85]

There are problems defining depressive illness in PD since many standardised tests are affected by the physical symptoms of PD. Autonomic symptoms are more common in elderly PD patients and can be associated with depression and anxiety. The psychomotor retardation of PD can be confused with depression. The differential diagnosis of dPD is very wide and can include states of grief, demoralisation, adjustment disorders, major mood disorders, minor depression and depressive symptoms not amounting to a diagnosis of depression (subsyndromal depression).[86]

It is not clear whether the symptoms of dPD differ from those of depression in persons without PD. The symptoms of depression in PD may be similar in nature to depression associated with executive dysfunction, termed by some as the depression executive dysfunction syndrome of later life, which is associated with a slow or poor response to antidepressants.[87] Some studies have suggested that patients with dPD have less guilt and sadness whereas others have shown no difference when compared with patients with major depression.[88,89] Although anhedonia, or the lack of ability to enjoy, may be a clinical feature of PD and a key symptom of dPD, not all studies have demonstrated this.[90] Tearfulness and emotionalism can occur in PD in a similar manner to stroke and must not be confused with depression. Confusion over the phenomenology and definition of dPD mean that diagnostic criteria are difficult to apply in practice. dPD probably represents a spectrum of mood disturbances from mood changes before PD motor symptoms through to depression associated with dementia.[86] The difficulty with definitions and diagnosis mean that it is important to better understand and define mood symptoms in PD and specific studies of the phenomenology are needed. For the present, clinicians should be aware of the difficulties in diagnosing mild depression and should have a low threshold for the diagnosis in PD.[72]

Epidemiology of depression in Parkinson's disease

The prevalence of dPD depends upon the definition used. Inclusive criteria give a higher figure than exclusive, specific criteria for major depression such as DSM IV diagnostic definitions of depression. A recent consensus meeting has tried to modify the DSM criteria for depression to be used specifically in dPD but these need validation and are used mainly in research.[86] The use of a simple standardised rating scale such as the Hamilton Depression Rating Scale (HDRS) or Geriatric Depression Scale (GDS-15) may aid assessment of patients, but may reflect the presence of depressive symptomatology rather than depressive illness.[91] The HDRS is based on a structured interview whereas the self-rated GDS takes five minutes to complete, has been validated against the HDRS and is used commonly in UK practice in older patients.[92] In a community study using the GDS as a screening tool, the prevalence of depression was 64% in patients and 34% in carers.[4] Other community studies using DSM-IV criteria for medical mood disorder reported much lower frequencies of 3–8%.[93] In a meta-analysis of 52 studies containing 5000 subjects, the prevalence of minor depression was 44%, major depression 11.8% and anxiety 25.3%.[94] Most studies show the prevalence for dPD to be around 40%, with major depression in 10% of patients and minor or subsyndromal depression in 30%. Depression is often unrecognised. In a survey of 1000 patients, 50% reported depressive symptoms but only 1% identified themselves as depressed.[95] This may be because people do not believe themselves to be depressed unless they feel sad. Similarly doctors can miss depression, with one study showing only a 35% diagnostic accuracy.[96] Minor depression can lead to major depression in 11% of cases over a year and major depression will lead on to minor depression in 33% of cases and will remain chronic in the majority of cases.[97] Age, psychosis and dPD increase mortality with a relative risk of 2.7 in dPD compared with those without depression, with the increased risk not due to suicide.[6]

There is a complex relationship between dPD and cognitive impairment, with depressed patients having impaired memory and cognitive impairment. dPD is a risk factor for dementia. Depression and dementia combined may represent a subtype of PD.[98] Defining and diagnosing dPD in the presence of dementia are problematic since most rating scales are unsuitable. The Cornell scale for depression in dementia has been used in research but takes 30 minutes to administer and may not be practical for screening in clinical practice.[79]

Aetiology of depression in Parkinson's disease

Many possible associations of dPD have been studied (*see* Table 6.5). Depression can precede the onset of motor symptoms and may represent early pathology in the brainstem linking to the limbic system.[12]

TABLE 6.5 Depression in Parkinson's disease: associations and aetiology

Associated conditions	Organic features	Psychosocial features
• Anxiety	• Biochemical changes	• Similar prevalence to other chronic diseases
• Psychosis	• Familial aggregation/ genetic predisposition	• No relation to PD severity
• Cognitive impairment	• Mesencephalic changes on sonography and MRI	• No relation to PD progression
• Sleep disturbance	• ERP changes	• Related to handicap
• Female	• PET scan studies	• Multifactorial
• ? Younger	• Produced by deep-brain stimulation	• Response to cognitive therapy
• Akinesia/postural instability and gait disorder (PIGD)	• Motor fluctuation	
• Motor fluctuation	• Response to rTMS, ECT and drugs	
• Right hemi-PD	• Early Braak stages	

There is some evidence for a laterality of mood with studies showing more depression in right hemi-PD.[99] Transcranial magnetic stimulation of the dominant hemisphere may improve mood.[100] More severe akinesia, gait disorders and motor fluctuation may increase depression. There is conflicting evidence as to whether psychosis or cognitive impairment are associated with depression. Studies comparing dPD with depression without PD have shown similar cognitive deficits in both conditions, with reduced verbal fluency and attention deficits in depression and problems of abstract reasoning and set shifting in dPD.[101] Patients with depressive pseudodementia respond to cueing in a similar manner to PD patients with subcortical dementia, which suggests that similar neural pathways are involved.[102] Some studies have shown that increasing age is a risk factor for dPD. Other studies suggest that the increased handicap and difficulties with social adjustment associated with having PD at a young age increase the risk of depression. Women are proportionately more likely to suffer dPD.

It is still unclear how much the dPD is due to the biology of the disease or is the result of psychosocial effects of chronic disease. An organic basis for depression is supported by studies showing a possible familial aggregation of unipolar depression and PD[103] and other studies showing abnormalities of the serotonin transporter gene, though the latter is still controversial.[104] The early pathological stages of PD (Braak stage 1&2) before the onset of motor symptoms may be associated with depression and anxiety.[12] Depression is more pronounced in 'off' periods, possibly due to the deregulation of the locus caeruleus similar to that found in rapid cycling bipolar affective disorder.[99] Noradrenergic deficiency and cell loss in the locus caeruleus may be associated with the bradyphrenia and attention deficits of PD. Dopamine deficiency in basal ganglia, orbitofrontal and limbic circuits is associated in animal studies with dysfunction of the reward system. This can lead to anhedonia or the reduced experience of reward seen in PD. Serotonergic abnormalities in the medial raphé projection to the diencephalon and limbic areas may produce the psychomotor retardation of PD and depression. PET studies of dPD have shown reduced cortical serotonin (5HT) binding and reduced limbic noradrenaline and dopamine but no correlation with basal ganglia dopamine levels.[105] Marked sleep disturbance is associated with dPD, with findings of abnormalities of melatonin and circadian rhythm in fluctuating PD being similar to those in non-PD depression.

In addition to these neurochemical disturbances, abnormalities of the mesencephalon on MRI and transcranial ultrasound, frontal cortical under-activity on PET scans, and reduced caudate metabolism all suggest an organic basis for dPD.[99] Cerebrovascular disease is an important determinant in the aetiology of depression[106] especially in the elderly, and may also be an important contributory factor to the development of depression in the elderly PD patient.

The possible neuroanatomical relationship between depression and the basal ganglia was emphasised by a description of acute severe depression brought on by deep-brain stimulation. In this case, stimulation of the left subthalamic nucleus improved symptoms of PD, but additional stimulation of the left substantia nigra evoked unequivocal depressive symptoms.[107] This case raises the possibility of specific neural pathways in the brain for mood, in addition to motor functions.[108] Depressed patients are more likely to develop PD than they are to develop osteoarthitis or diabetes, suggesting some common underlying aetiological factors.[109] At diagnosis, 9.2% of PD patients have a background history of depression compared with 4% of controls, again suggesting a link between depression and PD.[110]

There is, however, considerable disadvantage and handicap associated with a chronic neurological disorder. There is no good evidence for a direct correlation between disease severity and depression. Some workers have gone so far as to suggest a mainly psychosocial model for depression in PD.[111] A particular pattern of negative beliefs and worries described as metacognitive style may increase the risk of dPD.[112]

It is difficult to attribute functions of the human mind to purely neurochemical and structural changes, and intuitively it seems most likely that dPD has a major organic predisposition interacting with psychosocial factors influencing its presentation.

Management of depression in Parkinson's disease

Although the management of dPD has not been well studied, some of the principles can be summarised using the acronym 'CALM' (*see* Table 6.6) and applied through an algorithm (*see* Figure 6.3). It is important to consider both PD-related and non-PD-related factors. PD-related factors include reviewing and managing disease severity; motor symptoms; cognitive impairments; other disease-related psychopathology, and reviewing psychiatric side effects and fluctuating response to medications. Non-PD-related factors, often forgotten by physicians, include obtaining insights into previous psychiatric history, family history, temperament, coping styles, social resources and life events which all contribute to the aetiology of depression and may also significantly affect its management. A screening tool and a severity rating such as the GDS are useful in identifying depression and monitoring treatment. A clinical assessment of severity of depression, graded mild, moderate and severe may help with management decisions, with severe depression including affective psychosis, severe biological symptoms or suicidal ideas.

TABLE 6.6 The management of depression in Parkinson's disease: 'CALM'

Carer support	Counselling for patient and carer. Assessment of carer stress and depression
Cognition	Role for cognitive behaviour therapy
Assessment	Regular interdisciplinary assessment including diagnosis and severity of depression, associated cognitive impairment, exclude pseudodementia, psychosis, motor and mood fluctuation, ADL and social function
Liaison	Psychogeriatric referral if resistant or severe. Close liaison between primary healthcare team and specialists
Medical	Optimise dopaminergic therapy. Appropriate antidepressant. Avoid TCA. Careful use of SSRI monitoring motor function. Combined re-uptake inhibitors SNRI and especially NaSSA may prove beneficial. ECT effective in severe depression

Talking therapies for depression in Parkinson's disease

Provision of support, advice and counselling to both patients and carers may be combined with antidepressant therapy. A clear explanation that depression is a common intrinsic part of PD is needed in order for patients and carers to accept appropriate help and treatment. Cognitive therapy (CBT) can benefit mild or moderate depression

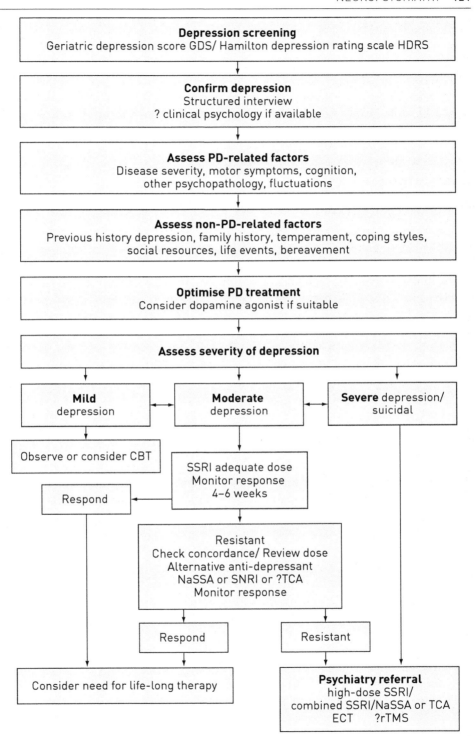

FIGURE 6.3 Suggested medical management of dPD.

in the elderly but there have only been small open studies of CBT in dPD.[113] Support groups held through PD clinics or the Parkinson's Disease Society can provide an informal form of group therapy. Counselling and support can be provided for patients and carers by social workers and counsellors with a special interest in PD, or through the welfare officer of the local Parkinson's Disease Society. The PD nurse specialists have a key role in the provision and co-ordination of these support services in the management of depression.

Drug treatments of depression in Parkinson's disease

Dopaminergic treatment

The first option in the drug treatment of dPD is to ensure optimal dopaminergic treatment. Mood elevation and anxiety reduction can be demonstrated using levodopa infusions, and therefore smoothing out fluctuations may be important in the control of dPD.[114] Optimisation of dopaminergic therapy could include the addition of a non-ergot dopamine agonist. Direct-acting dopamine agonists acting on the D3 receptors in the limbic system (e.g. pergolide, pramipexole) may have an antidepressant effect, and this may be due partly to an effect on psychomotor retardation. Pramipexole has compared favourably with sertraline in one trial.[115] More studies of the efficacy of pramipexole in dPD are now being undertaken.

Catechol-O-methyl transferase (COMT) inhibitors may have a similar effect through enhancement of dopaminergic transmission and reduction in motor fluctuation, but this has not been studied in trials.

Older reviews suggested that selegeline may be effective;[99] however, later evidence-based reviews have not confirmed this and the consensus is that selegeline is not very effective as an antidepressant in dPD.

Serotonin re-uptake inhibitors

A favourable side-effect profile means many clinicians use SSRI antidepressants as the first-line treatment in PD, although trial evidence for efficacy of these drugs in PD is based mainly on open studies.[117] There is a theoretical risk of increased parkinsonism with SSRI antidepressants, and some case reports exist of akathisia, tardive dyskinesia and dystonia, but there is no clinical evidence that these effects are significant.[118] The concerns about possible increased suicide risk need to be considered, especially when treating younger patients. The pattern of liver enzyme induction varies from one SSRI to another, and this may influence the choice of drug. There is no trial evidence that the SSRI antidepressants help symptoms of low mood outside a depressive illness in PD.

Combined re-uptake inhibitors

The noradrenaline and serotonin combined re-uptake inhibitors may have a role in dPD. They have yet to show advantages over SSRI drugs, and there is limited experience in PD. Venlafaxine, a serotonin and noradrenaline re-uptake inhibitor (SNRI), has an anxiolytic effect with a rapid onset of action in the elderly at 1–2 weeks.[119] These effects have not been demonstrated in dPD, but may be due to combined actions on serotonin and noradrenaline (which occur at higher doses) and an ability to titrate the dose rapidly. There is concern about cardiac and hypertensive side effects with higher doses or overdoses of venlafaxine, which needs to be prescribed under specialist supervision if used in high doses. Updated prescribing advice should be considered before prescription.[120]

Mirtazepine, a derivative of mianserin, is a noradrenaline and specific serotonin antidepressant (NaSSA) and may also have a rapid onset of action.[119] Antidepressant actions of NaSSA are produced through increasing noradrenaline levels by antagonism of pre-synaptic α_2 autoreceptors and by indirect enhancement of serotonin neurotransmission by 5-HT_1 receptors. Theoretically this profile of neurotransmitter action may be useful in dPD, reducing both depression and motor symptoms.[121] Mirtazepine has a sedative effect and may produce weight gain which can sometimes be used to good effect in dPD. It is possible that serotonergic manipulation could lead to hallucinosis in PD, and there are case reports of psychosis possibly induced by mirtazapine and SSRIs.[122]

Other drugs include reboxetine, which is a selective noradrenaline re-uptake inhibitor and which may cause insomnia, increased sweating and dry mouth, nefazodone, which has SSRI actions with additional theoretically beneficial 5-HT_2 antagonism and has fewer side effects, and duloxetine which is a balanced combined re-uptake inhibitor of 5HT and noradrenaline. Although these newer antidepressants have attractive profiles in combining 5HT and noradrenergic actions, there are only a few uncontrolled reports using reboxetine or nefazodone and no studies of duloxetine in dPD.

Tricyclics

A recent evidenced-based review suggested that amitriptyline should be considered in the non demented dPD patient.[73] Tricyclic antidepressants (TCA) were prescribed widely in dPD because of the belief that the anticholinergic effect may also help the motor symptoms. Desimipramine can increase tremor in PD, but other studies show that imipramine is most effective in patients with rigidity.[116] Nortriptyline may improve depressive symptoms in PD. In elderly patients, the anticholinergic side effects of these drugs, including confusion, hallucinosis, urinary retention, blurred vision, faecal impaction and dry mouth, reduce their tolerability. Since anticholinergic drugs are now avoided by most experts in the treatment of PD, tricyclic antidepressants are usually reserved for situations where other antidepressants have failed.

Other drug treatments

Moclobamide, a reversible monoamine oxidase A (MAOA) inhibitor, was considered as an option in resistant depression in PD. It has a combined effect on serotonin and noradrenaline and possibly other transmitters. In clinical practice in patients without PD, moclobamide is only a weak antidepressant and used rarely.

An ideal antidepressant in dPD would combine inhibition of re-uptake of dopamine, serotonin and noradrenaline with no hypertensive effect. To this end, some workers have combined MAOA inhibition with MAOB inhibition, showing enhanced antidepressant activity with no hypertensive effect.[123] Resistant depression may benefit from higher doses of SSRI in some patients in whom there may be rapid metabolism of these drugs. Such a high-dose regime has not been studied in dPD and is only weakly supported by trial evidence outside PD.[124] The combination of an SSRI in the day and mirtazepine at night may also be useful in resistant depression but has not been studied in dPD.

Non-pharmacological therapy of depression in Parkinson's disease

ECT has been shown to be effective in the treatment of depression, motor fluctuations and drug-induced mania. Motor symptoms, especially rigidity, have been shown to respond and relapse more quickly than depression, the response being greater in the elderly.[99,125,126] In a randomised controlled trial, repetitive transcranial magnetic stimulation (rTMS) has been shown to improve dPD to the same extent as fluoxetine.[127] rTMS induces electrical activity in the brain by repetitive activation of a surface electromagnet. The effects on depression may last only two weeks, and concurrent antidepressants are needed. In future, rTMS may be a useful alternative to ECT since it has a more focal effect, reducing adverse cognitive symptoms and avoiding the need for a general anaesthetic, in addition to improving motor function. Stimulation over the motor cortex can reduce motor slowing and improve cognition in elderly PD patients. rTMS requires further evaluation, but has a promising future role in the treatment of depression in PD.[99,100]

Summary of management of depression in Parkinson's disease

There is insufficient evidence from randomised controlled trials of the safety or efficacy of any antidepressant in dPD.[72,73] In a meta-analysis of the treatment of dPD patients compared with elderly depressed patients without PD, the newer antidepressants were well tolerated in dPD, but controlled treatment trials were almost non-existent. dPD patients may benefit less from antidepressant treatment, particularly SSRI, than do elderly patients without PD. The meta-analysis showed a positive effect for depression treatment in dPD whether with active drug or placebo.[128] A large placebo effect due to the expectation of reward may be found in other situations in PD and this may be due to placebo-induced dopamine or serotonin release in depression.[129] This placebo effect may be an important consideration in future strategies for the management of dPD and emphasises the need for placebo-controlled trials.

In the absence of substantial evidence, the management of dPD should be tailored to the individual and in particular to their co-existing therapy.[72]

One approach to dPD is to consider cognitive therapy, if available, in mild cases (*see* Figure 6.3). From the drug treatment point of view, the first step is to optimise dopaminergic therapy and to consider the use of a dopamine agonist if the patient is suitable. If there is no improvement, give a trial of at least six weeks of adequate doses of antidepressant with careful monitoring of the patient's mood and motor function. The presence of anxiety may influence the choice of a more sedative antidepressant such as mirtazepine, or an appropriate selective serotonin re-uptake inhibitor (SSRI). There is a small risk of producing a serotonin syndrome (hyperpyrexia, agitation, confusion) when selegeline is combined with tricyclics or SSRI antidepressants.[72] The response to an antidepressant is best reviewed after 4–6 weeks of a therapeutic dose. If there is no response after this period, a change of dose or of antidepressant can be considered. Some workers have suggested a cascade of antidepressant treatment, utilising a different group every six weeks until there is a response. In resistant cases, high doses or combined therapy may be needed. Future clarification of the efficacy of different antidepressant groups in dPD may allow the clinician to choose the most effective drug at the outset, avoiding the need for frequent change in therapy. Two or more episodes of depression have been considered an indication for long-term treatment, but the chronic nature of dPD suggests that lifelong therapy may be needed in most cases.

Referral to a psychiatrist should be considered if there is a severe depression with psychosis – especially if insight is lost, if there is medication failure in chronic depression, or if there are suicidal ideas. The development of suicidal ideas or life-threatening complications, such as refusal to eat, should be taken seriously, and electroconvulsive therapy (ECT) may be considered.

Mood disorders in Parkinson's disease – anxiety

Symptoms of anxiety are common in PD, occurring in at least 25% of patients often preceding the onset of motor symptoms.[130] Anxiety symptoms can be classified into social phobia, panic disorder, generalised anxiety or an obsessive–compulsive disorder. Anxiety may also be part of a depressive illness and can be helped by appropriate sedative antidepressant therapy. A review of sleep is important since anxiety can be associated with sleep disturbance and excessive day-time sleepiness.[131]

Increasing anxiety may be a manifestation of cognitive changes in PD, when new situations or changes from regular routine feel threatening to patients who are cognitively less flexible. Anxiety can also be a drug-induced side effect, occurring at peak dose or in an 'off' period or associated with mood fluctuations.[132]

For these reasons, it is important to take a good history from patients and carers in order to ascertain the cause of anxiety in PD. Anxiety can be measured using the Hospital Anxiety and Depression Scale (HADS).[91]

Restlessness at peak dose can be severe, with mental over-activity and, rarely, the development of mania. This may be a dopaminergic phenomenon, since dopamine agonists have been reported to produce mania in the absence of PD.

Explanation, support, advice and relaxation exercises, combined with appropriate pharmacotherapy are the mainstays of treatment of anxiety in PD. SSRI antidepressants, mirtazepine, trazodone, small doses of benzodiazepines and, only rarely, low–dose atypical neuroleptics could be used in cases of severe anxiety. Cognitive behaviour therapy and anxiety management by clinical psychologists may also have a role.

Impulse control disorders in PD

Dopamine dysregulation syndrome

Mood disorders in PD encompass major depression at one extreme and sensation-seeking behaviours or impulse control disorders at the other, with many patients presenting a mixed picture. Dopaminergic pathways link ventral tegmental areas of the brain via the basal ganglia to the frontal cortex. These pathways are involved in the derivation of pleasure, energy and drive. It is understandable that some patients derive excessive pleasure and abnormal drive from the stimulation of this system by dopaminergic drugs – the dopamine dysregulation syndrome (DDS). In its full form, this syndrome is relatively rare (2–4%) but can be extremely disruptive. Milder forms of dopamine dysregulation are common in clinical practice. DDS is more common in males (80%), particularly those with young-onset PD who have well-tolerated dyskinesias, previous mood disorders, novelty-seeking personality traits, and previous alcohol abuse, but it can also occur in older patients.[133]

Patients may self-medicate with large doses of dopaminergic drugs and become resistant to suggestions that doses should be lowered. These patients may develop abnormal repetitive pointless motor behaviours known as punding and may develop restlessness and the urge to go 'walkabout'. Punders are usually younger, with poor sleep, may spend long periods pursuing hobbies and may have more dyskinesia.[134] Patients can develop pathological gambling or shopping and lose large sums of money.[135] Abnormal sexual drive can develop, including hypersexuality, use of pornography or internet sites, transvestitism and aberrant sexual behaviour sometimes leading to prosecution. Although hypersexual behaviour increases with higher doses of dopaminergic medication, there is no relationship with any functional improvement brought about by these doses. The process of negotiating lower doses of dopaminergic drugs with such patients is extremely difficult. Short-term prescriptions or supervision of medication may need to be considered. Apomorphine should certainly be avoided. Atypical neuroleptics or mood stabilisers such as carbamazepine may be needed in some patients. Psychotherapy or behaviour therapy may be considered where these are available.

Patients should now be warned that dopaminergic drugs (especially dopamine agonists) may be associated rarely with abnormal behaviour including hypersexuality and gambling.[135] This is stated on the patient information sheets for dopamine agonists.

Sexual dysfunction

Sexual dysfunction is common in PD. Issues of sexuality may be overlooked or avoided in elderly people, who may be less willing to respond to direct questions on sexual matters in quality-of-life assessment tools. Impotence may be due to side effects of drugs such as antidepressants, or part of the disease. Hypersexualism can be a peak-dose phenomenon and can lead to complaints from the partner of unreasonable sexual demands. Sometimes unwelcome thoughts or behaviours are intrusive and similar in nature to thought patterns in obsessive-compulsive disorders. Hypersexualism is not associated with cognitive changes at peak dose and the cause in not well understood. Priapism due to levodopa has been reported and was noticed more in the days of high-dose treatment. Loss of libido is common, but less well recognised and has been reported to be a problem in women.[136]

The PD nurse specialist may be able to provide counselling and advice to patients and partners. This may be best undertaken in the patient's own home rather than in clinic. In hypersexuality, doses of dopaminergic drugs may need to be reduced, which requires careful negotiation. Atypical antipsychotics may be useful in low doses. Anti-androgens such as cyproterone acetate have been used in a small number of cases.

Psychosis

Psychotic symptoms indicate a separation from reality with the formation of beliefs and sensations without any basis in reason or sensory stimuli. In some respects the use of the term *psychosis* for the abnormal experiences in PD is incorrect. Patients can have illusions or visual hallucinations without being deluded or psychotic. It is important to distinguish between hallucinosis and the deluded non-affective psychosis which usually arises in association with hallucinosis.

Hallucinations are perceptions in any sensory modality occurring without external sensory stimuli. Many of the 'hallucinations' in PD are actually visual misinterpretations or illusions since they do have a sensory stimulus.

There is a gradation of severity of symptoms ranging from minor illusions, through vivid dreams, to frank psychosis, with patients often progressing down a 'neuropsychiatric slippery slope', one type of symptom increasing the likelihood of the next (*see* Figure 6.4). Although this progression is debatable, it is clear that once elderly patients start to hallucinate, the hallucinations can be very difficult to eliminate, and become permanent in 80% of patients.[137] Risk factors for hallucinosis include cognitive impairment, dementia, advanced disease, visual impairment, increased age, the use of some anti-parkinsonian drugs and sleep disturbance.[138] Changes of visual contrast and colour perception which occur in PD may contribute to hallucinosis.[139] Recurrent hallucinations are thought to be due to dopaminergic and serotonergic over-activity with cholinergic, and possibly glutamergic, under-activity.[140,141] The pathological cause of visual hallucinations is now thought to be nerve-cell loss and Lewy-body pathology in the ventral-temporal regions of the brain with involvement of both the dorsal and

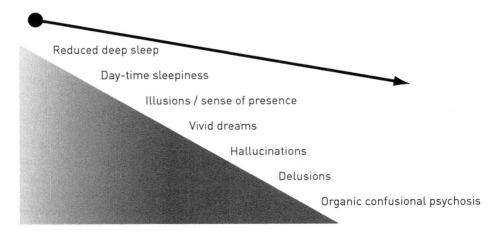

Reduced deep sleep

Day-time sleepiness

Illusions / sense of presence

Vivid dreams

Hallucinations

Delusions

Organic confusional psychosis

FIGURE 6.4 The neuropsychiatric 'slippery slope'.

ventral visual pathways in their generation.[138] Recurrent visual hallucinations may be associated with the co-existence of attentional and visual perceptive deficits, due to cholinergic deficits in the lateral frontal cortical connections with the visual pathways system.[142] These deficits may lead to over-activity of the visual system which produces a positive visual percept.[143] The presence of visual hallucinations is helpful in the differentiation of PD from other non-Lewy-body causes of parkinsonism.[138]

Psychosis implies the presence of delusions, which are false unshakable beliefs which cannot be understood from the individual's social and cultural background. Delusions are less common than hallucinations but occur only rarely in the absence of hallucinations. They are often associated with visuo-auditory hallucinations and with REM sleep behaviour disorder. Psychosis may occur in predisposed individuals who have a limbic predominance of Lewy bodies and increased limbic sensitivity to dopaminergic stimulation.[138] Psychosis is more likely to occur in association with a lower MMSE score or a family history of dementia.[144]

Epidemiology of psychosis in Parkinson's disease

There may be two groups of patients with hallucinosis or psychosis: patients with 'early-onset' hallucinations associated with motor fluctuations and large doses of medication, and those with late-onset hallucinations associated with cognitive impairment.[137] Pre-existing cognitive impairment and hallucinosis may be made worse by the use of direct-acting dopamine agonists, and elderly patients should be assessed carefully before prescribing these drugs. During the first five years following diagnosis, 30% of patients will develop hallucinosis or psychosis, with up to 50% developing psychosis some stage during their illness.[137] When considered over the total disease time course and expressed as a percentage, the median time of onset of hallucinations is more than 75%, with an increased risk associated with cognitive impairment, autonomic dysfunction and older age of disease onset.[138]

Clinical presentation of psychosis of Parkinson's disease

The first sign of developing hallucinosis or psychosis may be vivid dreams, illusions of shapes in shadows or patterns, or a transient passage of an object or coloured shape across the vision (visual transient).[145] There may be a peculiar sense of presence in the room. This sense of presence, and other strange experiences which people find difficult to describe within normal sensory experiences, can be described as extracampine hallucinations. These may progress to stereotyped, non-threatening visual hallucinosis in a clear sensorium. Hallucinations are visual, vivid and vital (living), including images of people who may be small (Lilliputian syndrome). They may occur in the evening and at night, in the shadows, in patterns on the furniture and carpets, and are often seen through windows or in mirrors. A few patients seem to have long-standing limited stereotyped 'benign hallucinations', which hardly interfere with function and which probably relate to the maintenance of insight. It is clear that hallucinations follow a malignant course in over 90% of cases and the term *benign hallucination* may not be helpful.[146] Hallucinations become intrusive when patients start to act upon them, by laying extra places at table or beating off non-existent intruders. Patients may then develop systematic delusions surrounding the hallucinations, and lose their ability to distinguish reality. Older patients have more complex and more inclusive delusional systems, possibly due to failure of inhibitory mechanisms in the ageing brain.[147] There are some rare reports of delusional misidentification in PD, in which the misidentification of a near relative is associated with secondary delusions. This may be due to the coexistence of psychosis and frontal lobe impairment.[148] Morbid jealousy is common, especially in males, when images of intruders are misinterpreted. A more serious form of hallucinosis is evidenced by the development of mixed visual, auditory and tactile hallucinations. These may be frightening, with visions of animals or insects, and occur throughout the day and night. This is an organic confusional psychosis and is similar to delirium tremens. Improvement using physostigmine suggests a cholinergic deficit as the basis for these hallucinations. Forty per cent of patients with recurrent visual hallucinations also experience some form of auditory hallucination.[137] The voices are external, talking in the first or second person, are separate from the visual hallucinations which are usually silent, and do not have any affective component.[149] Patients can experience tactile hallucinations, either in association with or separate from the visual hallucinosis.

Diagnosis and assessment

The severity of the psychosis and the degree of disruption to normal life need to be assessed. There is no gold standard for the diagnosis of psychosis in PD and no properly validated clinical diagnostic scale.[73] A simple hallucination severity scale can be used in clinic[150] (*see* Table 6.7) or, possibly, the Parkinson's psychosis questionnaire.[151] Other scales, such as the Neuropsychiatric inventory and the Brief psychiatric rating scale, are used mainly in research. Assessment should clarify whether hallucinosis is associated with delusions. It is important to assess cognition, mood and motor function.

TABLE 6.7 A Parkinson's disease hallucinosis score

Symptom	Score
None	0
Vivid dreams, illusions, sense of presence	1
Dreams encroaching on waking hours, occasional tolerable visual hallucinations	2
Regular evening and night-time intrusive visual hallucinations	3
Disturbing visual, auditory or tactile hallucinations, occur day and night, delusions	4

Management of psychosis

The principles of the management of psychosis can be summarised using the acronym 'ERA' (*see* Table 6.8). The management of non-affective psychosis in PD has been reviewed in the full version of the NICE guideline which summarised advice into a useful clinical algorithm (*see* Figure 6.5).[72] Carers often experience more distress than patients, particularly because the hallucinations tend to be worse in the evening or at night, giving poor sleep. Careful explanation should be given to the patient and carer, since not all hallucinations require treatment. Inter-current illness as a cause for delirium should be ruled out. Sensory regulation is important, with avoidance of vivid patterns and provision of adequate lighting to reduce shadows. Drug therapy may need to be reduced in a stepwise manner, removing the most hallucinogenic drugs

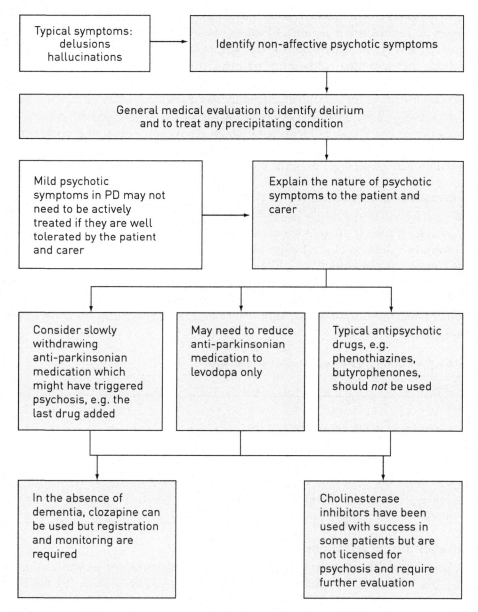

FIGURE 6.5 Medical management of psychosis and hallucinosis in PD.

TABLE 6.8 The principles of management of Parkinson's disease psychosis: 'ERA'

Exclude delirium	Screen for inter-current physical illness
Explain to carer	Worries the carer more than the patient!
Reduce sensory and deprivation sensory overload	Adequate lighting, avoid excessive patterned furniture and fittings
Reduce drugs	Cautiously, in a stepwise fashion
Anti-psychotics	Careful use of quetiapine or clozapine. Monitor ECG, cognitive and motor function. Do not use traditional antipsychotics
Acetylcholinesterase inhibitors	Careful use monitoring cognition and motor function

first until finally the minimum L-Dopa (levodopa) dose required for motor function is used (*see* Figure 6.6).[150] It is possible that COMT inhibitors cause less hallucinosis than the direct-acting dopamine agonists, and many clinicians would opt for COMT inhibitors as adjunctive therapy for control of motor wearing-off in patients with previous hallucinosis or cognitive impairment. Subcutaneous apomorphine may allow a reduction in doses of other drugs, with a consequent reduction in hallucinosis, although evidence for this effect is controversial. Occasionally, where these strategies have been ineffective, specific antipsychotics may be needed. Hallucinosis may be associated with serotonin (5-HT) over-activity and with a cholinergic deficit centrally. Successful management of psychotic symptoms in PD may rely on a multi-target approach to restore neurotransmitter imbalances, rather than focusing exclusively on the dopaminergic dysfunction.[152] Small open-label studies have shown efficacy of many agents, including the anti-emetic ondansetron (5-HT$_3$ antagonist), but the utility of these in clinical practice is limited. Typical neuroleptics must not be used since they may cause catastrophic deterioration in motor function.[72] Atypical neuroleptics are prescribed commonly but must be used in the smallest possible dose. In practice, the atypical neuroleptics risperidone and olanzapine can cause sedation, deterioration in cognition and worsening motor function.[153] There are additional concerns over increased risk of stroke in patients with dementia and stroke risk factors. Quetiapine may be better tolerated, but is a weaker antipsychotic agent and has yet to be proven effective in randomised placebo-controlled trials.[72,154] Clozapine is the most studied antipsychotic in PD; is effective in reducing psychosis, anxiety, motor fluctuation and hypersexuality,[155] and has been recommended in the NICE guidelines.[72] It is now licensed for use in the UK subject to registration with a monitoring scheme. Initially weekly blood tests need to be performed to minimise the small risk of agranulocytosis.

All atypical neuroleptics cause prolongation of the QT interval on ECG, especially in elderly patients. An ECG must be performed prior to therapy, and it is advisable to re-check the ECG at regular intervals. Atypical neuroleptics tend to accumulate in the elderly and therefore the doses used must be as small as possible with careful observation of the effects on motor and cognitive symptoms. Cessation of antipsy-

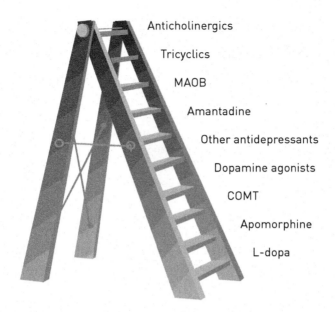

Anticholinergics

Tricyclics

MAOB

Amantadine

Other antidepressants

Dopamine agonists

COMT

Apomorphine

L-dopa

FIGURE 6.6 Stepwise drug reduction – psychosis and hallucinosis.

chotics can lead to a rebound psychosis and therefore, once these drugs are established chronic treatment is usually required.[156] Cholinesterase inhibitors may be warranted in dementia with psychosis, since enhancement of cholinergic activity may improve both cognition and psychosis.[72] Clinical experience suggests that cholinesterase inhibitors should be considered early in the management since they may help avoid unnecessary dopaminergic reduction or use of atypical neuroleptics. Where an acute psychotic breakdown occurs, there is not sufficient time to titrate cholinesterase inhibitors to an effective dose and the acute situation may need to be managed with atypical neuroleptics. Cholinesterase inhibitors should be prescribed under the supervision of a specialist who can monitor cognition, motor function and the severity of psychosis. ECT has been used to treat psychosis in PD in a small number of patients with serious resistant psychosis.

Cognition and movement in PD

There is an intricate relationship between cognition and movement in PD. Studies of specific goal–directed movements show that PD patients can produce rapid movements, but these tend to be inaccurate. This inaccuracy is counteracted in most circumstances by utilising visual direction, which causes slowing of movement. It has been postulated that some of the slowness of movement and hypokinesia in PD may be due to the adoption of a cautious cognitive strategy, in order to overcome the inaccuracy of movement.[157] In increasingly complex grasping tasks, however, PD patients do not adopt the normal cautious strategy of widening the hand with increasingly demanding tasks, but persist with hypometric hand grasp movements.[158]

In simple tasks, difficulty in initiating movement is due to cortical under-activation or poor preparation for movement. In more complex tasks, poor performance is due to a cognitive deficit in set shifting, with an inability to adopt appropriate strategies.[159] Increasingly severe cognitive deficits due to prolonged processing time are associated with increasing motor disability.[160] PET scan studies have shown that impairment of self-initiated movement is associated with under-activation of the dorsolateral prefrontal cortex.[16] With increasing motor severity, patients demonstrate frontal dysfunction, with poor verbal fluency and difficulty with divided attention. This can be seen in practice with patients demonstrating difficulty walking and talking at the same time. Regulation of gait variability and rhythmicity is an automatic process that does not demand attention in healthy adults. In patients with PD, however, this ability becomes attention-demanding and worsens when subjects perform secondary tasks. Moreover, the association between executive function and gait variability suggests that a decline in executive function in PD may exacerbate the effects of dual tasking on gait, potentially increasing fall risk.[161] Competition for attention through additional activities, decreased executive function, depression, fatigue, and impaired balance will increase difficulty in walking for PD subjects.[162]

In PD there are deficits of set shifting in both cognitive and motor tasks, with set shifting being the primary role of the basal ganglia. Movement may be a consequence of constant shifting of postural sets.[163] Regulation of the force of muscles is necessary in order to control the point at which opposing muscle groups reach equilibrium, and shifting this equilibrium point along a desired trajectory produces movement. A deficit of set shifting, and consequent force regulation, may be responsible for some of the motor syndrome of PD. Movement may be divided into separate sensory-motor-cognitive actions, with the basal ganglia playing a critical role in preparing, initiating and suppressing these actions.[163] Such theories unify cognition and movement, and explain the interaction between the cognitive and motor syndromes seen in PD.

This relationship between cognition and movement in PD has important implications for therapy (*see* Chapter 14). Function may be improved by encouraging attentional strategies to anticipate movement.[164] These strategies may allow movement to be produced by less automatic and more conscious attentional motor pathways,[164] such as the cerebellar-lateral premotor cortex pathways which develop compensatory over-activity in PD. Dopaminergic medication may have differential effects on some aspects of cognition and movement in PD since withdrawal of dopaminergic medication produces deterioration in delayed response tasks separate from motor deterioration but no changes in spatial learning.[165]

Psychiatry of other multisystem degenerations

The psychopathology of other conditions causing parkinsonism reflects the relative distribution of pathological changes in the basal ganglia, frontal, limbic and cortical regions of the brain.

Multiple system atrophy (MSA) causes extensive cell loss and gliosis in the striatum, basal ganglia, brainstem and cerebellum. There are no clear cognitive differences between patients with MSA and PD. One study has suggested that PD patients have more depression and anxiety, while MSA patients have more blunting of affect, which may reflect neuronal loss in the caudate and ventral striatum which are part of the lateral orbitofrontal and limbic circuits.[166] Motor function, autonomic function and depression are most linked with health-related quality of life in MSA.[167]

Patients with progressive supranuclear palsy (PSP) present with subjective complaints of forgetfulness and loss of concentration. PSP patients show symptoms compatible with lesioned orbitofrontal and medial frontal circuits.[168] Apathy, social withdrawal and loss of independence are associated with dysexecutive syndrome, with marked planning difficulties, reflecting extensive involvement of subcorticofrontal circuits.[169] Relative sparing of the raphé nucleus and locus caeruleus may reduce the occurrence of depression compared with PD. Emotional lability is common, but psychosis is rare in PSP. Quality of life in PSP may be related to depression associated with cognitive decline.[170] Subcorticofrontal dementia leads to a delay in initiation of thoughts, perseveration, reduced verbal fluency and dissociation between normal storage and impaired retrieval of information. Patients with PSP are more reliant on external environmental stimuli for behaviour (environmental dependence), which may be due to a lack of frontal control. Patients need to be given adequate time to respond to questions, and may respond to cueing to improve memory.

Patients with corticobasal degeneration (CBD) have more depression and irritability, but less apathy than those with PSP.[171] Patients may demonstrate cognitive abnormalities reflecting cortical disease including apraxias, alien hand, visual and sensory neglect. Gesture problems are said to be specific for CBD. Visuospatial function is intact in MSA, mildly impaired in PSP and significantly impaired in CBD, suggesting differential distribution of object-based and spatial functions in the brain.[172] Using the Addenbrookes Cognitive Examination (ACE-R) as a screening tool, there is more cognitive deterioration in patients with CBD than there is in those with PSP, with no deterioration in the case of patients with MSA.[173] Rarely, corticobasal syndrome can be due to motor neurone disease (MND), which itself can be associated with parkinsonism. MND may prove to be a multisystem disease and a cause of frontotemporal dementia.

Movement disorders in psychiatric illness

Movement disorders in psychiatric conditions can be primary – due to the disease itself, or secondary – due to treatment. Primary abnormalities are now difficult to separate from the effects of drug treatment. Patients with untreated schizophrenia can demonstrate dyskinesias (15%), extrapyramidal signs (10%), catatonia (rare) and abnormalities of voluntary movement such as mannerisms and stereotypic movements.[174] Catatonic patients become immobile, rigid, mute, resist movement and refuse nutrition. Rarely, catatonia can be a feature of severe depression. Stereotypes and mannerisms, including repetitive hand rubbing and rocking, can be seen in depressed elderly patients and in dementia. Most commonly, movement disorders are secondary to drug treatment, particularly neuroleptics. Increasing age, female sex, organic brain disease, long-term treatment and rapid withdrawal can predispose to the development of tardive movement disorders, the most common of which is tardive dyskinesia (TD). TD is caused most commonly by typical neuroleptics and, although the risk appears to be declining, it is not yet clear whether, in the long term, this may prove to be a problem with atypical neuroleptics.[175] TD can be very difficult to treat, with the best treatment being prevention by avoidance of precipitating medications. Atypical neuroleptics, used as alternative agents, may occasionally reduce the dyskinesia. With continued withdrawal of the causative drug, 33% of patients may improve over two years though there is a lack of comparative trials of continuation compared with cessation of neuroleptics.[176] There is insufficient evidence to support the use of other treatments for TD including benzodiazepines and calcium channel blockers.[177,178] Only rarely, with severe disability, should dopamine-depleting agents be used (tetrabenazine, starting with 12.5 mg). In elderly patients prochlorperazine and metaclopramide, used for nausea and dizziness, are common causes of tardive dyskinesia. Other drug-induced movements include dystonia, akathisia, parkinsonism and rarely tics and myoclonus. Drug-induced parkinsonism is more common with increasing age and disability.[179] Positron emission tomography (PET) studies reveal that an approximate 65% blockade of the D2 receptors is required for typical antipsychotics to be efficacious, but a blockade of 75–80% results in acute extrapyramidal side effects. Drugs which rapidly dissociate from the D2 receptor, such as atypical neuroleptics, are less likely to cause parkinsonism, alterations in prolactin or tardive dyskinesia.[180] Drug-induced parkinsonism is more common with the typical neuroleptics but can occur with atypical neuroleptics particularly when used in high doses[181] and can be clinically indistinguishable from idiopathic PD. Brain imaging with dopamine active transport scans (DAT) helps to determine whether the parkinsonism is entirely drug-induced or an exacerbation of subclinical PD.[182] An exacerbation of subclinical PD may require the use of levodopa, occasionally in association with continued low-dose atypical neuroleptics, in patients with continuing problematic psychosis. The routine use of anticholinergic agents for patients on neuroleptics is not recommended. Tremors, dystonias and extrapyramidal signs have also been reported with antidepressants, including TCA and SSRI agents.[183] Close liaison between the physician and psychiatrist is essential in the management of these disorders in order to avoid conflicting advice.

Conclusions

Professionals, carers and patients need to be aware of the intimate relationship between the cognitive, emotional and motor components of PD and related disorders. The recognition, assessment and management of psychiatric problems in PD are important in order to improve the quality of life of both patients and carers. Brief assessments of mood, cognition, executive function and perception may aid management, and help patients, carers and families to adjust to impairments in these areas. Close co-operation between the primary healthcare team and specialist interdisciplinary team is important at all stages of the disease.

REFERENCES

1 Parkinson J. *An Essay on the Shaking Palsy. 1817*. Published Macmillan Magazines and the Parkinson's Disease Society of the United Kingdom, London; 1992.

2 Berrios GE. *The History of Mental Symptoms*. Cambridge: Cambridge University Press; 1996.

3 Hobson P, Holden A, Meara J. Measuring the impact of Parkinson's disease with the Parkinson's disease quality of life questionnaire. *Age Ageing*. 1999; **28**: 341–6.

4 Meara J, Mitchelmore E, Hobson P. Use of the GDS-15 geriatric depression scale as a screening instrument for depressive symptomatology in patients with Parkinson's disease and their carers in the community. *Age Ageing*. 1999; **28**: 35–8.

5 Goetz CG, Stebbins GT. Mortality and hallucinations in nursing home patients with advanced Parkinson's disease. *Neurology*. 1995; **45**: 669–71.

6 Hughes TA, Ross HGF, Mindham RH, *et al*. Mortality in Parkinson's disease and its association with dementia and depression. *Acta Neurol Scand*. 2004; **110**(2): 118–23.

7 Heikkila VM, Turkka J, Karpelanen J, *et al*. Decreased driving ability in people with Parkinson's disease. *J Neurol Neurosurg Psychiatry*. 1998; **64**: 325–30.

8 Foltynie T, Brayne CE, Robbins T, *et al*. The cognitive ability of an incident cohort of Parkinson's patients in the UK. The CamPaIGN study. *Brain*. 2004; **127**(Pt 3): 550–60.

9 Goetz CG. Historical background of behavioural studies in Parkinson's disease. In: Huber SJ, Cummings JL, editors. *Parkinson's Disease: neurobehavioural aspects*. New York & Oxford: Oxford University Press; 1992: 3–9.

10 Stern GM. Pre-morbid personality structure of patients with Parkinson's disease. In: Wolters EC, Scheltens P, editors. *Mental Dysfunction in Parkinson's Disease*. Amsterdam: Vrije Universiteit; 1993: 103–17.

11 Chaudhuri KR, Yates L, Martinez-Martin P. The non-motor symptom complex of Parkinson's disease: a comprehensive assessment is essential. *Curr Neurol Neurosci Rep*. 2005; **5**(4): 275–83.

12 Heberlein I, Ludin HP, Scholz J, *et al*. Personality depression and premorbid lifestyle in twin pairs discordant for Parkinson's disease. *J Neurol Neurosurg Psychiatry*. 1998; **64**: 262–6.

13 Ishihara L, Brayne C. What is the evidence for a premorbid parkinsonian personality: a systematic review. *Mov Disord*. 2006; **21**(8): 1066–72.

14 Williams DT, Ford B, Fahn S. Phenomenology and psychopathology related to psychogenic movement disorders. In: Weiner WJ, Lang AE, editors. *Behavioural Neurology of Movement Disorders. Advances in Neurology, Vol. 65*. New York: Raven Press; 1995: 231–58.

15 Lishman WA. *Organic Psychiatry: the psychological consequences of cerebral disorder*. Oxford: Blackwell Science; 1998.

16 Jahanshahi M, Jenkins H, Brown R, *et al*. Self-initiated versus externally triggered movements: an investigation using measurement of regional cerebral blood flow with PET and movement-related potentials in normal and Parkinson's disease subjects. *Brain*. 1995; **118**: 913–33.

17 Ben Amer H, Grosset D. SPECT imaging in the diagnosis and staging of parkinsonism. *CNS*. 1999; **2**: 9–12.

18 Stebbins GT, Goetz CG, Carrillo MC, *et al*. Altered cortical visual processing in PD with hallucinations. *Neurology*. 2004; **63**: 1409–16.

19 Hu MTM, Taylor-Robertson SD, Ray Chaudhuri K, *et al*. Evidence for a cortical dysfunction in clinically non-demented patients with Parkinson's disease: a proton MR spectroscopy study. *J Neurol Neurosurg Psychiatry*. 1999; **67**: 20–6.

20 Hodges JR. *Cognitive Assessment for Clinicians*. Oxford: Oxford University Press; 1994.

21 Saint-Cyr JA, Taylor AE, Nicholson K. Behaviour and the basal ganglia. In: Weiner WJ, Lang AE, editors. *Behavioural Neurology of Movement Disorders. Advances in Neurology, Vol. 65*. New York: Raven Press; 1995: 1–28.

22 Savage CR. Neuropsychology of subcortical dementias. *Psychiatr Clin North Am*. 1997; **20**: 911–31.

23 Rinne JO, Rummukainen J, Paljarvi L, *et al.* Dementia in Parkinson's disease is related to neuronal loss in the medial substantia nigra. *Ann Neurol.* 1989; **26**: 47–50.

24 Rascol O, Sabatini U, Fabre N, *et al.* The ipsilateral cerebellar hemisphere is overactive during hand movements in akinetic parkinsonian patients. *Brain.* 1997; **12** (Pt. 1): 103–10.

25 Dubois B, Defontaines B, Deweer B, *et al.* Cognitive and behavioural changes in patients with focal lesions of the basal ganglia. In: Weiner WJ, Lang AE, editors. *Behavioural Neurology of Movement Disorders. Advances in Neurology, Vol. 65.* New York: Raven Press; 1995: 29–42.

26 Dubois B, Pillon B. Cognitive deficits in Parkinson's disease. *J Neurol.* 1997; **224**: 2–8.

27 Weintraub D, Moberg PJ, Culbertson WC, *et al.* Evidence for impaired encoding and retrieval memory profiles in Parkinson disease. *Cogn Behav Neurol.* 2004; **17**(4): 195–200.

28 Hunt LA, Sadun AA, Bassi CJ. Review of the visual system in Parkinson's disease. *Optometry Vis Sci.* 1995; **72**: 92–9.

29 Owsley C, Ball K, McGwin G, *et al.* Visual processing impairment and risk of motor vehicle crash among older adults. *JAMA.* 1998; **279**: 1083–8.

30 Radford K, Lincoln N, Lennox G. The effects of cognitive abilities on driving in people with Parkinson's disease. *Disabil Rehabil.* 2004; **26**(2): 65–70.

31 Katzen HL, Levin BE, Llabre ML. Age of disease onset influences cognition in Parkinson's disease. *J Int Neurospychol Soc.* 1998; **4**: 285–90.

32 Wermuth L, Knudsen L, Boldsen J. A study of cognitive functions in young Parkinsonian patients. *Acta Neurol Scand.* 1996; **93**(1): 21–4.

33 Mahieux F, Fenelon G, Flahault A, *et al.* Neuro-psychological prediction of dementia in Parkinson's disease. *J Neurol Neurosurg Psychiatry.* 1998; **64**: 178–83.

34 Janvin CC, Larsen JP, Aarsland D, *et al.* Subtypes of mild cognitive impairment in Parkinson's disease: progression to dementia. *Mov Disord.* 2006; **21**(9): 1343–9.

35 Janvin C, Aarsland D, Larsen JP, *et al.* Neuropsychological profile of patients with Parkinson's disease without dementia. *Dement Geriatr Cogn Disord.* 2003; **15**(3): 126–31.

36 Burn DJ, Rowan EN, Allan LM, *et al.* Motor subtype and cognitive decline in Parkinson's disease, Parkinson's disease with dementia, and dementia with Lewy bodies. *J Neurol Neurosurg Psychiatry.* 2006; **77**(5): 585–9.

37 Mari-beffa P, Hayes AE, Machado L, *et al.* Lack of inhibition in Parkinson's disease: evidence from a lexical decision task. *Neuropsychologia.* 2005; **43**(4): 638–46.

38 Cheesman AL, Barker RA, Lewis SJ, *et al.* Lateralisation of striatal function: evidence from 18F-dopa PET in Parkinson's disease. *J Neurol Neurosurg Psychiatry.* 2005; **76**: 1204–10.

39 Foltynie T, Goldberg TE, Lewis SG, *et al.* Planning ability in Parkinson's disease is influenced by the CONT val158met polymorphism. *Mov Disord.* 2004; **19**: 885–91.

40 Swainson R, SenGupta D, Shetty T, *et al.* Impaired dimensional selection but intact use of reward feedback during visual discrimination learning in Parkinson's disease. *Neuropsychologia.* 2006; **44**(8): 1290–304.

41 Kulisevsky J, Garcia-Sanchez C, Berthier ML, *et al.* Chronic effects of dopaminergic replacement on cognitive function in Parkinson's disease: two year follow up study of previously untreated patients. *Mov Disord.* 2000; **15**: 613–26.

42 Kulisevsky J. The role of dopamine in Parkinson's disease-related cognitive impairment. In: Wolters EC, Berendse HW, Stam CJ, editors. *Mental Dysfunction in Parkinson's Disease III.* Amsterdam: Vrije Universiteit; 2006.

43 Vingerhoets G, Van der Linden C, Lannoo E, *et al.* Cognitive outcome after unilateral pallidal stimulation in Parkinson's disease. *J Neurol Neurosurg Psychiatry.* 1999; **66**: 297–304.

44 Funkiewiez A, Ardouin C, Caputo E, *et al.* Long term effects of biliateral subthalamic nucleus stimulation on cognitive function, mood and behaviour in Parkinson's disease. *J Neurol Neurosurg Psychiatry.* 2004; **75**(6): 834–9.

45 Hobson P, Meara J. The detection of dementia and cognitive impairment in a community population of elderly people with Parkinson's disease by use of the CAMCOG neuro-psychological test. *Age Ageing.* 1999; **28**: 39–43.

46 Ballard CG, Aarsland D, McKeith I, *et al.* Fluctuations in attention: PD dementia vs DLB with parkinsonism. *Neurology.* 2002; **59**(11): 1714–20.

47 McKeith IG, Dickson DW, Lowe J, *et al.* Diagnosis and management of dementia with Lewy bodies. *Neurology.* 2005; **65**: 1863–72.

48 Mosimann UP, Mather G, Wesnes KA, *et al.* Visual perception in Parkinson's disease dementia and dementia with Lewy bodies. *Neurology.* 2004; **63**: 2091–6.

49 Mosimann UP, Rowan EN, Partington CE, *et al.* Characteristics of visual hallucinations in Parkinson's disease dementia and dementia with Lewy bodies. *Am J Geriatr Psychiatry.* 2006; **14**: 153–60.

50 Gananalingham KK, Byrne EJ, Thornton A, *et al.* Motor and cognitive function in Lewy body dementia: comparison with Alzheimer's and Parkinson's diseases. *J Neurol Neurosurg Psychiatry.* 1997; **62**: 243–52.

51 Holmes C, Cairns N, Lantos P, *et al.* Validity of current clinical criteria for Alzheimer's disease, vascular dementia and dementia with Lewy bodies. *Br J Psychiatry.* 1999; **174**: 45–50.

52 Hurtig HI, Trojanowski JQ, Galvin J, *et al.* Alpha-synuclein cortical Lewy bodies correlate with dementia in Parkinson's disease. *Neurology.* 2000; **54**: 1916–21.

53 Harding AJ, Halliday GM. Cortical Lewy body pathology in the diagnosis of dementia. *Acta Neuropathol (Berl).* 2001; **102**(4): 355–63.

54 Janvin CC, Larsen JP, Salmon DP, *et al.* Cognitive profiles of individual patients with Parkinson's disease and dementia: comparison with dementia with Lewy bodies and Alzheimer's disease. *Mov Disord.* 2006; **21**(3): 337–42.

55 Mitchell S. Extrapyramidal features in Alzheimer's disease. *Age Ageing.* 1999; **28**: 401–9.

56 De Vos RAI, Jansen ENH, Yilmazer D, *et al.* Pathological and clinical features of Parkinson's disease with and without dementia. In: Perry R, McKeith I, Perry E, editors. *Dementia with Lewy Bodies.* Cambridge: Cambridge University Press; 1996: 255–67.

57 Mandal PK, Pettegrew JW, Masliah E, *et al.* Interaction between Abeta peptide and alpha synuclein: molecular mechanisms in overlapping pathology of Alzheimer's and Parkinson's in Dementia with Lewy body disease. *Neurochem Res.* 2006; **31**(9): 1153–62. Epub.

58 Aarsland D, Ballard CG, Halliday G. Are Parkinson's disease with dementia and dementia with Lewy bodies the same entity? *J Geriatr Psychiatry Neurol.* 2004; **17**(3): 137–45.

59 Tsuboi Y, Dickson DW. Dementia with Lewy bodies and Parkinson's disease with dementia: Are they different? *Parkinsonism Relat Disord.* 2005; **11**: S47–S51.

60 Burton EJ, McKeith IG, Burn DJ, *et al.* Progression of white matter hyperintensities in Alzheimer disease, dementia with Lewy bodies, and Parkinson disease dementia: a comparison with normal aging. *Am J Geriatr Psychiatry.* 2006; **14**(10): 842–9.

61 Burn DJ. Parkinson's disease dementia: what's in a Lewy body? *J Neural Transm Suppl.* 2006; **70**: 361–5.

62 Riekkinen M, Kejonen K, Jakala P, *et al.* Reduction of noradrenaline impairs attention and dopamine depletion slows responses in Parkinson's disease. *Eur J Neurosci.* 1998; **10**: 1492–535.

63 Leentjens AEG, Schloltissen B. The role of serotonin in Parkinson's disease cognitive dysfunction. In: Wolters EC, Berendse HW, Stam CJ, editors. *Mental Dysfunction in Parkinson's Disease,* 1st ed. Amsterdam: Vrije Universiteit; 2006.

64 Newhouse PE, Potter A, Levin ED. Nicotinic system involvement in Alzheimer's and Parkinson's diseases. *Drugs Ageing.* 1997; **11**: 206–28.

65 Mattila PM, Roytta M, Lonnberg P, *et al.* Choline acetytransferase activity and striatal dopamine receptors in Parkinson's disease in relation to cognitive impairment. *Acta Neuropathol (Berl).* 2001; **102**(2): 160–6.

66 Bohnen NI, Kaufer DI, Ivanco LS, *et al.* Cortical cholinergic function is more severely affected in parkinsonian dementia than in Alzheimer disease: an in vivo positron emission tomographic study. *Arch Neurol.* 2003; **60**: 1745–8.

67 Burns A, Lawlor B, Craig S, editors. *Assessment Scales in Old Age Psychiatry.* London: Dunitz; 1999.

68 Dubois B, Slachevsky A, Litvan I, *et al*. The FAB: a frontal assessment battery at bedside. *Neurology*. 2000; **55**(11): 1621–6.

69 Mathuranath PS, Nestor PJ, Berrios GE, *et al*. A brief cognitive test battery to differentiate Alzheimer's disease and frontotemporal dementia. *Neurology*. 2000; **55**(11): 1613–20.

70 Ferman TJ, Smith GE, Boeve BF, *et al*. DLB fluctuations: specific features that reliably differentiate DLB from AD and normal aging. *Neurology*. 2004; **62**(2): 181–7.

71 Inzelberg R, Bonuccelli U, Schechtman E, *et al*. Association between amantadine and the onset of dementia in Parkinson's disease. *Mov Disord*. 2006; **21**(9): 1375–9.

72 National Institute of Health and Clincal Excellence. *The Diagnosis and Management of Parkinson's Disease in Primary and Secondary Care*. NICE Clinical Guideline CG035. June 2006. NICE.org.uk

73 Miyasaki JM, Shannon K, Voon V, *et al*. Practice parameter: evaluation and treatment of depression, psychosis and dementia in Parkinson's disease. *Neurology*. 2006; **66**: 996–1002.

74 Emrie M, Aarsland D, Albanese A, *et al*. Rivastigmine for dementia associated with Parkinson's disease. *N Eng J Med*. 2004; **351**: 2509–18.

75 Poewe W, Wolters E, Emrie M, *et al*. Long-term benefits of rivastigmine in dementia associated with Parkinson's disease: an active treatment extension study. *Mov Disord*. 2006; **21**(4): 456–61.

76 Ballard C, Lane R, Barone P, *et al*. Cardiac safety of rivastigmine in Lewy body and Parkinson's disease dementias. *Int J Clin Pract*. 2006; **60**(6): 639–45.

77 Minett TS, Thomas A, Wilkinson LM, *et al*. What happens when donepezil is suddenly withdrawn? An open label trial in dementia with Lewy bodies and Parkinson's disease with dementia. *Int J Geriatr Psychiatry*. 2003; **18**(11): 988–93.

78 Scherder EJA. Pain in Parkinson's disease; its relationship to cognitive functioning. In: Wolters EC, Berendse HW, Stam CJ, editors. *Mental Dysfunction in Parkinson's Disease*. Amsterdam: Vrije Universiteit; 2006.

79 Alexopoulos GS, Abrams RC, Young RC, *et al*. Cornell scale for depression in dementia. *Biol Psychiatry*. 1988; **23**(3): 271–84.

80 Pluck GC, Brown RG. Apathy in Parkinson's disease. *J Neurol Neurosurg Psychiatry*. 2002; **73**(6): 636–42.

81 Marin RS, Biedrzycki RC, Firinciogullari S. Reliability and validity of the Apathy Evaluation Scale. *Psychiatry Res*. 1991; **38**(2): 143–62.

82 Starkstein SE, Mayberg HS, Preziosi TJ, *et al*. Reliability, validity, and clinical correlates of apathy in Parkinson's disease. *J Neuropsychiatry Clin Neurosci*. 1992; **4**(2): 134–9.

83 Schrag A. Quality of life and depression in Parkinson's disease. *J Neurol Sci*. 2006; **248**(1–2): 151–7.

84 Aarsland D, Larsen JP, Tanberg E, *et al*. Predictors of nursing home placement in Parkinson's disease: a population-based, prospective study. *J Am Geriatr Soc*. 2000; **48**(8): 938–42.

85 Menza M, Marin H, Kaufman K, *et al*. Citalopram treatment of depression in Parkinson's disease: the impact on anxiety, disability, and cognition. *J Neuropsychiatry Clin Neurosci*. 2004; **16**(3): 315–9.

86 Marsh L, McDonald WM, Cummings J, *et al*. Provisional diagnostic criteria for depression in Parkinson's disease: report of a NINDS/NIMH working group. *Mov Disord*. 2006; **21**(2): 148–58.

87 Alexopolous GS. Role of executive dysfunction in late-life depression. *J Clin Psychiatry*. 2003; **64** (suppl. 14): 18–23.

88 Ehrt U, Bronnick K, Leentjens AF, *et al*. Depressive symptom profile in Parkinson's disease: a comparison with depression in elderly patients without Parkinson's disease. *Int J Geriatr Psychiatry*. 2006; **21**(3): 252–8.

89 Merschdorf U, Berg D, Csoti I, *et al*. Psychopathological symptoms of depression in Parkinson's disease compared to major depression psychopathology. *Psychopathology*. 2003; **36**(5): 221–5.

90 Weintraub D, Cary MS, Stern MB, *et al*. Daily affect in Parkinson disease is responsive to life events and motor symptoms. *Am J Geriatr Psychiatry*. 2006; **14**(2): 161–8.

91 Lam RW, Michalak EE, Swinson RP, editors. *Assessment Scales in Depression, Mania and Anxiety.* Abingdon: Informa; 2005.

92 Weintraub D, Oehlberg KA, Katz IR, *et al.* Test characteristics of the 15-item geriatric depression scale and Hamilton depression rating scale in Parkinson disease. *Am J Geriatr Psychiatry.* 2006; 14(2): 169–75.

93 Tandberg E, Larsen JP, Aarsland D, *et al.* The occurrence of depression in Parkinson's disease: a community based study. *Arch Neurol.* 1996; 53: 175–9.

94 Miyawaki E, Meah T, Kormos D, *et al. Depression in Parkinson's Disease: a meta-analysis regarding severity.* Poster 588. Presented at 4th International Congress on Movement Disorders; 1996 June; Vienna, Austria.

95 Global Parkinson's Disease Survey Steering Committee. Factors impacting on quality of life in Parkinson's disease: results from an international survey. *Mov Disord.* 2002; 17(1): 60–7.

96 Shulman LM, Taback RL, Rabinstein AA, *et al.* Non-recognition of depression and other non-motor symptoms in Parkinson's disease. *Parkinsonism Relat Disord.* 2002; 8(3): 193–7.

97 Starkstein SE, Mayberg HS, Leiguarada R, *et al.* A prospective longitudinal study of depression, cognitive decline, and physical impairments in patients with Parkinson's disease. *J Neurol Neurosurg Psychiatry.* 1992; 55(5): 377–82.

98 Lewis SJ, Foltynie T, Blackwell AD, *et al.* Heterogeneity of Parkinson's disease in the early clinical stages using a data driven approach. *J Neurol Neurosurg Psychiatry.* 2005; 76(3): 343–8.

99 Tom T, Cummings JL. Depression in Parkinson's disease: pharmacological characteristics and treatment. *Drugs Ageing.* 1998; 12: 55–74.

100 Shajahan P, Ebmeier K. Transcranial magnetic stimulation: a treatment of the future? *Prog Neurol Psychiatry.* 1998; 2: 19–22.

101 Kuzis G, Sabe L, Tiberti C, *et al.* Cognitive functions in major depression and Parkinson's disease. *Arch Neurol.* 1997; 54: 982–6.

102 Coen RF, Kirby M, Swanwick GR, *et al.* Distinguishing between patients with depression or very mild Alzheimer's disease using the delayed word recall test. *Dementia Geriatr Cogn Disord.* 1997; 8: 244–7.

103 Fahim S, van Duijn CM, Baker FM, *et al.* A study of familial aggregation of depression, dementia and Parkinson's disease. *Eur J Epidemiol.* 1998; 14: 233–8.

104 Mossner R, Henneberg A, Schmitt A, *et al.* Allelic variation of serotonin transporter expression is associated with depression in Parkinson's disease. *Mol Psychiatry.* 2001; 6(3): 350–2.

105 Remy P, Doder M, Lees A, *et al.* Depression in Parkinson's disease: loss of dopamine and noradrenaline innervation in the limbic system. *Brain.* 2005; 128 (Pt 6): 1314–22.

106 Pohjasvaara T, Leppavuori A, Siira I, *et al.* Frequency and clinical determinants of post-stroke depression. *Stroke.* 1998; 29: 2311–7.

107 Bejjani BP, Damier P, Arnulf I, *et al.* Transient acute depression induced by high-frequency deep-brain stimulation. *N Eng J Med.* 1999; 340: 1476–80.

108 Yudofsky SC. Parkinson's disease depression and electrical stimulation of the brain. *N Eng J Med.* 1999; 340: 1500–2.

109 Nilsson FM, Kessing LV, Bolwig TJ. Increased risk of developing Parkinson's disease for patients with major affective disorder: a register study. *Acta Psychiatr Scand.* 2001; 104(5): 380–6.

110 Leentjens AF, Van den Akker M, Metsemakers JF, *et al.* Higher incidence of depression preceding the onset of Parkinson's disease: a register study. *Mov Disord.* 2003; 18(4): 414–8.

111 Brown R, Jahanshahi M. Depression in Parkinson's disease: a psychosocial viewpoint. In: Weiner WJ, Lang AE, editors. *Behavioural Neurology of Movement Disorders. Advances in Neurology, Vol. 65.* New York: Raven Press; 1995: 61–84.

112 Allott R, Wells A, Morrison AP, *et al.* Distress in Parkinson's disease: contributions of disease factors and metacognitive style. *Br J Psychiatry.* 2005; 187: 182–3.

113 Cole K, Vaughan FL. The feasibility of using cognitive behaviour therapy for depression associated with Parkinson's disease: a literature review. *Parkinsonism Relat Disord.* 2005; 11(5): 269–76.

114 Maricle RA, Nutt JG, Valentine RJ, *et al*. Dose response relationship of levodopa with mood and anxiety in fluctuating Parkinson's disease: a double-blind placebo-controlled study. *Neurology*. 1995; **45**: 1757–60.

115 Barone P, Scarzella L, Marconi R, *et al*. Pramipexole versus sertraline in the treatment of depression in Parkinson's disease. *J Neurol*. 2006; **253**: 555–61.

116 Silver JM, Yudofsky SC. Drug treatment of depression in Parkinson's disease. In: Huber SJ, Cummings JL, editors. *Parkinson's Disease: neurobehavioural aspects*. New York & Oxford: Oxford University Press; 1992: 240–54.

117 Meara RJ, Bhowmick BK, Hobson JP. Safety and efficacy of sertraline in the treatment of depression concomitant to Parkinson's disease. *J Psychopharmacol*. 1998; **12** (3 suppl. A): A19.

118 Lynd LD, Gerber PE. Selective serotonin reuptake inhibitor induced movement disorders. *Ann Pharmacother*. 1998; **32**: 692–8.

119 Montgomery SA. New developments in the treatment of depression. *J Clin Psychiatry*. 1999; **60** (suppl. 14): 10–15; discussion 31–5.

120 Updated prescibing advice for venlafaxine. At www.mhra.gov.uk

121 Bierbrauer J. Motor signs in Parkinson's disease are altered by serotonergic and noradrenergic transmission levels. *Mov Disord*. 1998; **13** (suppl. 2): P1.155.

122 Normann C, Hesslinger B, Frauenknecht S, *et al*. Psychosis during chronic levodopa therapy triggered by the new antidepressive drug mirtazapine. *Pharmacopsychiatry*. 1997; **30**: 263–5.

123 Steur ENHJ, Ballering LAP. Moclobamide and selegeline in the treatment of depression in Parkinson's disease. *J Neurol Neurosurg Psychiatry*. 1997; **63**: 547.

124 Ruhe HG, Huyser J, Swinkels JA, *et al*. Dose escalation for insufficient response to standard-dose selective serotonin reuptake inhibitors in major depressive disorder. *B J Psychiatry*. 2006; **189**: 309–16.

125 Moellentine C, Rummans T, Ahlskog JE, *et al*. Effectiveness of ECT in patients with parkinsonism. *J Neuropsychiatr Clin Neurosci*. 1998; **10**: 187–93.

126 Fregni F, Simon DK, Pascual-Leone A. Non-invasive brain stimulation for Parkinson's disease: a systematic review and meta-analysis of the literature. *J Neurol Neurosurg Psychiatry*. 2005; **76**(12): 1614–23.

127 Fregni F, Santos CM, Myczkowski ML, *et al*. Repetitive transcranial magnetic stimulation is as effective as fluoxetine in the treatment of depression in patients with Parkinson's disease. *J Neurol Neurosurg Psychiatry*. 2004; **75**(8): 1171–4.

128 Weintraub D, Morales KH, Moberg PJ, *et al*. Anti-depressant studies in Parkinson's disease: a review and meta-analysis. *Mov Disord*. 2005; **20**(9): 1161–9.

129 de la Fuente-Fernandez R, Stoessl AJ. The placebo effect in Parkinson's disease. *Trends Neurosci*. 2002; **25**(6): 302–6.

130 Weisskopf MG, Chen H, Schwarzchikld MA, *et al*. Prospective study of phobic anxiety and risk of Parkinson's disease. *Mov Disord*. 2003; **18**(6): 646–51.

131 Wegelin J, McNamara P, Durso R, *et al*. Correlates of excessive daytime sleepiness in Parkinson's disease. *Parkinsonism Relat Disord*. 2005; **11**(7): 441–8.

132 Richard IH, Frank S, McDermott MP, *et al*. The ups and downs of Parkinson disease: a prospective study of mood and anxiety fluctuations. *Cogn Behav Neurol*. 2004; **17**(4): 201–7.

133 Evans AH, Lawrence AD, Potts J, *et al*. Factors influencing susceptibility to compulsive dopaminergic drug use in Parkinson disease. *Neurology*. 2005; **65**(10): 1570–4.

134 Evans AH, Katzenschlager R, Paviour D, *et al*. Punding in Parkinson's disease: its relation to the dopamine dysregulation syndrome. *Mov Disord*. 2004; **19**(4): 397–405.

135 Weintraub D, Potenza MN. Impulse control disorders in Parkinson's disease. *Curr Neurol Neurosci Rep*. 2006; **6**(4): 302–6.

136 Wermuth L, Stenager E. Sexual problems in young patients with Parkinson's disease. *Acta Neurol Scand*. 1995; **91**: 453–5.

137 Graham JM, Grunwald RA, Sagar HJ. Hallucinosis in idiopathic Parkinson's disease. *J Neurol Neurosurg Psychiatry*. 1997; **63**: 434–40.

138 Williams DR, Lees AJ. Visual hallucinations in the diagnosis of idiopathic Parkinson's disease: a retrospective autopsy study. *Lancet Neurol.* 2005; **4**(10): 605–10.

139 Pieri V, Diederich NJ, Raman R, Goetz CG. Decreased color discrimination and contrast sensitivity in Parkinson's disease. *J Neurol Sci.* 2000; **172**(1): 7–11.

140 Perry EK, Marshall E, Thompson P, *et al.* Monoaminergic activities in Lewy body dementia: relation to hallucinosis and extrapyramidal features. *J Neural Transm Park Dis Dement Sect.* 1993; **6**(3): 167–77.

141 Riederer P, Mehler-Wex C, Gerlach M. Biochemical basis of psychosis in Parkinson's disease. In: Wolters EC, Berendse HW, Stam CJ, editors. *Mental Dysfunction in Parkinson's Disease.* Amsterdam: Vrije Universiteit; 2006.

142 Collerton D, Perry E, McKeith I. Why people see things that are not there: a novel Perception and Attention Deficit model for recurrent complex visual hallucinations. *Behav Brain Sci.* 2005; **28**(6): 737–57.

143 Ffytche DH, Howard RJ. The perceptual consequences of visual loss: 'positive' pathologies of vision. *Brain.* 1999; **122** (Pt 7): 1247–60.

144 Paleacu D, Schechtman E, Inzelberg R. Association between family history of dementia and hallucinations in Parkinson disease. *Neurology.* 2005; **64**(10): 1712–5.

145 Fenelon G, Mahieux F, Huon R, *et al.* Hallucinations in Parkinson's disease: prevalence, phenomenology and risk factors. *Brain.* 2000; **123** (Pt 4): 733–45.

146 Goetz CG, Fan W, Leurgans S, *et al.* The malignant course of 'benign hallucinations' in Parkinson disease. *Arch Neurol.* 2006; **63**(5): 713–6.

147 Goetz CG, Wuu J, Curgian L, *et al.* Age-related influences on the clinical characteristics of new-onset hallucinations in Parkinson's disease patients. *Mov Disord.* 2006; **21**(2): 267–70.

148 Roane DM, Rogers JD, Robinson JH, *et al.* Delusional misidentification associated with parkinsonism. *J Neuropsychiatr Clin Neurosc.* 1998; **10**: 194–8.

149 Inzelberg R, Kiperwasser S, Korczyn AD. Auditory hallucinations in Parkinson's disease. *J Neurol Neurosurg Psychiatry.* 1998; **64**: 533–5.

150 Hindle JV. Psychiatric problems in Parkinson's disease. *Geriatr Med.* 1999; **29**: 37–43.

151 Brandstaedter D, Speiker S, Siebert U, *et al.* Development and evaluation of the Parkinson Psychosis Questionnaire: a screening-instrument for the early diagnosis of drug-induced psychosis in Parkinson's disease. *J Neurol.* 2005; **252**(9): 1060–6.

152 Papapetropoulos S, Mash DC. Psychotic symptoms in Parkinson's disease: from description to etiology. *J Neurol.* 2005; **252**(7): 753–64.

153 Graham JM, Sussman JD, Ford KS, *et al.* Olanzapine in the treatment of hallucinosis in idiopathic Parkinson's disease: a cautionary note. *J Neurol Neurosurg Psychiatry.* 1998; **65**: 774–7.

154 Parsa MA, Bastani B. Quetiapine in the treatment of psychosis in patients with Parkinson's disease. *J Neuropsychiatr Clin Neurosci.* 1998; **10**: 216–9.

155 Trosch RM, Frioedman JH, Lannon MC, *et al.* Clozapine use in Parkinson's disease: a retrospective analysis of a large multicentred clinical experience. *Mov Disord.* 1998; **13**: 377–82.

156 Fernandez HH, Trieschmann ME, Okun MS. Rebound psychosis: effect of discontinuation of antipsychotics in Parkinson's disease. *Mov Disord.* 2005; **20**(1): 104–5.

157 Brown RG, Jahanshahi M. Cognitive motor dysfunction in Parkinson's disease. *Neurology.* 1996; **36** (Suppl.1): 24–31.

158 Jackson GM, Jackson SR, Hindle JV. The control of bimanual reach-to-grasp movements in hemi-parkinsonian patients. *Experimental Brain Research.* 2000; **132**(3): 390–8.

159 Wascher E, Verlanger R, Vieregge P, *et al.* Responses to cued signals in Parkinson's disease – distinguishing between disorders of cognition and activation. *Brain.* 1997; **120**: 1355–75.

160 Hayashi R, Hanya N, Kurashima T, *et al.* Relationship between cognitive impairments, event-related potentials and motor disability scores in Parkinson's disease. *J Neurol Sci.* 1996; **141**: 45–8.

161 Yogev G, Giladi N, Peretz C, *et al.* Dual tasking, gait rhythmicity, and Parkinson's disease: which aspects of gait are attention demanding? *Eur J Neurosci.* 2005; **22**(5): 1248–56.

162 Rochester L, Hetherington V, Jones D, *et al.* Attending to the task: interference effects of functional tasks on walking in Parkinson's disease and the roles of cognition, depression, fatigue, and balance. *Arch Phys Med Rehabil.* 2004; **85**(10): 1578–85.

163 Hayes AE, Matthew CD, Keele SW, *et al.* Towards a functional analysis of the basal ganglia. *J Cogn Neurosci.* 1998; **10**: 178–98.

164 Cunnington R, Iansek R, Bradshaw JL. Movement-related potentials in Parkinson's disease: external cues and attentional strategies. *Mov Disord.* 1999; **14**: 63–8.

165 Fern-pollak L, Whone AL, Brooks DJ, *et al.* Cognitive and motor effects of dopaminergic medication withdrawal in Parkinson's disease. *Neuropsychologia.* 2004; **42**(14): 1917–26.

166 Fetoni V, Soliveri P, Testa D, *et al.* Affective symptoms in multiple system atrophy and Parkinson's disease: response to levodopa therapy. *J Neurol Neurosurg Psychiatry.* 1999; **66**: 541–4.

167 Schrag A, Geser F, Stampfer-Kountchev M, *et al.* Health-related quality of life in multiple system atrophy. *Mov Disord.* 2006; **21**(6): 809–15.

168 Aarsland D, Litvan I, Larsen JP. Neuropsychiatric symptoms of patients with progressive supranuclear palsy and Parkinson's disease. *J Neuropsychiatry Clin Neurosci.* 2001; **13**(1): 42–9.

169 Millar D, Griffiths P, Zermansky AJ, *et al.* Characterizing behavioral and cognitive dysexecutive changes in progressive supranuclear palsy. *Mov Disord.* 2006; **21**(2): 199–207.

170 Schrag A, Seai C, Davis J, *et al.* Health-related quality of life in patients with progressive supranuclear palsy. *Mov Disord.* 2003; **18**(12): 1464–9.

171 Litvan I, Cummings JL, Mega M. Neuropsychiatric features of corticobasal degeneration. *J Neurol Neurosurg Psychiatry.* 1998; **65**: 717–21.

172 Bak TH, Caine D, Hearn VC, *et al.* Visuospatial functions in atypical parkinsonian syndromes. *J Neurol Neurosurg Psychiatry.* 2006; **77**(4): 454–6.

173 Bak TH, Rogers TT, Crawford LM, *et al.* Cognitive bedside assessment in atypical parkinsonian syndromes. *J Neurol Neurosurg Psychiatry.* 2005; **76**(3): 420–2.

174 Marsden CD. Motor disorders in schizophrenia. *Psychol Med.* 1982; **12**: 13–5.

175 Tarsy D, Baldessarinini RJ. Epidemiology of tardive dyskinesia: is risk declining with modern antipsychotics? *Mov Disord.* 2006; **21**(5): 589–98.

176 Soares-Weisser K, Rathbone J. Neuroleptic reduction and/or cessation and neuroleptics as specific treatments for tardive dyskinesia. *Cochrane Database Systemic Review.* 2006 Jan 25; (1): CD000459.

177 Bhoopathi P, Soares-Weisser K. Benzodiazepines for neuroleptic-induced tardive dyskinesia. *Cochrane Database Systemic Review.* 2006; (3): CD000205.

178 Soares-Weisser K, Rathbone J. Calcium channel blockers for neuroleptic-induced tardive dyskinesia. *Cochrane Database Systemic Review.* 2004; (1): CD000206.

179 Noves K, Lui H, Holloway RG. What is the risk of developing parkinsonism following neuroleptic use? *Neurology.* 2006; **66**(6): 941–3.

180 Seeman P. Atypical antipsychotics: mechanism of action. *Can J Psychiatry.* 2002; **47**(1): 27–38.

181 Rochon PA, Stukel TA, Sykora K, *et al.* Atypical antipsychotics and parkinsonism. *Arch Intern Med.* 2005; **165**(16): 1882–8.

182 Lorberboym M, Treves TA, Melamed E, *et al.* [^{123}I]-FP/CIT SPECT imaging for distinguishing drug-induced parkinsonism from Parkinson's disease. *Mov Disord.* 2006; **21**(4): 510–4.

183 Kompoliti K. Drug-induced and iatrogenic neurological disorders. In: Goetz CG, Pappert EJ, editors. *Textbook of Clinical Neurology.* Philadelphia: WB Saunders; 1999: 1123–52.

7

Autonomic dysfunction

ROSE ANNE KENNY

Introduction

Autonomic symptoms in Parkinson's disease (PD) were first reported in 1817 by James Parkinson himself. He described abnormalities of salivation and sweating, and dysfunction of the alimentary tract and urinary bladder.

Patients rarely volunteer symptoms of autonomic disturbance in clinic, and perhaps because of this, there has been little interest in autonomic dysfunction in PD until recent years. Demonstration of the importance of dysautonomia in the aetiology of falls,[1] and possibly cognitive dysfunction,[2] in the non-parkinsonian elderly has, however, led to a recent resurgence of interest in this area.

This chapter will cover the differential diagnosis of dysautonomia in PD, and explain the investigations used to measure autonomic function in both clinical and research settings. The clinical implications of dysautonomia in PD and current, and potentially future, treatment options will be discussed.

Classification of autonomic dysfunction in parkinsonian patients

Autonomic dysfunction is due to primary (where the aetiology is not known) and secondary (where the lesion has been defined or where there are definite associations with other diseases, syndromes or medications) disorders. The primary and secondary causes of autonomic dysfunction in parkinsonian patients are listed in Table 7.1.

TABLE 7.1 Classification of autonomic disorders in the elderly

I. PRIMARY AUTONOMIC FAILURE

A) Chronic
- Pure autonomic failure
- Multiple System Atrophy
  - with parkinsonian features
  - with cerebellar and pyramidal features
  - with multiple features (combination of above)
- Parkinson's disease with autonomic failure
- Lewy body dementia

B) Acute or Subacute dysautonomias

II. SECONDARY AUTONOMIC FAILURE OR DYSFUNCTION

A) Central
- Brain tumours, especially of the third ventricle or posterior fossa
- Multiple sclerosis
- Syringobulbia

B) Spinal
- Spinal transverse myelitis
- Transverse myelitis
- Syringomyelia
- Spinal tumours

C) Peripheral
- Afferent
  - Guillain-Barré syndrome
  - tabes dorsalis
  - Holmes-Adie syndrome
- Efferent
  - diabetes mellitus
  - amyloidosis
  - surgery (such as splanchnicectomy)

II. SECONDARY AUTONOMIC FAILURE OR DYSFUNCTION (CONT.)
D) Miscellaneous
• Autoimmune and collagen disorders
• Renal failure
• Neoplasia
• Human immunodeficiency virus infection
III. DRUGS (see Table 7.2)
IV. NEURALLY MEDIATED SYNCOPE
• Vasovagal syncope
• Carotid sinus hypersensitivity
• Swallow syncope
• Situational syncope

Adapted and modified from: Mathias[86,87]

Primary autonomic disturbance

There are three primary causes of autonomic dysfunction in patients with definite extrapyramidal signs: idiopathic PD with autonomic failure, multiple system atrophy (MSA) and Lewy body dementia. It is important to distinguish between these syndromes, since treatment and prognosis differ markedly between them.

1 Idiopathic PD with autonomic failure

Symptoms of autonomic impairment are common in PD. Use of structured question-naires has demonstrated that up to 90% of PD subjects have at least one autonomic symptom, compared with 43% of age-matched controls.[3] Increased salivation, constipation and orthostatic dizziness are particularly prominent in PD.[4] High scores on autonomic symptom questionnaires do not, unfortunately, distinguish reliably between subjects with and without objective evidence of autonomic failure.[5]

When objective measures of autonomic dysfunction are utilised, abnormalities are frequently detected in PD patients. Difficulty in distinguishing idiopathic PD from other parkinsonian syndromes has, in the past, constituted a major problem in accurately defining prevalence of dysautonomia in the disease. The introduction of standardised diagnostic criteria for PD has improved diagnostic accuracy, and reports since the introduction of these guidelines continue to suggest that between 50% and 80% of subjects have objective evidence of autonomic involvement.[6,7,8] Variation in methods used to assess autonomic function may account for most of the variability in prevalence figures. Measures of parasympathetic dysfunction, such as heart rate variability, may be more sensitive than simple orthostatic blood pressure recording, and may therefore account for an apparent earlier onset of parasympathetic over sympathetic involvement in PD.[9,10]

Autonomic dysfunction in PD is associated with increasing age.[11,12] There are conflicting reports regarding the relationship of autonomic impairment with PD disease duration or motor severity.[11,13] Despite evidence in non-parkinsonian elderly people, current evidence does not support a causative association of autonomic impairment with falls in PD.[14,15]

The association of autonomic impairment with cognitive decline in PD is an area of current interest. We have recently demonstrated an association of impaired attention and visual memory with orthostatic hypotension in PD.[16] Whether this association is causative and related to episodic cerebral hypoperfusion,[17,18,19] or associative and related to distribution of Lewy body pathology, particularly neurodegenerative pathology involving the anterior cingulate gyrus, is currently unclear.[20]

2 Multiple system atrophy (MSA)

A syndrome of chronic autonomic failure associated with the parkinsonian features of rigidity, tremor and akinesia was first described by Shy and Drager in 1960.[21] There are three major clinical groups within the definition of multiple system atrophy (MSA):

a. *Parkinsonian form* – 20% of cases. Extrapyramidal features with autonomic failure. May indicate striatonigral degeneration.

b. *Cerebellar form* – 20% of cases. Cerebellar and/or pyramidal features. Pathology indicates olivopontocerebellar atrophy/degeneration.

c. *Multiple form* – 60% of cases. Combination of parkinsonian and cerebellar or pyramidal features. Multiple neuronal system degeneration.

MSA is difficult to distinguish from PD: between 7% and 22% of patients considered to have PD in life have neuropathological features of MSA on post-mortem studies.[22]

In general, early and profoundly symptomatic autonomic involvement suggests a diagnosis of MSA rather than PD. A relatively symmetrical extrapyramidal presentation, rapid disease progression, early-onset rapid eye movement sleep behaviour disorder, sleep apnoea, involuntary day-time sighing, characteristic hypophonic but strained speech and a poor response to dopaminergic therapy are also helpful diagnostic features of MSA.[23]

Differentiating MSA from PD with autonomic involvement is important, as the prognosis for each of these conditions is very different. Patients with MSA have a median life expectancy of only 6.8 years from diagnosis.[24] Clinical features continue at present to be the principle factors upon which the diagnosis of MSA versus PD is based, but characteristic MRI appearances,[25] cardiac MIBG scintigraphy[24] and sphincter EMG abnormalities[26,27] are also useful additional features.

3 Dementia with Lewy bodies (DLB)

This clinical syndrome was originally described by the Newcastle group in 1989:[28] it accounts for 5–10% of patients in PD brain banks[29] and 12–27% of dementia in the elderly.[30]

Guidelines for clinical and pathological diagnosis were published in 1996[30] and have been found to be specific but not particularly sensitive for detecting DLB on clinical grounds.[31] The majority of patients have a dominant syndrome of cognitive impairment frequently characterised by fluctuations in cognitive performance, episodic confusion, visual and – less often – auditory hallucinations and delusions. The extrapyramidal features tend to be mild and occur late although they are usually levodopa responsive. Less often patients present with classical levodopa-responsive PD often followed by early development of dementia. Other features are unexplained falls, early gait impairment, myoclonus, weight loss, REM sleep disorders, supranuclear gaze palsy and marked sensitivity to neuroleptics.

Pathologically widespread Lewy bodies are seen in the brainstem and other cortical areas. Diffuse amyloid plaques are found in two-thirds of cases, while neurofibrillary tangles are seen less often.

Dysautonomia is common in DLB, with carotid sinus hypersensitivity, orthostatic hypotension or vasovagal syncope demonstrable in 77% of patients.[32] Overall patients with LBD have a sixfold higher prevalence of neurocardiovascular instability than the normal elderly population. As with the dysautonomia associated with PD, it is currently unclear whether this neurocardiovascular instability represents a cause or a consequence of the neurodegenerative process, although the association of MRI deep white matter hyperintensities with magnitude of orthostatic blood pressure drop in DLB has been cited as supporting a causative role of dysautonomia in the dementing process.[33]

Secondary causes of autonomic failure

Antiparkinsonian medications and other drugs may interfere with autonomic function (*see* Table 7.2). With the introduction of levodopa in the 1970s it became accepted clinical dogma that dopaminergic medications were *the* cause of orthostatic hypotension in PD. There is certainly evidence that levodopa,[34] or levodopa in combination with selegeline,[35] exacerbates the tendency towards orthostatic hypotension, but recent investigators have demonstrated that disease duration, severity and patient age are more important factors in the development of autonomic dysfunction than the dose of levodopa given.[36]

TABLE 7.2 Drugs, chemicals and toxins that cause or exacerbate autonomic symptoms in Parkinson's disease

I. DECREASING SYMPATHETIC ACTIVITY
Centrally acting
• Clonidine
• Methyldopa
• Reserpine
• Barbiturates
• Anaesthetics
Peripherally acting
• Sympathetic neuron (guanethidine, bethanidine)
• α-Adrenoceptor blockade (phenoxybenzamine, prazosin)
• β-Adrenoceptor blockade (propranolol, timolol)

II. INCREASING SYMPATHETIC ACTIVITY

- Amphetamines
- Releasing norepinephrine (tyramine)
- Uptake blockers (imipramine)
- Monoamine oxidase inhibitors (trancypromine)
- β-Adrenoceptor stimulants (isoproterenol)

III. DECREASING PARASYMPATHETIC ACTIVITY

- Antidepressants (imipramine)
- Tranquilisers (phenothiazines)
- Antidysrhythmics (disopyramide)
- Anticholinergics (atropine, probanthine)
- Toxins (botulinum)

IV. INCREASING PARASYMPATHETIC ACTIVITY

- Cholinomimetics (carbachol, bethanechol, pilocarpine, mushroom poisoning)
- Anticholinesterases
  - Reversible carbonate inhibitors (pyridostigmine, neostigmine)
  - Organophosphorus inhibitors (parathion)

V. MISCELLANEOUS

- Alcohol, thiamine (vitamin B$_1$) deficiency
- Vincristine
- Perhexilene maleate
- Thallium, arsenic, mercury
- Cyclosporin

Adapted from: Mathias[86,87]

Autonomic dysfunction in parkinsonian patients may also result from an associated disorder known to cause autonomic neuropathy, e.g. amyloidosis, diabetes mellitus (*see* Table 7.1).

A careful assessment for secondary causes is an important component of the investigation and management of parkinsonian patients with autonomic symptoms.

Features of autonomic dysfunction in PD

Autonomic symptoms are very common in PD[3,37] (*see* Table 7.3).

Cardiovascular features

Orthostatic hypotension (OH) is a cardinal feature of autonomic dysfunction. Symptoms may be non-specific with generalised weakness and lethargy. Dizziness, syncope and falls may result from cerebral ischaemia. Between 10% and 58% of patients with PD have OH.[7,8] Dizziness is a more common symptom in those with OH than in those without OH, but as an isolated symptom it lacks the necessary sensitivity or specificity to reliably distinguish subjects with and without objective evidence of dysautonomia.[5] The characteristic 'coat-hanger' ache is a common symptom,[38] whilst chest discomfort, spinal cord ischaemia and calf claudication may also occur.

Whilst falls are frequent in PD, motor disability and postural instability seem to be more important direct risk factors for falls than orthostatic hypotension or other cardiovascular factors.[15,39]

TABLE 7.3 Reported frequency of autonomic symptoms and signs in patients with Parkinson's disease derived from two studies (n= 178)

Symptoms	% of frequency
Orthostatic hypotension	21–58
Urgency	14– 5
Urinary incontinence	2
Sialorrea	55
Dysphagia	9–22
Constipation	43–72
Seborrhea	61
Sweating	13
Heat/cold intolerance	22
Impotence	20–60

From: Martignoni et al.[37] and Singer et al.[3]

Gastrointestinal features

Sialorrhea and dysphagia, although common in late PD, are not regarded as features of true autonomic dysfunction but rather a manifestation of hypokinesia with resultant poverty of automatic swallowing. Both symptoms respond to dopaminergic therapy.

Constipation is seen in 61–73% of patients compared with 28% of age-matched controls.[40] In 46% of patients, constipation predates the first motor manifestations. Constipation may be associated with megacolon,[41] pseudo-obstruction or volvulus.

Constipation in PD is probably multifactorial in origin; decreased motor activity, poor oral food and fluid intake and anticholinergic medications all contribute to the problem, but slowing of intestinal motility secondary to degeneration of parasympathetic nerves in the vagal nucleus, myenteric plexus and submucosal plexus of the gastrointestinal tract is likely to be the principle factor underlying prolonged colonic transit time.[42,43]

Dysynergy of the anal sphincter at defecation may also contribute to constipation in PD. Several authors have described paradoxical contraction of the voluntary sphincters during defecation leading to marked difficulties with rectal evacuation.[44] A dystonic phenomenon, sometimes responsive to dopaminergic medication, has been proposed to explain this finding.[45]

The relative importance of sphincter dysynergy over generalised delayed colonic transit time in the pathogenesis of constipation in PD is currently unclear.[46]

Genitourinary features

Function of the urinary tract is often impaired in MSA at an early stage. This is caused by a combination of detrusor hyperreflexia and sphincter denervation/reinervation leading to urgency, frequency, incontinence and difficulty initiating voiding. Sphincteric denervation is caused by progressive cell loss in the motor nuclei of the striated sphincters in segments S2–S4 of the spinal cord.[47]

Isolated detrusor hyperreflexia is more common in PD than in MSA.[27] This may be exacerbated by dopaminergic medication[48] and can be treated with anticholinergic medication. In older patients, other factors, including prostatic hypertrophy in the male, and pelvic floor dysfunction in the female, are often initially and erroneously considered to cause urinary urgency and frequency.

Erectile and ejaculatory failure occur in 20–60% of patients with PD.[3] Psychogenic and other factors may contribute to the problem.

Thermoregulatory disturbance

Whilst hyperhidrosis or excessive sweating is frequently cited as a feature of autonomic disturbance in PD, it is related to 'off' periods with tremor and is felt by many authors to represent an appropriate thermoregulatory response to increased muscle activity. Patients with true autonomic failure exhibit hypohidrosis and anhidrosis with defective temperature regulation.[49]

Investigation of autonomic function

Tables 7.4 and 7.5 indicate the battery of tests which may be performed to investigate the patient with autonomic failure. In practice, extensive testing will only be required in a few patients: most of the tests necessary to confirm autonomic dysfunction are non-invasive and relatively simple to carry out. We will discuss those tests most frequently used, with particular note of the effects of ageing upon them, and then discuss those of particular relevance to current research into the pathophysiology underlying autonomic dysfunction in PD.

Postural challenge testing: active stand and head-up tilt

Orthostatic hypotension is defined as a 20 mm Hg fall in systolic blood pressure or to less than 90 mm Hg on standing for three minutes.[50] A two-minute stand is adequate to demonstrate reproducible OH in elderly subjects. Some definitions of OH have included a 10 mm Hg fall in diastolic blood pressure in the diagnostic criteria. In practice there is no correlation between diastolic pressure drops and orthostatic symptoms; the principle focus therefore remains systolic blood pressure change.

Whilst manual blood pressure measurement may be a useful screening test in a busy clinic, phasic beat-to-beat blood pressure recording using digital photoplethysmography (Portapres©) is more accurate in detecting transient but symptomatic orthostatic change. Care must be taken to ensure that the arm (sphygmomanometer) or hand (Portapres©) is maintained at the level of the heart on standing to avoid the hydrostatic effect of a column of blood giving a falsely elevated reading.

TABLE 7.4 Investigations of autonomic dysfunction in Parkinson's disease

Cardiovascular	
Physiological	Head-up tilt; Active stand; Valsalva manoeuvre
	Pressor stimuli – isometric exercise, cold pressor, mental arithmetic
	Heart rate responses – deep breathing, hyperventilation, standing, head-up tilt, 30:15 ratio.
	Carotid sinus massage
	Liquid meal
Biochemical	Plasma noradrenaline – supine and standing; urinary catecholamines; plasma renin activity and aldosterone
Pharmacological	Noradrenaline: α-receptors, vascular
	Isoprenaline: β-receptors, vascular and cardiac
	Tyramine: pressor and noradrenaline response
	Edrophonium: noradrenaline response
	Atropine: parasympathetic cardiac blockade
Sweating	Central regulation – increase of core temperature by 1° C
	Sweat gland response – intradermal acetylcholine, quantitative sudomotor axon reflex test (Q-SART), spot test
Gastrointestinal	Barium studies, video cinefluoroscopy, endoscopy, gastric emptying studies
Renal function	Day and night urine volumes, sodium and potassium excretion
Urinary tract	Urodynamic studies, intravenous urography, ultrasound examination, sphincter electromyography
Sexual function	Penile plethysmography
	Intracavernosal papaverine
Respiratory	Laryngoscopy
	Sleep studies to assess apnea/oxygen desaturation
Eye	Schirmer's test
	Pupil function – pharmacological and physiological

Source: Adapted from Mathias and Bannister[88]

Orthostatic blood pressure changes are not always reproducible. The effect of recumbent posture on the renin–angiotensin system and atrial natriuretic peptide levels, with resultant decrease in plasma volume, results in a higher level of reproducibility of OH with repeated morning recordings. Postprandial hypotension may coexist with OH[51] thus measurements taken between 30 and 90 minutes after a meal or glucose load may also have a higher diagnostic yield. Measurements are more likely to be reproducible in patients with abnormal autonomic function.[52]

Failure of the heart rate to rise in the presence of a substantial fall in blood pressure is indicative of a baroreflex abnormality, as in sympathetic or parasympathetic failure.

TABLE 7.5 Cardiovascular autonomic function tests: age-related normal values

	Normal values (age < 65 years)	Normal values (age > 65 years)
Tests of parasympathetic function		
Valsalva ratio		
(ratio of longest R-R interval within 20 beats after the manoeuvre and shortest R-R interval during the manoeuvre)	>1.10	>1.12
30:15 ratio		
(heart rate variability following standing)	>1.00	>1.06
Heart rate variability with deep breathing		
(5 seconds inspiration, 5 seconds expiration: difference between mean maximum and minimum heart rates over 6 cycles)	> 10 beats per minute	>1 beats per minute
Tests of sympathetic function		
Cold Pressor Test		
(DBP rise following contact with ice)	>10 mm Hg rise	>4 mm Hg rise
Phase 4 Valsalva SBP overshoot		>5 mmHg
Systolic blood pressure response to standing	>20 mm Hg fall	>20 mm Hg fall

Source: Ewing and Clarke[53]

Cardiovascular autonomic function test battery[53]

Resting heart rate is determined mainly by vagal tone which decreases on standing with consequent increase in the heart rate of 11–29 beats per minute. There is a biphasic response with maximum heart rate reached at around the 15th beat after standing, slowing to a relatively stable rate around the 30th beat. A comparison of the R-R intervals measured at these times yields the 30:15 ratio. A reduction in 30:15 ratio is indicative of parasympathetic dysfunction. The integrity of vagal outflow is further assessed by the variability of the heart rate to deep breathing.

Placing one hand in ice water, mental stress (e.g. serial 7 test) and isometric exercise such as sustained handgrip, result in increased systemic blood pressure. The afferent pathways involved in these stresses (pain, central command, muscle receptors) are distinct from the afferent pathways of the arterial baroreflex. In subjects with evidence of disturbances in control of systemic blood pressure during orthostatic stress or Valsalva straining, a rise suggests that efferent sympathetic pathways are functioning.

The cold pressor test is most easy to apply to elderly subjects. Subjects are rested in the semi-recumbent position. Responses are measured before and during immersion of one hand in ice water for one minute. The changes in blood pressure during the last 10 seconds of the test are compared with baseline values. A blood pressure rise of 10–15 mm Hg in systolic blood pressure and of 10 mm Hg in diastolic blood pressure is considered to be a normal response.

The response to isometric exercise can be assessed using sustained handgrip. The maximum voluntary contraction is first determined using a handgrip dynamometer, or measuring the maximum pressure of mercury attained when squeezing the bulb of a sphygmomanometer. Handgrip is then maintained at 30% of that maximum for as long as possible, up to five minutes. Blood pressure is measured three times before and at one-minute intervals during handgrip. The result is expressed as the difference between the highest diastolic blood pressure during the handgrip exercise and the mean of the three resting diastolic blood pressure readings. A rise in diastolic blood pressure of less than 10 mm Hg is regarded as abnormal.

The Valsalva manoeuvre tests the integrity of the entire baroreflex pathway. The heart rate is recorded with an electrocardiogram at the bedside as the patient breathes forcibly into a mercury manometer, sufficient to elevate the column to 40 mm Hg for 10–15 seconds. This allows the ratio of the longest R-R interval during the manoeuvre to the shortest R-R interval after the manoeuvre to be calculated.

There is an age-related decline in the heart rate and blood pressure variability as measured with this test battery.[54,55] We have defined 'age-related' normal values for subjects over 65 years, taking a normal range as within two standard deviations of the mean for healthy elderly controls. These values are listed in Table 7.5.

The American Diabetic Association requires the presence of only one abnormal value on two occasions to diagnose autonomic dysfunction.[56] The high, but unexplained, number of abnormal tests in asymptomatic healthy elderly volunteers has led us to use more stringent criteria for those over 65, requiring three or more abnormal tests before a diagnosis of autonomic failure is made.

In a recent series in our unit, 78% of patients with PD and OH had autonomic failure using age-related parameters of cardiovascular control.[57] Despite making allowances for age, practical problems can cause difficulties in interpretation of cardiovascular autonomic function tests in parkinsonian patients. Bradykinetic subjects may take longer to stand, complicating interpretation of the 30:15 ratio, and standardisation of depth of breathing and Valsalva effort can be difficult in frail individuals.

Biochemical and pharmacological techniques

Biochemical and pharmacological investigations are sometimes used in researching dysautonomia in PD, but are rarely required in the clinical setting. Resting values of blood pressure, heart rate and plasma noradrenaline and adrenaline are normal in both lying and standing position in newly diagnosed untreated patients with PD. Subjects with PD and OH have reduced baseline plasma noradrenaline levels with supersensitivity to exogenous noradrenaline and up regulation of peripheral alpha receptors,[58] suggesting that post-synaptic sympathetic dysfunction develops during the course of the disease. The reduction in yohimbine- (pre-synaptic alpha-2 antagonist) induced noradrenaline release in patients with PD and OH compared with that in those without OH and in controls supports this view.[59]

The growth hormone (GH) response to the central alpha agonist clonidine attracted attention in the early 1990s as a possible tool to distinguish MSA from

PD. Normal subjects show an 8–10 mU/l rise in GH following a 2 mcg/kg dose of intravenous clonidine.[60] In subjects with multiple system atrophy and central autonomic failure, this response is lost.[61] Early reports suggested that the response is preserved in idiopathic PD,[62] but subsequent investigations have demonstrated that whilst this test shows 100% sensitivity for MSA the response in PD is more variable, making this insufficiently specific as a tool to distinguish PD from MSA.[63]

Neurophysiology

In MSA degeneration of sacral anterior horn cells in Onuf's nucleus results in denervation and reinervation of the urethral and anal sphincters with characteristic resultant EMG changes.[64] In PD sphincter EMG is usually normal in the early stages of the disease, but neurogenic change can occur and thereby reduce the specificity of the test as a means of distinguishing PD from MSA.[27,65] In addition, the invasive nature of this test limits its use in clinical practice.

Imaging

Neuroimaging techniques can be useful in helping to distinguish between PD with autonomic features and MSA, but such techniques do not objectively quantify or explain the nature of any autonomic disturbance.

Characteristic changes in the pons can sometimes be seen in MSA with magnetic resonance imaging[25] whilst positron emission tomography (PET) has shown some promise in helping distinguish MSA from PD but is still primarily a research tool.[66,67]

Cardiac radiolabelled metaiadobenzylguanidine (^{123}I-MIBG) scanning has recently been shown to be a relatively non-invasive investigation which may help distinguish PD from MSA. This analogue of norepinephrine is taken up by functioning postganglionic sympathetic neurons. Uptake is markedly reduced in patients with PD but normal in MSA.[68,69] Whilst the test has a high sensitivity for PD, the specificity is limited in the early stages of the disease.[70]

Management of symptomatic autonomic dysfunction
Orthostatic hypotension

Orthostatic hypotension is probably the most common and disruptive symptom of autonomic dysfunction in the parkinsonian patient. Although impressive falls in blood pressure may be recorded during autonomic assessment, currently the treatment of orthostatic hypotension is not thought necessary unless the patient is symptomatic. If a relationship between repeated hypotensive insults and cognitive decline is confirmed, the approach to asymptomatic OH may change.

Initial treatment of OH is non-pharmacological: 'conservative' advice to avoid sudden postural change; the wearing of elastic stockings, and elevation of the head of the bed at night, can be surprisingly effective (see Table 7.6). The patient's medication chart should be reviewed carefully and medications which exacerbate a hypotensive tendency should be withdrawn if possible.

TABLE 7.6 'Conservative' methods for the control of orthostatic hypotension in parkinsonian patients

Method	Comment
Avoidance of sudden head-up positional change, and straining at stool	Most likely to be effective in the morning following nocturnal polyuria
Avoidance of large meals and alcohol	Postprandial hypotension may aggravate problems. Alcohol vasodilates
Adequate fluid and salt intake	Maintenance of plasma volume
Avoidance of excessive heat	Loss of intravascular volume and cutaneous vasodilatation
Elevation of bed-head 20–30 degrees at night	Reduces salt and water loss, via reduced renal arterial pressure and increased renin
Elastic stockings, abdominal binders	Attempt to reduce venous pooling. Many patients find them uncomfortable
Awareness of vasoactive/hypotensive drug side effects when prescribing	Even minor changes of an agent may cause major changes via supersensitivity. The combination of levodopa with selegiline may have particularly potent hypotensive effects and should be avoided. Psychotropic drugs may also have significant cardiovascular effects

Fludrocortisone is often the initial drug of choice when treating orthostatic hypotension. It has multiple pharmacological actions, including plasma volume expansion, reducing natriuresis and sensitising remaining alpha adrenoceptors to noradrenaline. A dose of 0.1–0.2 mg is the usual starting dose. A study of six parkinsonian patients with symptomatic OH showed effective reduction in orthostatic symptoms with 0.05–0.2 mg fludrocortisone.[71] Unfortunately fludrocortisone is poorly tolerated in the long term in older patients with hypotensive disorders; up to 33% discontinue treatment within five months of commencement.[72] Supine hypertension, peripheral oedema and hypokalaemia are common side effects.

Alpha receptor agonists such as midodrine may have some role in the treatment of debilitating orthostatic hypotension.[73] Supine hypertension and peripheral vasoconstriction are particular problems in the elderly. Midodrine can be prescribed under general licence in the USA but is prescribed on a named patient basis only in the UK.

DDAVP (Desmopressin) is a synthetic antidiuretic hormone analogue, which can be given via intramuscular or intranasal routes. It acts on the renal tubules as a potent antidiuretic reducing nocturnal polyuria and thereby raising morning blood pressure. Treatment requires careful monitoring, with water intoxication and hyponatraemia a problematic side effect, especially in the elderly. A pilot trial of triglycl-lysine-vasopressin in patients with Parkinson's disease and OH resulted in a 25% increase in supine blood pressure but minimal reduction in blood pressure change during head-up tilt.[74]

Erythropoietin (EPO) is used in some centres in the USA for the treatment of symptomatic OH in PD. EPO has a direct effect on blood volume through the effects on red cell synthesis, but increase in haemoglobin binding of nitric oxide, thereby reducing its vasodilatory effect, is thought to be the principle mechanism of the pressor effect.[75] Acetylcholinesterase inhibition with pyridostigmine reduces orthostatic hypotension and symptoms of postural dizziness in a small number of patients with PD, acting potentially through augmentation of sympathetic cholinergic ganglion transmission.[76] Larger trials are needed before this could be considered for use in a clinical setting.

Recommended drug treatments in the treatment of OH are listed in Table 7.7.

TABLE 7.7 Drug treatments used in the management of orthostatic hypotension

Proposed mode of action/class	Drugs used
Sympathomimetic vasoconstrictor	
• Direct-acting	Midodrine, phenylephrine, clonidine
• Indirect acting	Tyramine with monoamine oxidase type A inhibitors (e.g. tranylcypramine)
	Pyridostigmine
Preventing vasodilatation	
• Prostaglandin synthetase inhibitors	Indomethacin, flurbiprofen
• Dopamine receptor blockade	Metoclopramide, domperidone
• Beta$_2$ adrenoceptor blockade	Propranolol
Increasing cardiac output	Pindolol, prenalterol
Reducing salt loss/blood volume expansion	Fludrocortisone, erythropoietin
Reducing nocturnal polyuria – vasopressin V$_2$ receptor agonists	Desmopressin (DDAVP)
Reducing postprandial hypotension	
• Adenosine receptor blockade	Caffeine
• Gut peptide release inhibitors	Octreotide (SMS 201-995)

Constipation

Constipation in PD will often respond to dietary and drug manipulations. Osmotic laxatives are effective at reducing colonic transit time and alleviating the symptom of constipation.[77]

Cisapride, a prokinetic agent, was effective for constipation in PD,[78] but is currently unavailable because of an associated risk of cardiac conduction defects. Alternative prokinetic agents include domperidone and the new 5-HT4 receptor agonists, tegaserod and mosapride citrate. Domperidone is an effective prokinetic agent in the upper gastrointestinal tract,[79] but has been shown to have little effect on the lower gastrointestinal slow transit times in PD. The 5-HT4 receptor agonists facilitate intestinal motility by facilitating release of acetylcholine from enteric cholinergic neurons. A small study in patients with MSA and PD has suggested a beneficial effect of mosapride on constipation.[80]

There are other potentially useful prokinetic agents, which are yet untested in PD. The prostaglandin E1 analogue misopostol increases the number of bowel movements per week in subjects with idiopathic constipation,[81] but has not yet been assessed in PD. Experimental studies have shown that neurotrophic factors may promote survival of gastrointestinal neurons and promote motility in subjects with other neurodegenerative conditions,[82] but the effect in PD is again unknown.

Anal sphincter dysynergy sometimes responds to dopaminergic medication – for example, a dose of dispersible levodopa taken just before defecation or apomorphine.[44] Botulinum toxin injection of the striated pelvic floor musculature can also be effective treatment, leading to reversible weakness of the external sphincter and improved rectal emptying.[83]

Urinary frequency, incontinence and impotence

Urinary frequency and urge incontinence can sometimes be managed with cholinergic agents such as oxybutinin or tolterodine, but some care must be taken with the prescription of such agents which may precipitate deterioration in cognitive function in some individuals.[84] Erectile dysfunction can be effectively managed with phosphodiesterase inhibitors,[85] but care must be taken in subjects with significant and symptomatic orthostatic hypotension.

Conclusions

➤ Autonomic dysfunction accounts for significant cardiovascular, gastrointestinal and genitourinary co-morbidity in PD, and may also be associated with an accelerated risk of cognitive decline.

➤ Drugs and coexistent diseases may contribute to autonomic symptoms.

➤ Numerous tests are available to investigate the presence and severity of autonomic dysfunction in parkinsonian patients. In practice, simple and non-invasive tests of cardiovascular function such as active stand, autonomic function test battery and head-up tilt are easiest to interpret and to incorporate into the PD clinic assessment. The effect of ageing upon these parameters should be carefully considered.

➤ Biochemical, pharmacological and imaging techniques are still primarily research tools.

➤ Treatment options for autonomic problems in PD have advanced in recent years. Some approaches remain experimental at present, but offer further hope for the future.

REFERENCES

1 Richardson DA, Bexton RS, Shaw FE, *et al*. Prevalence of cardioinhibitory carotid sinus hypersensitivity in patients 50 years or over presenting to the accident and emergency

department with 'unexplained' or 'recurrent' falls. *Pacing Clin Electrophysiol.* 1997; **20** (3 Pt 2): 820–3.

2 Kenny RA, Kalaria R, Ballard C. Neurocardiovascular instability in cognitive impairment and dementia. *Ann N Y Acad Sci.* 2002; **977**: 183–95.

3 Singer C, Weiner WJ, Sanchez-Ramos JR. Autonomic dysfunction in men with Parkinson's disease. *Eur Neurol.* 1992; **32**(3): 134–40.

4 Siddiqui MF, Rast S, Lynn MJ, *et al.* Autonomic dysfunction in Parkinson's disease: a comprehensive symptom survey. *Parkinsonism Relat Disord.* 2002; **8**(4): 277–84.

5 Allcock LM, Kenny RA, Burn DJ. Clinical phenotype of subjects with Parkinson's disease and orthostatic hypotension: autonomic symptom and demographic comparison. *Mov Disord.* 2006; **21**(11): 1851–5

6 Awerbuch GI, Sandyk R. Autonomic functions in the early stages of Parkinson's disease. *Int J Neurosci.* 1994; **74**(1–4): 9–16.

7 Allcock LM, Ullyart K, Kenny RA, *et al.* Frequency of orthostatic hypotension in a community based cohort of patients with Parkinson's disease. *J Neurol Neurosurg Psychiatry.* 2004; **75**(10): 1470–1.

8 Senard JM, Rai S, Lapeyre-Mestre M, *et al.* Prevalence of orthostatic hypotension in Parkinson's disease. *J Neurol Neurosurg Psychiatry.* 1997; **63**(5): 584–9.

9 Camerlingo M, Aillon C, Bottacchi E, *et al.* Parasympathetic assessment in Parkinson's disease. *Adv Neurol.* 1987; **45**: 267–9.

10 Ludin SM, Steiger UH, Ludin HP. Autonomic disturbances and cardiovascular reflexes in idiopathic Parkinson's disease. *J Neurol.* 1987; **235**(1): 10–5.

11 Reid JL, Calne DB, George CF, *et al.* Cardiovascular reflexes in Parkinsonism. *Clin Sci.* 1971; **41**(1): 63–7.

12 Martin R, Manzanares R, Molto JM, *et al.* Cardiovascular reflexes in Parkinson disease. *Ital J Neurol Sci.* 1993; **14**(6): 437–42.

13 Meco G, Pratesi L, Bonifati V. Cardiovascular reflexes and autonomic dysfunction in Parkinson's disease. *J Neurol.* 1991; **238**(4): 195–9.

14 Wood B, Walker R. Parkinson's disease: characteristics of fallers and non-fallers. *Age Ageing.* 2001; **30**(5): 423–4.

15 Gray P, Hildebrand K. Fall risk factors in Parkinson's disease. *J Neurosci Nurs.* 2000; **32**(4): 222–8.

16 Allcock LM, Tordoff S, Hildreth T, *et al.* Orthostatic hypotension in Parkinson's disease: association with cognitive decline? *Int J Geriatr Psychiatry.* 2006; **21**(8): 778–83.

17 Viramo P, Luukinen H, Koski K, *et al.* Orthostatic hypotension and cognitive decline in older people. *J Am Geriatr Soc.* 1999; **47**(5): 600–4.

18 Burton EJ, Kenny RA, O'Brien J, *et al.* White matter hyperintensities are associated with impairment of memory, attention, and global cognitive performance in older stroke patients. *Stroke.* 2004; **35**(6): 1270–5.

19 Passant U, Warkentin S, Minthon L, *et al.* Cortical blood flow during head-up postural change in subjects with orthostatic hypotension. *Clin Auton Res.* 1993; **3**(5): 311–8.

20 Matsui H, Udaka F, Miyoshi T, *et al.* Three-dimensional stereotactic surface projection study of orthostatic hypotension and brain perfusion image in Parkinson's disease. *Acta Neurol Scand.* 2005; **112**(1): 36–41.

21 Shy GM, Drager GA. A neurological syndrome associated with orthostatic hypotension: a clinical-pathologic study. *Arch Neurol.* 1960; **2**: 511–27.

22 Hughes AJ, Daniel SE, Kilford L, *et al.* Accuracy of clinical diagnosis of idiopathic Parkinson's disease: a clinico-pathological study of 100 cases. *J Neurol Neurosurg Psychiatry.* 1992; **55**(3): 181–4.

23 Quinn NP. How to diagnose multiple system atrophy. *Mov Disord.* 2005; **20** (Suppl. 12): S5–S10.

24 Ben-Shlomo Y, Wenning GK, Tison F, *et al.* Survival of patients with pathologically proven multiple system atrophy: a meta-analysis. *Neurology.* 1997; **48**(2): 384–93.

25 Kraft E, Schwarz J, Trenkwalder C, *et al*. The combination of hypointense and hyperintense signal changes on T2-weighted magnetic resonance imaging sequences: a specific marker of multiple system atrophy? *Arch Neurol.* 1999; **56**(2): 225–8.

26 Wenning GK, Kraft E, Beck R, *et al*. Cerebellar presentation of multiple system atrophy. *Mov Disord.* 1997; **12**(1): 115–7.

27 Giladi N, Simon ES, Korczyn AD, *et al*. Anal sphincter EMG does not distinguish between multiple system atrophy and Parkinson's disease. *Muscle Nerve.* 2000; **23**(5): 731–4.

28 Perry RH, Irving D, Blessed G, *et al*. Clinically and neuropathologically distinct form of dementia in the elderly. *Lancet.* 1989; **1**(8630): 166.

29 Hughes AJ, Daniel SE, Blankson S, *et al*. A clinicopathologic study of 100 cases of Parkinson's disease. *Arch Neurol.* 1993; **50**(2): 140–8.

30 McKeith IG, Galasko D, Kosaka K, *et al*. Consensus guidelines for the clinical and pathologic diagnosis of dementia with Lewy bodies (DLB): report of the consortium on DLB international workshop. *Neurology.* 1996; **47**(5): 1113–24.

31 Litvan I, Bhatia KP, Burn DJ, *et al*. Movement Disorders Society Scientific Issues Committee report: SIC Task Force appraisal of clinical diagnostic criteria for Parkinsonian disorders. *Mov Disord.* 2003; **18**(5): 467–86.

32 Ballard C, Shaw F, McKeith I, *et al*. High prevalence of neurovascular instability in neurodegenerative dementias. *Neurology.* 1998; **51**(6): 1760–2.

33 Ballard C, O'Brien J, Barber B, *et al*. Neurocardiovascular instability, hypotensive episodes and MRI lesions in neurodegenerative dementia. *Alzheimer's Reports.* 1999; **2** (Suppl. 1): 554.

34 Calne DB, Brennan J, Spiers AS, *et al*. Hypotension caused by L-dopa. *BMJ.* 1970; **1**(694): 474–5.

35 Churchyard A, Mathias CJ, Boonkongchuen P, *et al*. Autonomic effects of selegiline: possible cardiovascular toxicity in Parkinson's disease. *J Neurol Neurosurg Psychiatry.* 1997; **63**(2): 228–34.

36 Orskov L, Jakobsen J, Dupont E, *et al*. Autonomic function in parkinsonian patients relates to duration of disease. *Neurology.* 1987; **37**(7): 1173–8.

37 Martignoni E, Pacchetti C, Godi L, *et al*. Autonomic disorders in Parkinson's disease. *J Neural Transm Suppl.* 1995; **45**: 11–9.

38 Bleasdale-Barr KM, Mathias CJ. Neck and other muscle pains in autonomic failure: their association with orthostatic hypotension. *J R Soc Med.* 1998; **91**(7): 355–9.

39 Wood BH, Bilclough JA, Bowron A, *et al*. Incidence and prediction of falls in Parkinson's disease: a prospective multidisciplinary study. *J Neurol Neurosurg Psychiatry.* 2002; **72**(6): 721–5.

40 Korczyn AD. Autonomic nervous system screening in patients with early Parkinson's disease. In: Przuntek HRP, editor. *Early Diagnosis and Preventive Therapy in Parkinson's Disease.* Vienna, New York: Springer; 1989: 41–8.

41 Caplan LH, Jacobson HG, Rubinstein BM, *et al*. Megacolon and volvulus in Parkinson's disease. *Radiology.* 1965; **85**: 73–9.

42 Wakabayashi K, Takahashi H, Ohama E, *et al*. Lewy bodies in the visceral autonomic nervous system in Parkinson's disease. *Adv Neurol.* 1993; **60**: 609–12.

43 Singaram C, Ashraf W, Gaumnitz EA, *et al*. Dopaminergic defect of enteric nervous system in Parkinson's disease patients with chronic constipation. *Lancet.* 1995; **346**(8979): 861–4.

44 Mathers SE, Kempster PA, Law PJ, *et al*. Anal sphincter dysfunction in Parkinson's disease. *Arch Neurol.* 1989; **46**(10): 1061–4.

45 Mathers SE, Kempster PA, Swash M, *et al*. Constipation and paradoxical puborectalis contraction in anismus and Parkinson's disease: a dystonic phenomenon? *J Neurol Neurosurg Psychiatry.* 1988; **51**(12): 1503–7.

46 Jost WH, Eckardt VF. Constipation in idiopathic Parkinson's disease. *Scand J Gastroenterol.* 2003; **38**(7): 681–6.

47 Konno H, Yamamoto T, Iwasaki Y, *et al*. Shy-Drager syndrome and amyotrophic lateral sclerosis: cytoarchitectonic and morphometric studies of sacral autonomic neurons. *J Neurol Sci.* 1986; **73**(2): 193–204.

48 Uchiyama T, Sakakibara R, Hattori T, *et al*. Short-term effect of a single levodopa dose on micturition disturbance in Parkinson's disease patients with the wearing-off phenomenon. *Mov Disord*. 2003; **18**(5): 573–8.

49 De Marinis M, Stocchi F, Testa SR, *et al*. Alterations of thermoregulation in Parkinson's disease. *Funct Neurol*. 1991; **6**(3): 279–83.

50 Atkins D, Hanusa B, Sefcik T, *et al*. Syncope and orthostatic hypotension. *Am J Med*. 1991; **91**(2): 179–85.

51 Robinson BJ, Johnson RH, Lambie DG, *et al*. Autonomic responses to glucose ingestion in elderly subjects with orthostatic hypotension. *Age Ageing*. 1985; **14**(3): 168–73.

52 Ward C, Kenny RA. Reproducibility of orthostatic hypotension in symptomatic elderly. *Am J Med*. 1996; **100**(4): 418–22.

53 Ewing DJ, Clarke BF. Diagnosis and management of diabetic autonomic neuropathy. *BMJ*. (Clin Res Ed) 1982; **285**(6346): 916–8.

54 Low PA, Opfer-Gehrking TL, Proper CJ, *et al*. The effect of aging on cardiac autonomic and postganglionic sudomotor function. *Muscle Nerve*. 1990; **13**(2): 152–7.

55 Kaijser L, Sachs C. Autonomic cardiovascular responses in old age. *Clin Physiol*. 1985; **5**(4): 347–57.

56 Report and recommendations of the San Antonio conference on diabetic neuropathy. Consensus statement. *Diabetes*. 1988; **37**(7): 1000–4.

57 Allcock LM, Dey AB, Gibb I, *et al*. Neurohumoral responses to cardiovascular and pharmacological stimuli in Parkinson's disease with orthostatic hypotension and age-related orthostatic hypotension. *Age Ageing*. 1999; **28** (Suppl. 2): 106.

58 Senard JM, Valet P, Durrieu G, *et al*. Adrenergic supersensitivity in parkinsonians with orthostatic hypotension. *Eur J Clin Invest*. 1990; **20**(6): 613–9.

59 Senard JM, Rascol O, Durrieu G, *et al*. Effects of yohimbine on plasma catecholamine levels in orthostatic hypotension related to Parkinson disease or multiple system atrophy. *Clin Neuropharmacol*. 1993; **16**(1): 70–6.

60 Alba-Roth J, Losa M, Spiess Y, *et al*. Interaction of clonidine and GHRH on GH secretion in vivo and in vitro. *Clin Endocrinol*. (Oxf) 1989; **30**(5): 485–91.

61 Thomaides TN, Chaudhuri KR, Maule S, *et al*. Growth hormone response to clonidine in central and peripheral primary autonomic failure. *Lancet*. 1992; **340**(8814): 263–6.

62 Kimber JR, Watson L, Mathias CJ. Distinction of idiopathic Parkinson's disease from multiple-system atrophy by stimulation of growth-hormone release with clonidine. *Lancet*. 1997; **349**(9069): 1877–81.

63 Tranchant C, Guiraud-Chaumeil C, Echaniz-Laguna A, *et al*. Is clonidine growth hormone stimulation a good test to differentiate multiple system atrophy from idiopathic Parkinson's disease? *J Neurol*. 2000; **247**(11): 853–6.

64 Eardley I, Quinn NP, Fowler CJ, *et al*. The value of urethral sphincter electromyography in the differential diagnosis of parkinsonism. *Br J Urol*. 1989; **64**(4): 360–2.

65 Libelius R, Johansson F. Quantitative electromyography of the external anal sphincter in Parkinson's disease and multiple system atrophy. *Muscle Nerve*. 2000; **23**(8): 1250–6.

66 Burn DJ, Sawle GV, Brooks DJ. Differential diagnosis of Parkinson's disease, multiple system atrophy, and Steele-Richardson-Olszewski syndrome: discriminant analysis of striatal 18F-dopa PET data. *J Neurol Neurosurg Psychiatry*. 1994; **57**(3): 278–84.

67 Brooks DJ, Ibanez V, Sawle GV, *et al*. Differing patterns of striatal 18F-dopa uptake in Parkinson's disease, multiple system atrophy, and progressive supranuclear palsy. *Ann Neurol*. 1990; **28**(4): 547–55.

68 Iwasa K, Nakajima K, Yoshikawa H, *et al*. Decreased myocardial ^{123}I-MIBG uptake in Parkinson's disease. *Acta Neurol Scand*. 1998; **97**(5): 303–6.

69 Braune S, Reinhardt M, Bathmann J, *et al*. Impaired cardiac uptake of meta-[^{123}I] iodobenzylguanidine in Parkinson's disease with autonomic failure. *Acta Neurol Scand*. 1998; **97**(5): 307–14.

70 Nagayama H, Hamamoto M, Ueda M, *et al*. Reliability of MIBG myocardial scintigraphy in the diagnosis of Parkinson's disease. *J Neurol Neurosurg Psychiatry*. 2005; 76(2): 249–51.

71 Hoehn MM. Levodopa-induced postural hypotension: treatment with fludrocortisone. *Arch Neurol*. 1975; 32(1): 50–1.

72 Hussain RM, McIntosh SJ, Lawson J, *et al*. Fludrocortisone in the treatment of hypotensive disorders in the elderly. *Heart*. 1996; 76(6): 507–9.

73 Low PA, Gilden JL, Freeman R, *et al*. Efficacy of midodrine for neurogenic orthostatic hypotension: reply. *JAMA*. 1997; 278(5): 388.

74 Rittig S, Arentsen J, Sorensen K, *et al*. The hemodynamic effects of triglycyl-lysine-vasopressin (Glypressin) in patients with parkinsonism and orthostatic hypotension. *Mov Disord*. 1991; 6(1): 21–8.

75 Hoeldtke RD, Streeten DH. Treatment of orthostatic hypotension with erythropoietin. *N Eng J Med*. 1993; 329(9): 611–5.

76 Singer W, Opfer-Gehrking TL, McPhee BR, *et al*. Acetylcholinesterase inhibition: a novel approach in the treatment of neurogenic orthostatic hypotension. *J Neurol Neurosurg Psychiatry*. 2003; 74(9): 1294–8.

77 Eichhorn TE, Oertel WH. Macrogol 3350/electrolyte improves constipation in Parkinson's disease and multiple system atrophy. *Mov Disord*. 2001; 16(6): 1176–7.

78 Jost WH, Schimrigk K. Cisapride treatment of constipation in Parkinson's disease. *Mov Disord*. 1993; 8(3): 339–43.

79 Soykan I, Sarosiek I, Shifflett J, *et al*. Effect of chronic oral domperidone therapy on gastrointestinal symptoms and gastric emptying in patients with Parkinson's disease. *Mov Disord*. 1997; 12(6): 952–7.

80 Liu Z, Sakakibara R, Odaka T, *et al*. Mosapride citrate, a novel 5-HT4 agonist and partial 5-HT3 antagonist, ameliorates constipation in parkinsonian patients. *Mov Disord*. 2005; 20(6): 680–6.

81 Soffer EE, Metcalf A, Launspach J. Misoprostol is effective treatment for patients with severe chronic constipation. *Dig Dis Sci*. 1994; 39(5): 929–33.

82 A controlled trial of recombinant methionyl human BDNF in ALS: The BDNF Study Group (Phase III). *Neurology*. 1999; 52(7): 1427–33.

83 Albanese A, Maria G, Bentivoglio AR, *et al*. Severe constipation in Parkinson's disease relieved by botulinum toxin. *Mov Disord*. 1997; 12(5): 764–6.

84 Perry EK, Kilford L, Lees AJ, *et al*. Increased Alzheimer pathology in Parkinson's disease related to antimuscarinic drugs. *Ann Neurol*. 2003; 54(2): 235–8.

85 Zesiewicz TA, Helal M, Hauser RA. Sildenafil citrate (Viagra) for the treatment of erectile dysfunction in men with Parkinson's disease. *Mov Disord*. 2000; 15(2): 305–8.

86 Mathias CJ. Disorders of the autonomic nervous system. In: Bradley WG, Fenichel OM, Marsden CD, editors. *Neurology in Clinical Practice*. Boston: Butterworth-Heinemann; 1991: 1661–85.

87 Mathias CJ. Orthostatic hypotension: causes, mechanisms, and influencing factors. *Neurology*. 1995; 45 (4 Suppl. 5): S6–11.

88 Mathias CJ, Bannister R. Investigation of autonomic disorders. In: Bannister R, Mathias CJ, editors. *Autonomic Failure: a textbook of clinical disorders of the autonomic nervous system*. Oxford: Oxford University Press; 1992: 255–90.

8

Oral problems: speech, diet and oral care

LIZZY MARKS, KAREN HYLAND AND JANICE FISKE

UPDATED FOR SECOND EDITION BY LIZZY MARKS

Introduction

The purpose of this chapter is to highlight the importance of the roles of the speech and language therapist, dietician and dentist in the team approach to the management of the person with Parkinson's disease.

Communication problems

Clinical relevance

Speech, swallowing and drooling difficulties are responsible for some of the most embarrassing, upsetting and socially isolating effects of Parkinson's disease (PD). The first section of this chapter will address practical aspects of assessment and management of these difficulties from the speech and language therapist's viewpoint.

Incidence of communication problems and access to speech and language therapy

Logemann, et al.[1] identified that 89% of patients with PD experience voice and speech problems. These symptoms become more prevalent as the disease progresses. Speech and language therapists commonly report that people with PD tend to seek advice only when the deficits markedly interfere with everyday life. Oxtoby[2] found that 4% of people with PD are referred to a speech and language therapist. The National Institute of Health and Clinical Excellence (NICE) guidelines[3] state that speech and language therapy should be available for all people with PD and appropriate referral activated at diagnosis and at each regular review. This will be documented in the patient's notes. Speech and language therapy may involve focusing on improving vocal loudness; for example, by using the Lee Silverman Voice Treatment®[4] teaching strategies to optimise speech intelligibility and by ensuring that an effective means of communication is available throughout the disease, including the use of assistive technologies.

Features and assessment

In 1969, Darley, et al.[5] analysed the hypokinetic dysarthric speech of PD and defined it in terms of problems with respiration, phonation (voice), articulation, and prosody (the variations in rate, pitch and loudness that lend the individual their unique emphasis and interest in verbal expression).

More recently Marigliani, et al.[6] described four groups of speech deficits:
1. voice
2. fluency
3. articulation
4. language and cognition.

The characteristics of the four main groups are detailed below, and can be used to identify the predominant communication disorder as part of a functional assessment.

Voice

The main features of voice problems in PD include:
➤ reduced respiratory support for speech
➤ reduced voice volume
➤ harsh, breathy, whispery or gurgly voice quality
➤ limited or reduced ability to signal intonation
➤ disturbed resonance, often hypernasal.

Additional clinical observations include: (i) reduced attempts to communicate due to poor initiation, motivation and the degree of effort required; and (ii) a lack of awareness of a soft voice.

Fluency

The main features of fluency include:
- a 'stuttering-like' speech pattern
- a large number of pauses
- the listener's impression of hurried speech
- sound, syllable or word repetitions
- initial word blocks and initiation difficulties.

Additional clinical observations of fluency are that: (i) it can result in non-functional communication; and (ii) effort, anxiety and frustration are exhibited by the patient.

Articulation

The main feature of articulation problems is:
- imprecise and inaccurate articulatory movements for intended speech.

Additional clinical observations of articulation are that: (i) it can result in non-functional communication; and (ii) the patient has poor perception of his/her own speech pattern.

Language and cognition

The main features of language and cognition include:
- a reduction in general cognitive function
- disturbed auditory comprehension
- poor topic maintenance
- reduced initiation of conversation
- inappropriate cessation of sentences
- disrupted thought sequencing, which is reflected in the content of the conversation
- limited eye contact, facial expression and body language
- decreased insight and self-monitoring skills
- an increased dependence on the support person in conversation.

Additional clinical observations of language and cognition are that: (i) the support person reports an altered quality of conversation, and sometimes also 'personality changes'; (ii) they also report an impression of reduced motivation to converse on the part of the patient; and (iii) high levels of support person stress related to the altered conversational skills.

Assessment

The Parkinson's Disease Society publishes case history and assessment forms for use by speech and language therapists.[8] Ramig *et al.*,[4] in the *Lee Silverman Voice Treatment Guide*, provide various reproducible case history and initial assessment forms for use by a speech and language therapist trained and certified by the LSVT® Foundation. Formal dysarthria assessments available include the *Frenchay Dysarthria Assessments*

(Pamela Enderby, College Hill Press, San Diego, CA, USA, 1980), and the *Assessment of Intelligibility of Dysarthric Speech* (Yorkston and Beukleman, 1981; available from Taskmaster Ltd, Morris Road, Leicester, LE2 6BR, UK: Taskmaster@webleicester. co.uk). The coexistence of other age-related factors or medical disorders can influence assessment,[7] the ability to participate in therapy, and its outcome. Examples include reduced vision, hearing, respiratory disease and stroke.

Management of communication problems

The primary aim is to teach straightforward strategies to encourage conscious attention to speech production.[6] The speech and language therapist may start by explaining the mechanism of speech production and how it is affected by PD, using diagrams of the vocal tract. The goals will be made explicit and focus attention on a specific aspect of communication; for example, to produce a voice that is loud enough for a person to hear from a distance.

For fluency difficulties, the strategy to say 'one word at a time' can be helpful. Teaching methods of slowing down the rate of speech can help articulation difficulties. This may include 'exaggerate beginnings, middles and ends of words', or teaching pausing between words and phrases. Some patients report benefit from sucking sweets or lozenges while speaking. This may be due to an increase in conscious attention to speech, caused by the presence of an object in the mouth. However, any sweets used in this way must be sugar free, or they will jeopardise oral health.

The individual's speech and swallowing may be affected by the timings of medication. Patients may need to consider seeing people and making telephone calls when they know they will be at their best, in order to avoid fatigue and frustration.

Performing two tasks simultaneously – such as walking and speaking – may be problematic as one or both activities can become compromised. This is likely to be due to conscious attention being directed mainly to the content of the spoken message.

Teaching the family and/or carer what is taught to the patient is central to ensuring improved carry-over of the strategy provided in the clinical setting. The majority of patients require constant prompting and this support is crucial to the therapy outcome.

Lee Silverman Voice Treatment® programme

This treatment method was developed as it was noted that traditional speech and language therapy focusing on articulation and rate had a limited or inconsistent effect.[9] The rationale is based on there being a high incidence of disordered voice in PD, which has a major role in decreased intelligibility. Also, a problem with self-perception and monitoring leads to reduced vocal volume. In addition, it is known that intensive treatment that focuses on voice has been sucessful.[10] It uses the principles of exercise science, skill acquisition and motor learning. Its use has been supported in the NICE guidelines.[3] It has five essential treatment concepts.

1. Voice focus – the patient only has to think about use of a loud voice. This maximally impacts on other aspects of speech production. It allows maximum change with minimum cognitive effort.

2. High effort – multiple repetitions.
3. Intensive treatment – sixteen treatment sessions over a four-week period.
4. Calibration – the patient knows and accepts the amount of effort to consistently increase vocal loudness to a level that is within normal limits.
5. Quantification – measurements of duration, volume and fundamental frequency are taken throughout each treatment session.

The idea of 'calibration' is embedded in each treatment session. The patient recognises the need for increased loudness. Then he or she is convinced that louder voice is normal and that it has a positive impact on daily communicaton. Next, he or she becomes comfortable with using a louder voice. The clinician works to build daily increments of calibration via a hierarchy of tasks, carry-over exercises and homework. Ramig *et al.* demonstrate that 90% of patients improve from pre- to post-treatment and approximately 80% of patients maintain these improvements for up to two years after treatment. The patient can purchase a DVD or video to use at home during and after treatment to facilitate homework and continue to maintain the benefits of treatment after it has drawn to an end. The treatment is delivered by a clinician trained and certified by the LSVT® Foundation. Courses are run annually in the UK and can be found via the webiste www.lsvt.org.

Augmentative and alternative communication systems

Some individuals may benefit from equipment to facilitate their speech and writing. Such equipment can be costly, and patients' needs also change over time.[8] A speech and language therapist can offer advice on where to go for assessment, advice and funding or loaning of equipment, as well as the appropriate support to use the aid.

Commonly used aids include the following.

➤ An alphabet or communication board to clarify words or specific letters. This can be provided by the therapist and made in conjunction with the patient and their family and/or carers, tailored to the individual's needs.

➤ A portable computer with speech output. For example, the Lightwriter SL35 has optional features of a 'keyguard' for those with tremor and a portable printer (*see* Figure 8.1). For further information, contact Toby Churchill Ltd, 20 Panton Street, Cambridge, CB2 1HP (Tel: 01223 576117). www.toby-churchill.com

➤ A voice amplifier for use in conversations and on the telephone. For further information, see suppliers such as Kapitex Healthcare Ltd, Kapitex House, 1 Sandbeck Way, Wetherby, West Yorkshire, LS22 7GH (Tel: 01937 580796). www.kapitex.com

➤ A pacing board may be used to assist people with dysfluent speech to break the message into smaller units. This is a rectangular wooden block, measuring approximately 35 cm by 9 cm, which is divided into five equal blocks. The individual points to each section in turn while speaking, so as to break the phrase down into manageable units.

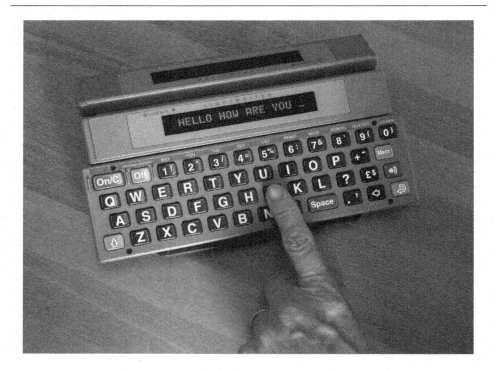

FIGURE 8.1 'Lightwriter' communication aid with speech synthesis.

Swallowing problems

The following section focuses on the practical issues relating to the investigation and management of swallowing disorders in PD. NICE guidelines[3] highlight the importance of referring to a speech and language therapist for 'review and management to support the safety and efficiency of swallowing and to minimise the risk of aspiration'.

Clinical relevance

Research shows that up to 94% of people with PD experience a degree of dysphagia.[11] Swallowing problems in PD may result in the following:

➤ weight loss and malnutrition
➤ dehydration
➤ aspiration pneumonia and bronchopneumonia, which is a common cause of death in PD
➤ high levels of anxiety during each meal for both the patient and carer
➤ disturbed intake of medication(s)
➤ reduced social contact.

Additional complications in managing the patient may be that: (i) the presence of dysphagia is not always apparent to either the person with PD, the caregiver or the team; and (ii) aspiration may be silent, with no obvious signs of coughing or choking after swallowing.[6] Thus, the speech and language therapist's detailed evaluation is an important element of the team's assessment.

Assessment

Assessment of the three phases of the swallowing process (oral, pharyngeal and oesophageal) needs to be tailored to the individual's needs. Among the various methods of investigation that may be used, the following merit discussion.

Detailed case history

A detailed case history is normally obtained from the patient and/or the caregiver by the speech and language therapist. In 1965, Eadie and Tyrer[12] identified that only 2% of patients reported dysphagic problems, even though specific questioning revealed that 50% of them experienced dysphagic symptoms. Therefore, it is important to ask the right questions to elicit information regarding oro–motor and associated features.

Oro-motor features[3]

These include:

➤ drooling of saliva; this may occur when the person opens their mouth to eat or drink, or it may be constant
➤ difficulty swallowing tablets or capsules due to reduced tongue control, which leads to difficulty manipulating and clearing tablets from the mouth
➤ a 'gurgly' voice quality; this is the strongest indicator of risk of aspiration
➤ coughing before, during or after swallowing
➤ 'choking' episodes
➤ 'discomfort' or 'sticking' with swallowing
➤ regurgitation of food via the nose
➤ oesophageal reflux; if present, this may lead to increased pharyngeal secretions and hence aspiration.

Associated features

These include:

➤ an increased time taken to complete a meal
➤ nocturnal coughing or choking; this is indicative of difficulty in managing saliva
➤ an ability to self-feed; a note should be made of how much assistance is needed, and when
➤ whether the patient prefers to eat and drink during the 'on' (active) or 'off' (inactive) phase of fluctuating parkinsonian symptoms
➤ whether there is any weight loss
➤ whether the food needs to be cut up into smaller pieces
➤ a 'fear' of swallowing
➤ a reduced appetite; this may be exacerbated by reduced oesophageal motility
➤ a history of chest infections.

Observation of eating/drinking

Observation should be made of eating habits, especially meal duration. If the patient is taking more than 45 minutes to complete his/her meal due to fatigue, the food may become unappetising when cold. The presence of drooling should also be noted.

Prepharyngeal symptoms

Symptoms to be identified include:
- impaired head and neck posture
- upper limb dysmotility
- jaw rigidity
- impulsive feeding behaviour
- impaired amount regulation
- fatigue.

Oral features

These include tongue tremor, repetitive 'tongue pumping', reduced bolus formation or control and an increased time being taken for manipulation of the food bolus in the mouth.

Pharyngeal features

These include difficulty initiating the swallow reflex, delay in triggering of the swallow reflex, and pooling in the pyriform sinuses or valleculae. If pills are retained here, delivery of medications may be erratic.

Laryngeal features

These include reduction in laryngeal closure and laryngeal elevation, as well as reduced or slow epiglottal lowering. Penetration and/or aspiration (sometimes silent) is indicated by voice change or coughing, which may occur a number of minutes after swallowing.

Videofluoroscopy

A modified barium videofluoroscopy might be performed: first, to identify the specific areas of breakdown in the swallowing process; second, to try out rehabilitation strategies; and third, to demonstrate the effectiveness of these techniques. All patients must undertake a 'bedside or clinical' evaluation before a videofluoroscopy is performed. There are several points to consider before performing a videofluoroscopy.[13]
- It involves transport and/or porters to arrive at the videofluoroscopy suite, and therefore also the potential for waiting and fatigue.
- It takes place in an unfamiliar setting; these artificial conditions are unlike any other 'meal'.
- Do you want to assess the patient while 'on' or 'off', or both? This can create additional stress.
- Positioning can be difficult and uncomfortable for the patient.
- The taste of barium can affect the swallow.

➤ It is not representative of an entire meal.
➤ The duration of exposure to radiation may be several minutes.
➤ The total time needed for the investigation can be extensive. It can can take about two hours to set up and perform the videofluoroscopy, analyse the video, write the report, and then inform the patient and team of the results and recommendations.
➤ The cost of an investigation that potentially involves many professionals may be high.

Videofluoroscopy can be helpful in some instances, particularly for research purposes. However, it only offers a 'snapshot' in time and the patient may be more likely to aspirate due to the stress of the situation, which may switch them 'off' as they walk into the room, and so the results are not representative of their abilities.

Fibre-optic endoscopic evaluation of swallowing (FEES)

This may be carried out jointly by a speech and language therapist and an ear, nose and throat surgeon, either in the out-patient department or at the bedside. Use of the technique has been clearly described.[14] A nasoendoscope is passed through the nose and down into the pharynx, to hover above the larynx. This permits a direct view of the larynx and pharynx while the patient is swallowing food and drink. Penetration and aspiration of the food or drink through the vocal cords can be observed, and any pooling or residue above the cords is commented on, as this may lead to potential aspiration. FEES also permits the identification of any defects in the larynx, pooling of saliva in the hypopharynx, and any mass lesions that may be causing obstruction. The technique is not appropriate for people with dyskinesia, due to the delicate nature of the nasoendoscope's fibres.

Cervical auscultation

This non-invasive, highly portable, low-cost technique uses a stethoscope held against the neck at the junction of the cricoid cartilage and the trachea, to help detect aspiration for the occurrence of the breath and the swallow sounds before and after swallowing, by listening. Bosma[15] described the signals from the normal swallow as being associated with two discrete and perceptually distinct sounds – the 'Initial Discrete Sound' and the 'Final Discrete Sound'. Abnormal sounds would be:
➤ change in respiratory rate
➤ no/delayed/weak expiratory puff
➤ no/early apnoea
➤ no swallow sounds
➤ only one 'click' or 'burst'
➤ indistinct sound
➤ sound out of place.

Many other investigators have explored this approach.[17,18,19] The technique requires training, and is an adjunct to the speech and language therapist's assessment.

Pulse oximetry

The oxygen saturation of the bloodstream is measured with a probe attached to the patient's fingertip. Measurements can be taken before, during and after swallowing. If aspiration is occurring, the respiratory rate will increase and the percentage of oxygen in the blood will fall.[20]

This technique is particularly helpful in a ward environment as an adjunct to the speech and language therapist's clinical evaluation, and also as a management strategy for monitoring swallowing function.

Drawing the results together

The members of the multidisciplinary team need to use one another's skills during the ongoing assessment period, and must also ensure that they share results. Next, they explain the results and their implications to the patient and his/her carer. From here, they formulate an agreed management plan with the patient and caregiver and offer consistent reinforcement of one another's advice, as well as monitoring its effectiveness.

Management

The prime considerations in the management of swallowing problems in PD are as follows.

1. Airway protection – the ability to prevent food or drink entering the trachea, as safety is a paramount consideration.
2. Nutrition – can the person consume sufficient calories?
3. Hydration – can the person take in sufficient fluid?
4. Raising the patient's and carer's awareness of their problems.
5. Management strategies to address specific problems experienced by each individual patient, e.g. difficulty swallowing pills.
6. Regular monitoring, and modifying advice as appropriate by all members of the multidisciplinary team.

Explanation of dysphagia

The starting point for management of dysphagia is an explanation of the normal swallowing mechanism, using pictures of oral, pharyngeal and oesophageal stages, and how PD affects swallowing.

Positioning and posture

The characteristic stooped posture of PD, combined with impaired lip seal and tongue movement, leads to reduced oral retention of food and saliva.[21] In more advanced disease, positioning the person upright and then maintaining this during a meal is not always easy. Speech and language therapists need to work closely with physiotherapists and occupational therapists on mealtime seating. Tilting chairs, which allow the head and neck to be maintained in an upright position, may be helpful.

Another strategy during swallowing is the chin tuck towards the chest. This widens the vallecular space and increases the chance that the bolus will hesitate in the valleculae while waiting for the swallow to be fully triggered, rather than falling into the airway. Posterior spoon placement may help to reduce oral transit times.

Consistency and temperature of food and fluids

To reduce the problem of the bolus dissipating in the oral and pharyngeal cavities, the food should be cohesive and require only two to three chews before swallowing. It is vital to consider 'lubricity' and aesthetics when helping people modify their diet. Purée is generally not recommended, as it is nutritionally less beneficial, gives insufficient sensory feedback, and is aesthetically less pleasing.

Other recommendations include avoiding mixed textures, anything with pips, seeds, bones, skin or anything that is stringy. Thickened fluids have a slower rate of flow than thin fluids; they are therefore easier to control and less likely to spill into the pharynx before triggering of the swallow reflex. Two consistencies of thickened fluids are commonly used, depending on the severity of the dyspahgia: syrup thick and custard thick. Pre-thickened fluids in these consistencies are available on prescription. Thickening powder (also available on presciption) is often more palatable in fruit juice and squash rather than in tea or plain water. A chilled bolus is found to trigger a swallow reflex more promptly as it adds stimulation to the sensory receptors in the mouth.[22]

Rate

Self-feeding – when physically feasible – is the main goal for most people, using adapted cutlery if indicated. If not allowed to self-feed, the person loses out on kinaesthetic feedback obtained when lifting the cup or spoon to the lips. Self-feeding may help initiation and rhythm, which is disrupted if fed by another person.

If the patient tends to overfill his/her mouth and tends to forget to swallow, loading the spoon and then passing it to them to feed themself is often helpful. Verbal cueing is an extremely important strategy. If there is a similar problem with drinks, verbal cues to take one small sip at a time and assisting the patient to put the glass down between mouthfuls, is of benefit. Saying, '1-2-3-SWALLOW' may assist those with problems initiating.

Having smaller portions more frequently, for example six per day, is psychologically advantageous and motivating. This is because: (i) patients feel under less pressure to finish a large portion in the same length of time, and therefore can enjoy the meal more; and (ii) they will not be left feeling hungry if they do not finish one large meal in a fixed time segment.[22]

Reflux and oesophageal dysfunction

In 1965, Eadie and Tyrer[23] found that 54% of people with PD over a two-year period reported oesophageal reflux. The irritation caused by reflux may lead to an increase in oral and pharyngeal secretions, and hence aspiration. Similarly, reduced oesophageal motility may contribute to reduced appetite. Remaining upright for 30 minutes after a meal is therefore desirable.

Medication

The timing of meals shortly after administration of levodopa/carbidopa medications may also improve swallowing and prevent aspiration.[24] Generally patients prefer to be 'on' rather than 'off', and this may be at the expense of their swallowing function, especially if they are very dyskinetic.

For difficulties with swallowing tablets, it may help to:

➤ place the tablet on the centre of the tongue
➤ reduce distractions
➤ use verbal cues, such as '1-2-3-SWALLOW'
➤ take several mouthfuls of thickened fluid to moisten the mouth and pharynx before taking the medication
➤ have medication that is dispersible or in a sugar-free elixir or as a subcutaneous injection.

Insight and cueing

The basis of self-modification is insight and the ability to self-monitor. Management needs to include carer education, as patients may not be able to modify their swallowing behaviour reliably, and may require external cueing.

This ensures that the task is given conscious attention. For example, a cue card (*see* Figure 8.2) showing the instructions can be read silently by the person with PD, or mentally rehearsed.[3] Alternatively, a carer or staff member can read the card.[6]

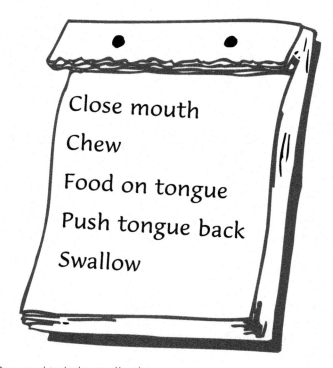

FIGURE 8.2 Cue card to help swallowing.

Difficulty managing simultaneous tasks

Meal times should be sociable, but it is also necessary to encourage the person with PD to concentrate on swallowing, when pausing between conversational turns, such as talking and listening.

Reducing environmental distractions

This is also beneficial, particularly for people with cognitive change. For example, turn off the radio or television during meals.

Weight loss

Dysphagia does not account for the weight loss completely. Jankovic *et al.*[25] stated that it may be related to hypothalamic dysfunction, though there may be other reasons. A dietician may recommend oral supplements – such as Fortifresh™, Enlive™, Ensure™, Maxijul™ – or non-oral routes such as nasogastric or gastrostomy feeding tubes.

The decision to start alternative feeding regimens must be based on a range of factors. These include the patient's and carer's wishes, documented evidence of the need for alternative feeding, and also a risk/benefit analysis (if it is recommended). Short-term feeding via a nasogatric tube may be helpful in re-establishing a drug regimen (RCP–CC guidelines). In some cases, longer-term enteral feeding via a gastrostomy may be recommended in combination with oral feeding if the individual is not meeting their nutrition and hydration needs orally, or is spending a major part of the day trying to eat and drink, and experiencing recurrent chest infections.

The timing of the introduction of this strategy needs to be discussed as a team. If the patient and carer opt for this treatment they will require counselling prior to insertion from a nutrition link nurse and/or dietician regarding management of the tube at home, as well as training to manage it confidently. A discharge planning meeting with all involved can smooth the transition from hospital to home.

Drooling

Bateson *et al.*[26] found that drooling and difficulty swallowing saliva are reported by 78% of people with PD. Drooling has been attributed to 'hypersalivation', but studies have shown that people with PD secrete similar amounts of saliva as do age-matched controls. The cause of the problem is pooling of saliva in the mouth due to reduced swallow frequency, coupled with a head-down posture and reduced oral muscular control.

Drooling is embarrassing to the individual, may result in soiling of clothes and contributes to low self-esteem. It can cause angular chelitis (sore cracks at the corners of the mouth) due to candidal infection. Oral and dental problems can exacerbate drooling and recent onset of drooling may be associated with an acute dental problem.

The NICE Guidelines[3] recommend referral to a speech and language therapist for full assessment of swallowing function. The speech and language therapist can provide advice on use of behavioural management techniques to encourage regular saliva swallows, e.g. 'swallow hard before starting to talk', lip seal and swallowing exercises. One such behaviour modification approach involves increasing the person's awareness of swallowing saliva and drooling using a combination of monitoring charts and external cueing using a portable metronomic brooch which acts as an auditory cue to swallowing.[27]

There is anecdotal evidence that some individuals find that chewing sugar-free gum or sucking on a sugar-free sweet facilitates triggering of the swallowing reflex and thus may help to assist with reducing drooling.

Other interventions include sublingual 1% atropine ophthalmic solution twice daily[28] (limited by side effects); botulinum toxin A injections into the parotid and sub-mandibular salivary gland under ultrasound control,[29] and parotid radiotherapy (unilateral or bilateral). The latter technique is not recommended as it can lead to a permanent dry mouth and all its associated problems. Additionally, irreversible damage to the blood vessels of bone in the irradiated area occurs. If, at a later date, it is necessary to extract teeth in this area, there is a major risk of osteoradionecrosis (a form of osteomyelitis).

Other useful equipment

The 'swallow reminder' brooch

This is a simple brooch-style device that 'beeps' at regular intervals to remind the user to swallow. Measuring 37 mm diameter by 22 mm thick, it is powered by a watch-style battery, and is available from Winslow, Goyt Side Road, Chesterfield, Derbyshire S40 2PH (0845 230 2777). www.winslow-cat

The Pat Saunders one-way straw

This drinking straw has a valve that prevents the liquid from falling to the bottom of the straw once it has been sucked up. It is useful in reducing fatigue and ingestion of excessive quantities of air through a straw, which causes pain and discomfort. It is available from Nottingham Rehab Supplies, Findel House, Excelsior Road, Ashby De La Zouch, Leicestershire, LE65 1NG (Tel: 0845 120 4522). www.nrs-uk.co.uk

The 'Kapi-cup'

This is a lightweight cup that is shaped to allow drinking without having to tilt the head back. The nose cut-out enables easy delivery, allowing the chin tuck position (*see* Figure 8.3). It is available from Kapitex Healthcare Ltd, Kapitex House, 1 Sandbeck Way, Wetherby, West Yorkshire, LS22 7GH (Tel: 01937 580796). www.kapitex.com

Parkinson's disease and diet

Clinical relevance

Parkinson's disease can have a major effect on food intake and nutritional status. The key issues with regard to achieving and maintaining optimal nutrition are outlined below, and appropriate remedial action described.

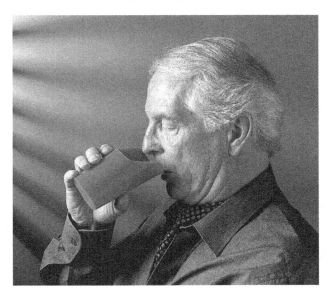

FIGURE 8.3 Use of the 'Flexicup', with chin-tuck position.

A healthy weight

In 1992, significant malnutrition was found among elderly individuals with PD,[30] while in 1995 Beyer *et al.*[31] reported that patients with PD appear to be at greater nutritional risk than a matched population. PD patients have lower body mass index (BMI), lower triceps skinfold thickness (TSF), and lower percentage ideal body-weight (IBW). The weight loss may result from reduced energy intake (*see* Table 8.1), an increased energy expenditure (*see* Table 8.2), or a combination of both factors. Research showed that under-nutrition is present in people with PD, and becomes more prevalent in the later stages of the disease.[32]

By virtue of its effect on muscular movement, PD has widespread effects on eating, swallowing and bowel function, and consequently also affects the nutritional status and oral health of the individual. Social isolation, loss of self-esteem and depression increase the risk of developing malnutrition and dental disease, especially when high-sugar snacks and drinks replace well-balanced meals.

Nutrition

The key issues in the dietary management of PD are to achieve optimal nutrition and energy balance; address swallowing difficulties in collaboration with other multidisciplinary team members; maintain good oral health, and reduce the problems of constipation. To assist patients and their carers to understand the diet-related problems associated with PD, the Dieticians in Neurological Therapy (DINT) and Nutrition Advisory Group for the Elderly (NAGE) Special Interest Groups of the British Dietetic Association have collaborated with the Parkinson's Disease Society to produce the booklet, *Parkinson's and Diet*. Effective multidisciplinary treatment with constant review of patients' needs can improve the quality of life and delay the need

TABLE 8.1 Factors affecting weight loss – reduced energy intake

- poor appetite (often associated with medication)
- sensory change (loss of food smell and taste)
- nausea/vomiting
- dysphagia
- feeling full
- poorly fitting dentures
- dementia
- depression

Physical and social factors

- difficulty in accessing food, i.e. shopping when mobility is affected
- difficulty in cooking
- difficulty in handling eating utensils
- increased length of time to eat a meal, which goes cold and becomes unappetising
- increased anxieties about eating and drinking, i.e. conveying food from the plate to the mouth, food scattering, loss of lip seal causing drooling, excess salivation, and inability to retain fluids and semi-solids in the mouth

TABLE 8.2 Factors affecting weight loss: increased energy expenditure

As a result of:

- dyskinesia (primarily associated with loss of body fat rather than muscle bulk)
- tremor
- jerky movements

TABLE 8.3 Main elements of a nutrition risk-assessment tool

- eating patterns and habits, including ethnic and cultural behaviour
- food likes and dislikes, with any known digestive problems and current appetite
- height, weight and trends in weight, i.e. loss/gain usually over the past 3–12 months
- activity (dyskinesia/akinesia) and rest patterns
- medical and physical condition
- dental and oral health
- swallowing and chewing difficulties, and mouth condition
- other risk factors and socioeconomic circumstances

for institutional care. Simple screening and assessment tools can be used to detect and quantify nutritional status and identify persons at risk of malnutrition. The information gathered is assessed against specific criteria (*see* Table 8.3), and a 'score' is calculated. This process can be part of any screening strategy used by healthcare professionals working in hospitals, out-patient departments, day hospitals and community or home settings. Such an assessment identifies people who require nutrition support, thus facilitating appropriate referrals to the multidisciplinary team. The optimal multidisciplinary team includes doctor, nurse(s), physiotherapist, occupational therapist, speech and language therapist, dietician, dentist and pharmacist, together with the support of catering services and carers who are the providers of food and nourishment.[33]

Malnutrition can occur in individuals with PD, often as a deficiency of a particular nutrient or perhaps after a period of inadequate eating due to the physical problems related to the disease. The consequences of malnutrition include depression, apathy, fatigue, weakness, anorexia and anxiety, and these can be experienced by someone whose appearance is not significantly abnormal. Weight loss with muscle wasting and a loss of subcutaneous fat are typical physical signs of malnutrition. Vulnerable individuals have an increased risk of pressure sores with the loss of lean body mass and increased immobility; there is also an increased risk of general infection due to depressed cellular immunity.

Social isolation, physical disability, lack of good dentition and reduction of mobility, as well as dysphagia, all affect food intake and can lead to malnutrition. A lack of mobility may mean that it is difficult to purchase, carry and prepare food. A restricted income with competing demands will affect the type, quantity and quality of food purchased.

Nutritional support

Most persons identified as nutritionally at risk will require an individually prescribed regime, which is regularly monitored, reviewed and communicated between the patient, carers, dietician and other healthcare professionals.

The simplest way of providing nutrition support is to encourage the person to eat more. The provision of and access to small snacks and meals is not always easy. Patients should be advised to:

➤ eat little and often – they should try to have something to eat or a nourishing drink every two to three hours
➤ have snacks between meals, such as nibbles of cheese and crackers, a sandwich, or cereal and milk.

Although dieticians recommend three to four intakes of food each day, PD patients must try to achieve three meals and three snacks per day. Suggested between-meal snacks include:

➤ full-cream milk with plain biscuits such as cream crackers, or digestives
➤ milky tea or coffee with plain biscuits (e.g. rich tea)
➤ fresh or dried fruit such as satsuma, banana, prunes or apricots, with a milky drink
➤ high-fibre breakfast cereal with full-cream milk (and fresh or dried fruit)

> cubed or grated cheese with buttered crackers
> smooth peanut butter with or without buttered crackers.

Patients who are not able to eat or drink quantities sufficient to match their identified nutritional needs require nutritional supplements. A nutritional supplement is any item given in addition to the ordinary or usual diet in order to increase energy and/or nutrient intake of an inadequately nourished person. Nutrition support can be varied and diverse, and includes:
> food enrichment
> the addition of energy, e.g. glucose polymer
> the addition of nutritional supplements, e.g. energy-dense, protein-enriched beverages and desserts
> artificial feeding, e.g. enteral nutrition, nasogastric/gastrostomy feeding for partial or total nutrition.

Enrichment of an ordinary food with another energy and/or nutrient-dense food that does not increase the volume of the meal might include:
> milk powder added to ordinary milk, and used for drinks, cereals, puddings and soups
> cream or grated cheese added to soup, potatoes, vegetables
> butter/margarine added to potatoes and vegetables.

If these feeds no longer improve the nutritional status of patients, prescription food or nutritional supplements are recommended in the short term, and diet therapy should be started. There is a wide range of nutrition support products, ranging from a 100% energy source (i.e. glucose polymer powder or syrup) to fruit juice or milk-based protein and energy-enhanced drinks with additional vitamins and minerals and milk-based desserts. The range of nutrition support products is extensive, and information on them and their use is easily obtained from dieticians.

To add variety, many of the manufacturers provide recipes and tips on use. The use of nutritional supplements needs to be monitored and is subject to regular review, particularly with regard to their impact on other food and fluid consumption, overall nutrition and dental health.

Enhancement of nutrition: supplement use
This can be achieved in several ways, including:
> sipping milk-based food-supplement drinks (rather than more acidic fruit-juice-based drinks) with food, at main meal times, or perhaps serving them frozen as 'ice-cream' dessert or sorbet
> adding Scandishake™ to full-cream milk and sipping this with meals; alternatively, it can be added to desserts such as custard, trifle, milk pudding or full-cream yoghurt
> encouraging savoury food supplements, such as Ensure™, Complan™, Buildup™, as soup with meals, or added to sauces on meat or fish dishes.

It is also possible to add cream and fats (e.g. oil, butter, margarine) to foods and drinks. Patients should also be encouraged to consume 2 litres of fluid every day.

Changes in the texture of food

The texture of food is very important to its palatability, and in general meals should consist of a variety of different textures. The texture of food needs to be modified if the person has:

➤ problems in the mouth, e.g. ill-fitting dentures
➤ problems with swallowing reflex, e.g. dysphagia.

Food textures are classified according to their ease of consumption (*see* Table 8.4).[34]

TABLE 8.4 A classification of food textures, with food examples[34]

Texture classification	Example of food
Hard	apple
Chewy	cooked meat
Soft	cake, bread/butter (no crust)
Liquid hard lump	muesli
Liquid soft lump	cornflakes and milk
Thickened soft lump	plain yoghurt and banana
Thickened hard lump	stew with chewy meat
Liquid	milk, water and orange juice
Slides down easily	butter, peanut butter, mousse

A patient with progressively worsening levels of dysphagia should be assessed for the following staged dysphagia diets:[35]

➤ a soft diet, e.g. using minced meat, flaked fish, soft fruit, vegetables and mashed potato (with food enrichment, i.e. butter/margarine, milk powder)
➤ a soft, smooth diet where food is soft and mashed, e.g. puréed meat with gravy, fish in sauce, mashed soft vegetables, soft mashed potatoes, milk pudding, fruit yoghurts (with food enrichment)
➤ a puréed diet (homogenised) where food is puréed using a blender and additional fluid is added, e.g. puréed meat, potato, vegetables and fruit, smooth yoghurt, mousse, ground rice pudding.

As the degree of restriction increases, so too does the likelihood of an inadequate intake. Puréed food becomes more dilute with added fluid, and often has a watery taste and unacceptable appearance. If a whole meal is liquidised together, the resulting mixture is often unappetising, bearing little resemblance in appearance or taste to the original, and this is not recommended. Commercial food moulds can be used to shape puréed vegetables, potatoes, meat and fish separately when being served. As the puréed diet is generally inadequate in energy (even if consumed), food and nutrition supplements are required to prevent malnutrition.

Fibre

Constipation

Many people with PD find constipation a problem, but this can be helped by: (i) increasing fluid intake; (ii) taking exercise; and (iii) increasing the intake of fibre-rich food.

Fibre works by absorbing fluid as it moves through the bowel, forming a soft stool that can be passed more easily. However, too much bulk with little fluid can increase constipation. People with PD tend to have a low fibre intake (11 grams treated; 14 grams untreated).

Increasing fibre intake

Fibre is found in cereal grains, seeds, nuts, fruit, vegetables and pulses, e.g. peas, beans and lentils. Loose bran, which can be added to food, is not recommended as it can lead to bloating and also reduces the absorption of vitamins and minerals. Increased fibre intake (>15 grams per day) should be achieved by:

➤ including high-fibre varieties of foods, e.g. wholemeal bread, whole-wheat pasta and brown rice; recipes can be adapted to use some wholemeal flour instead of all white
➤ including a breakfast cereal containing wheat, wheatbran or oats, e.g. Weetabix™, porridge or branflakes
➤ increasing the intake of all kinds of vegetables – raw/cooked, fresh/frozen; also, more peas, beans or lentils should be used
➤ increasing the intake of fruit – fresh, stewed, tinned or dried, e.g. prunes, or oranges but not bananas.

When increasing fibre intake, it is important to do so gradually in order to avoid bloating or flatulence. As a rule, one new fibre food should be introduced every three days.

Fluids

It is essential to drink plenty throughout the day, in order to help the fibre to do its work. People with PD and constipation tend to have a low fluid intake which may have preceded the motor symptoms. The aim should be to drink more than1.5 litres (8–10 cups, 6–8 mugs) every day.

Protein and lipids

High-protein meals may reduce the clinical response to levodopa because of their influence on drug absorption in the gastrointestinal mucosa. Large amounts of neutral amino acids (e.g. phenylalanine, tryptophan, tyrosine) may compete with levodopa and reducing its transfer across the blood–brain barrier. Protein may slow gastric emptying. As L-Dopa is not absorbed from the stomach, delayed gastric emptying may lead to a delayed response to medication with 'off' periods. Avoiding large protein meals and therefore decreasing neutral amino acids may improve clinical response to medication.

High-lipid meals may slow gastric emptying even more than protein. Decreasing lipid meals may promote gastric emptying and promoting absorption and improving efficacy of L-Dopa.

When symptom control on medication is not adequate, dietary manipulation is a possible option. Any dietary manipulation should be carried out under controlled conditions, since in some cases it is not in the patient's best interest to alter existing dietary patterns. Modifying lipids and protein intake could result in malnutrition, especially in older people. Healthy, motivated individuals can maintain an adequate intake of nutrients, yet modify their dietary protein and lipid intake, if they are educated, supported and advised by their state-registered dietician and PD team.

Vitamins, minerals and antioxidants

Eating a well-balanced diet will provide adequate levels of vitamins and minerals for most people. It is generally advised to increase the intake of foods containing fibre, valuable nutrients, vitamins and minerals, rather than buying expensive vitamin supplements. Some vitamins, when taken in large doses, can cause severe side effects. If a person is taking supplements with high doses of vitamin and minerals, or requires further advice on this matter generally, it is highly recommended that they see a state-registered dietician.

The production of free radicals may cause cellular damage, and is thought to play a part in the development of PD. Antioxidants, including vitamins A, C and E, can (in theory) inhibit free-radical production. Although many patients take supplementary anti-oxidants, there is no current evidence to suggest that these will alter the progression of PD. In a well-balanced diet, antioxidant intake should be adequate.

Teamwork

Comprehensive nutritional screening through referral to a multidisciplinary team will identify those individuals who require further assessment and possible nutritional support. Effective interdisciplinary working can improve nutrition. Each profession has its own knowledge base, skills and expertise, though this is not always recognised by other occupations. Working 'inter-professionally' across occupational boundaries will enable dieticians to share knowledge and experience of nutrition in PD, and also enable other team members to identify problems at an early stage.

Oral care
Clinical relevance

Parkinson's disease can have a profoundly adverse effect on oral health and oral healthcare. An understanding of the issues concerned help both the individual with PD and the dental team to work together, to minimise actual and potential oral problems. Poor oral health can endanger health, as the aspiration of saliva containing oral pathogens can cause bronchopneumonia.[36]

Access to dental services

In a review of the dental awareness and needs of PD patients, 71% of people with PD felt that dental care was extremely, or very, important.[37] The reviewers identified three major factors as barriers to obtaining dental care. The first two factors – cost and anxiety – are common to the general population. The third factor – access to dental premises – is related to the mobility problems of PD. Dental services need to take into account the current mobility of the individual and their likely mobility throughout the life of their disease process. This requires the consideration of: (i) the individual's access to the dental surgery while they remain ambulant and if they become confined to a wheelchair; (ii) the individual's best times of day for coping with dental care (often dictated by the pattern of their PD symptoms and medication); and (iii) the possible, eventual need for domiciliary (home-based) dental care.

People with PD need to be made aware of the importance of good oral healthcare as early as possible after their diagnosis. Those people who already have a general dental practitioner (GDP) should alert the dentist to their diagnosis and continue with regular dental care. People without a GDP, need to be put in contact with a dentist in the general dental service, the community dental service (CDS), or the hospital dental service, as appropriate. In the event that a local dentist cannot be found, the British Society for Disability and Oral Health (BSDH) may be able to advise.

Individuals are more amenable to dental treatment in the early stages of PD. At this point, they require the provision of high-quality, low-maintenance dental care. It is especially pertinent to put long-term preventive measures in place to minimise the need for further invasive dental treatment. It is important for the individual with PD and/or their carer to realise that the dental team understands both the process of PD and the problems associated with it; and that they are a part of their multidisciplinary care team.

Within this context, dental team members will find it particularly useful to liaise with the dietician, speech and language therapist and the PD nurse.

Communication

The progressive communication difficulties associated with PD can affect the ability to access dental services and to voice individual needs and wants.

Depression and cognitive change can further erode the individual's ability to communicate with the dental team and further affect their ability to co-operate for dental treatment.

Oral problems

The oral problems associated with PD have been described as:[33]

➤ xerostomia (dry mouth)
➤ burning mouth
➤ dental caries (decay)
➤ muscle control over dentures
➤ periodontal (gum) disease
➤ maintenance of oral hygiene.

Xerostomia

Dry mouth, due to a decreased quantity or quality (thick, ropey or frothy) of saliva, is commonly associated with PD and its associated drug treatment. Up to 55% of people with PD complain of a dry mouth. This compares with 3–5% of the total population and 20% of the elderly population.[37] Xerostomia is disadvantageous to:

➤ oral health, as it leads to an increased risk of caries, exacerbation of periodontal disease and poor denture control
➤ oral comfort, as it causes difficulty in talking, eating and swallowing, as well as burning mouth, and denture discomfort
➤ general health, due to dysphagia, reduced nutritional status and oesophageal injury from dietary acid
➤ quality of life, as a result of the combined effects of all of the above factors.

Burning mouth

Burning mouth (BM) is five times as commonly reported by people with PD (24%) than it is by the general population.[38] Within the general population, the associated continuous, burning sensation of the oral mucosa and/or tongue has been attributed to vitamin and mineral deficiencies; hormonal imbalances; xerostomia; candidal infections; denture design faults; parafunctional activity; depression and alexithymia (feelings of powerlessness to cope with circumstances or problems in dealing with feelings).[38]

In PD, BM seems to be associated with medication, depression and alexithymia. Clifford *et al.* believe that BM in PD could be particularly associated with levodopa medication which promotes parafunctional, purposeless chewing.[38] In their study, 77% of respondents and 96% of people with BM were taking levodopa and none of them had experienced BM before the onset of PD. BM is a distressing complaint, but is treatable in 70% of cases by identifying and treating the underlying cause. Where levodopa is the prime cause of BM, treatment is only possible if this medication can be changed. A high proportion of people with PD have BM that seems to go largely unreported and, consequently, untreated – possibly because people assume that it is a symptom of their condition which cannot be treated.[38] It is recommended that dentists and the multidisciplinary team enquire about BM when taking a history.

Dental caries (decay)

Elderly people with PD have been described as having significantly more teeth and less caries than a control group of corresponding age.[39] However, this statement is based on a sample of only 30 elderly, Swedish people with PD and cannot be considered representative of people with PD as a whole. Indeed, it is the author's (JF) experience and subjective opinion that elderly people with PD have an increased incidence of dental decay, particularly root caries which occur at the necks of the teeth. While tooth loss can have profound emotional effects on people,[40] for the person with PD it can also jeopardise their general health by compromising dietary selection and intake.

Aetiology of dental caries

This is determined by host factors, including susceptibility of the enamel, and also the flow rate and composition of the saliva, which has buffering, washing and remineralisation functions. Diet and plaque micro-organisms are also involved.[41] There is a direct relationship between dental caries and the intake of carbohydrates, particularly sucrose. The frequency of carbohydrate/sugar intake, rather than the amount consumed, is the important factor. The greater the number of intakes, the greater the risk of developing caries. Also, the stickiness and concentration of the sugars consumed have an influence. The main source of nutrition for oral bacteria, which adhere to the teeth as plaque, is carbohydrate in the saliva. The interaction between bacterial plaque and carbohydrate results in a fall in pH which causes demineralisation of the dental enamel and initiates the process of dental caries.

Several factors put people with PD at greater risk of developing dental caries. These include xerostomia; eating little and often; the long-term consumption of energy-enriched foods/drinks and the use of high-calorie dietary supplements to maintain body weight; dietary manipulation to increase the efficacy of levodopa as the restricted protein intake can lead to increased consumption of carbohydrate; the retention of pooled high-sugar foods and drinks in the mouth for long periods depending on the degree of dysphagia; and the difficulty of achieving good standards of daily oral hygiene.

It is important that the dietician and the dental team work together with the aim of achieving an improved nutritional intake and maintaining good oral health. Without collaboration, the dietary and dental advice given to the person with PD and their carer can be conflicting and confusing. There will be times when prioritising is necessary as part of the person's individual care plan.

Root caries

This occurs at the necks of the teeth; it can develop rapidly and is also very destructive (*see* Figure 8.4). The condition is often painless, and the first indication of its presence can be when an undermined crown of a tooth breaks off. The best treatment is to prevent it in the first place. For the person with PD, this involves advice about the following.

➤ Alleviating xerostomia by sipping water and avoiding acidic or fizzy drinks and encouraging the use of sugar-free or xylitol-containing chewing gum. Additionally, artificial saliva may be helpful for some people, particularly at meal times.[42]

➤ Ensuring measures to prevent dental disease are in place. This requires a partnership between the dental team, the person with PD and (if appropriate) their carer. The dental team can provide advice, support and the professional application of fluoride and chlorhexidine varnishes. The individual and/or the carer have to take responsibility for daily regimes such as the use of fluoride or chlorhexidine gels and tooth-brushing.

➤ Dietary guidelines which are compatible with national, nutritional guidelines for healthy eating in general and for maintaining body weight in particular. This is consistent with good oral health.

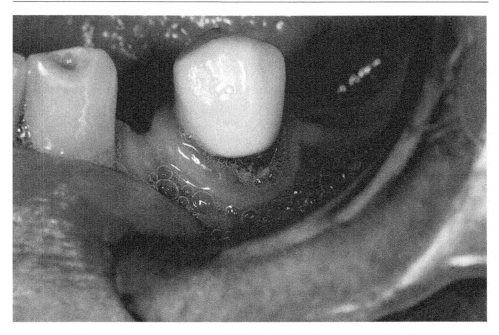

FIGURE 8.4 Root caries and associated 'frothy' saliva in a person with Parkinson's disease.

Muscle control over dentures

The success of wearing dentures depends, to a large extent, on the wearer's ability to control the dentures with their oral musculature. It also relies on the presence of an adequate amount and quality of saliva. Thick, 'ropey' or 'frothy' saliva in an abundant quantity has the same detrimental effect on denture retention as does dry mouth. The muscle inco-ordination, rigid facial muscles and xerostomia of PD conspire to jeopardise denture retention and control. This is particularly so in the case of complete upper and lower dentures and some acrylic (plastic) partial dentures. For some people this will mean they are not able to cope with dentures. Other people will require the use of a denture fixative/adhesive to increase denture retention and denture-wearing confidence.

A dentist providing a person with PD with replacement dentures would be prudent to consider using one of the copy/duplication techniques in order to retain the learned muscle control of familiar dentures. The individual should keep their old dentures since, even if these no longer fit well, they can provide the dentist with useful information which may contribute to easier adaptation to the new dentures.

Dentists planning to provide a person with PD with complete dentures for the first time might consider the use of overdentures (where strategic roots of teeth are left in the jaw bone and the denture sits over them) as they help to retain proprioception and maintain jaw control. For the person with early PD who requires dentures, consideration should be given to the possible role of dental implants or implant-retained overdentures. Although this is an expensive option, it may well be cost effective in the long term, providing the individual with security and helping to preserve their self-esteem and social contacts.

Periodontal (gum) disease

Poor oral hygiene leads to plaque accumulation. In the long term this can lead to periodontal disease, which has been categorised as:

➤ gingivitis – inflammation of the gums, giving them a red, swollen appearance and causing bleeding when they are brushed

➤ periodontitis – this develops from a pre-existing gingivitis, to destroy the supporting bone of the teeth, and leads to gum recession, loose teeth and tooth loss. Not every gingivitis develops into periodontitis.[43]

The degree of susceptibility of the individual and adequate removal of dental plaque on a daily basis are integral to the process. Xerostomia and refined carbohydrate intake contribute by reducing the capacity for oral clearance of food.

Maintenance of oral hygiene

The prevention of dental disease is the most important aspect of dental care for people with PD. Reduced muscle co-ordination, muscle rigidity and tremor mitigate against the individual's ability to achieve adequate plaque control. Maintaining independence for as long as possible is an important part of the general management of PD, and is to be encouraged in oral care wherever possible. Toothbrush handle adaptations, to improve the grip and manipulation of the brush, can help the person retain independence for teeth or denture cleaning (*see* Figure 8.5).

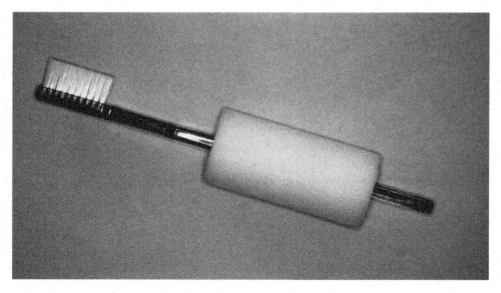

FIGURE 8.5 A small piece of polystyrene or rubber tubing can be used to improve the grip of a toothbrush handle.

An electric toothbrush can facilitate cleaning, particularly where manual dexterity is compromised. Some people find that the extra weight of an electric toothbrush helps to reduce hand and arm tremor. Dental gels, such as chlorhexidine and fluoride, and toothpastes can be used as normal. The use of mouthrinses should be avoided due to the increased risk of silent aspiration.

The recruitment of a family member or carer to supervise and provide support for daily oral hygiene measures is pertinent. If PD reaches the stage where the individual can no longer provide self-care, this person can be trained to take over the task. With advice and support from an empathetic dental team, many of the anxieties that carers experience in providing mouth care can be allayed. Finnerty, in association with the Parkinson's Disease Society of the UK, has addressed the issue of oral awareness in a useful booklet *Parkinson's and Dental Health*.[43]

Dental management

Appointments should be scheduled for the individual's best time of day. They should be as short and stress-free as possible, as anxiety and stress tend to increase tremor and dyskinesia. Asking the person to relax or to sit still is likely to increase involuntary movements, and is best avoided.

Individuals with PD should be assisted to the dental chair only as needed; however, the path to the chair should be cleared of obstacles. The person should be seated in and raised slowly from the dental chair in order to avoid problems with loss of balance or postural hypotension. On leaving the dental chair, the characteristic slow movements and shuffling gait of PD can make it difficult for the person to get moving. Reminding the person to 'take big steps' helps to initiate the walking process.

During operative dentistry, the control of the person's movements can be difficult. Jolly *et al.* advocate the use of mouth props (such as rubber bite blocks) during restorative procedures.[42] Additionally, these authors suggest that the person's head might be cradled in the operator's arm at the elbow to control head movements. This practice can help, though on occasion movements can be severe and this practice may lead to bruised ribs! Some days it may be best to abandon the treatment – which can be challenging to all concerned – in the hope that the next appointment will be on a 'less mobile' day.

While inhalational sedation using relative analgesia or intravenous sedation may help to control tremor, it may exacerbate the risk of aspiration as it depresses the (already impaired) swallow reflex. Care is required in the administration of local anaesthetic agents in order to avoid either damage to the patient or needle-stick injury to the operator as a result of random movements.

The person should not be reclined more than 45° in the dental chair because of potential difficulties such as triggering the swallow reflex and the risk of pulmonary aspiration of saliva and debris. Use of a rubber dam, with additional suction behind the dam to cope with salivary secretions, is recommended for restorative dentistry. The use of 'four-handed' (dental-nurse-assisted) dentistry and high-volume suction are advocated.

General principles for oral healthcare

The following guidelines are suggested as a way of attaining optimal oral healthcare for people with PD.

➤ Contact with a dentist as early as possible after the diagnosis of PD.

➤ Advise the person with PD of potential oral and denture problems and make available information on how to avoid or minimise these problems.

➤ Aim to maintain comfort, independence and self-esteem.

➤ Provide information and support to improve/maintain oral hygiene and oral comfort.

➤ Put rigorous preventive regimes in place.

➤ Provide high-quality, low-maintenance dental care in the early stages of the disease.

➤ Organise continuing care by arranging regular reviews at intervals tailored to meet the individual's needs.

The Parkinson's Disease Society leaflet carries the title 'Just a little more time'. This is one of the main requirements of people with PD in the dental setting. Good time management is an important feature of a successful dental practice. Sufficient time needs to be allocated for appointments to avoid the sense of rushing which will only delay communication further. The use of questions which require yes/no responses can both aid the flow of information and reduce the time taken to obtain it. The time required by some people with PD is best accommodated by the use of a salaried dental service.

Conclusions

A carefully taken case history and observation of eating and drinking are helpful forms of investigation for patients with PD. Management plans need to be formulated with the patients and carers, who benefit from awareness raising, regular support, reinforcement of strategies and monitoring, particularly within their own environments. Timely and effective intervention for swallowing disorders has the potential to reduce the occurance of aspiration pneumonia.

The dietician is the appropriate team member to assess, advise and monitor the nutritional status and dietary intake of people with PD, while the dental team advises on preventing dental disease, maintaining oral comfort and managing oral problems.

The speech and language therapist, the dietician and the dental staff are all important members of the PD multidisciplinary care team. They contribute unique and complementary aspects of care associated with PD and help to maintain the individual's self-esteem and quality of life.

REFERENCES

1 Logemann J, Fisher H, Boshes B, *et al.* Frequency and co-occurrence of vocal tract dysfunctions in the speech of a large sample of Parkinson patients. *J Speech Hearing Disord.* 1978; **42**: 47–57.

2 Oxtoby M. *Parkinson's Disease Patients and Their Social Needs.* London: Parkinson's Disease Society; 1982.

3 National Institute for Health and Clinical Excellence. *Guidelines on the Diagnosis and Management of Parkinson's Disease in Primary and Secondary Care.* NICE clinical guideline CG035. London: NICE; 2006, June. www.NICE.org.uk

4 Ramig L, Pawlas A, Countryman S. *The Lee Silverman Voice Treatment.* USA: National Center for Voice and Speech; 1995.

5 Darley F, Aronson A, Brown J. Differential diagnostic patterns of dysarthria. *J Speech Hearing Res.* 1969; **12**: 246–69.

6 Marigliani C, Gates S, Jacks D. Speech pathology and Parkinson's disease. In: Morris M, Iansek R, editors. *Parkinson's Disease: a Team Approach.* Australia: Southern Health Care Network; 1998: Chapter 7.

7 Scott S, Caird F, Williams B. *Communication in Parkinson's Disease.* London, Sydney: Croom Helm; 1985.

8 *Parkinson's and the Speech and Language Therapist.* London: The Parkinson's Disease Society, 215 Vauxhall Bridge Road, London, SW1V 1EJ, UK.

9 Green M. *The Voice and its Disorders.* London: Pitman Medical; 1980.

10 Scott S, Caird FL. Speech therapy for Parkinson's disease. *J Neurol Neurosurg Psychiatry.* 1983; **46**: 140–4.

11 Nilsson H, Ekberb O, Olsson R, *et al.* Quantitative assessment of oral and pharyngeal function in Parkinson's disease. *Dysphagia.* 1996; **11**(2): 69–70.

12 Eadie M, Tyrer J. Alimentary disorders in parkinsonism. *Austr Ann Med.* 1965; **14**: 13–22.

13 Groher M, Crary M. Glan Hafren NHS Trust. In: Dysphagia Conference; 1997 May; Cardiff: National Museum of Wales.

14 Langmore S, Schat K, Olson N. Fibreoptic endoscopic examination of swallowing safety: a new procedure. *Dysphagia.* 1988; **2**: 216–9.

15 Bosma J. Introduction to the Cervical Auscultation Workshop; 1992 April 22; Baltimore: Department of Pediatrics, University of Maryland.

16 Takahashi K, Groher M, Michi K. Methodology for detecting swallowing sounds. *Dysphagia.* 1994; **9**: 54–62.

17 Hamlet S, Penney D, Formolo J. Stethoscope acoustics and cervical auscultation of swallowing. *Dysphagia.* 1994; **9**: 63–8.

18 Chichero J, Murdoch B. The physiologic cause of swallowing sounds: answers from heart sounds and vocal tract acoustics. *Dysphagia.* 1998; **13**: 39–52.

19 Zenner P, Losinski D, Mills R. Using cervical auscultation in the clinical dysphagia examination in long-term care. *Dysphagia.* 1995; **10**: 27–31.

20 Sellars C, Dunnet C, Carter R. A preliminary comparison of videofluoroscopy of swallow and pulse oximetry in the identification of aspiration in dysphagic patients. *Dysphagia.* 1998; **13**: 82–6.

21 Scott A. The management of dysphagia in Parkinson's disease. *Austr Commun Q.* 1997; **Winter**: 30–1.

22 Groher M. *Dysphagia Diagnosis and Management,* 2nd ed. Boston: Butterworth-Heinemann; 1992.

23 Eadie M, Tyrer J. Radiological abnormalities of the upper part of the alimentary tract in parkinsonism. *Austr Ann Med.* 1965; **14**: 23–7.

24 Kirshner H. Disorders of the pharyngeal and esophageal stages of swallowing in Parkinson's disease. *Dysphagia.* 1997; **12**: 19–20.

25 Jankovic J, Wooten M, Van der Linden C, *et al*. Low body weight in Parkinson's disease. *South Med J*. 1992; **85**: 351–4.

26 Bateson M, Gibberd F, Wilson R. Salivary symptoms in Parkinson's disease. *Arch Neurol*. 1989; **39**: 1309–14.

27 Marks L, Turner K, O'Sullivan J, *et al*. Drooling in Parkinson's disease: a novel speech and language therapy treatment. *Int J Language and Communication Disord*. 2001; **36** (Suppl.): 282–7.

28 Hyson HC, Johnson AM, Jog MS. Sublingual atropine for sialorrhea secondary to parkinsonism: a pilot study. *Mov Disord*. 2002; **17**(6): 1318–20.

29 Sullivan JD, Bhatia KP, Lees AJ. Botulinum toxin A as a treatment for drooling saliva in PD. *Neurology*. 2000; **55**: 606–7.

30 Durrieu G, Llau M, Rascol D, *et al*. Parkinson's disease and weight loss: a study with anthropometric and nutritional status. *Clin Autonom Res*. 1992; **2**: 153–7.

31 Beyer PL, Palarino MY, Michalek D, *et al*. Weight change and body composition in patients with Parkinson's disease. *J Am Dietet Assoc*. 1995; **95**: 979–83.

32 Markus HS, Tomkins AM, Stern GM. Increased prevalence of undernutrition in Parkinson's disease and its relationship to clinical disease parameters. *J Neural Transm*. 1993; **5**: 117–25.

33 Hyland K, Fiske J, Mathews N. Nutritional and dental health management in Parkinson's disease. *Community Nurs*. 2000; **14**: 28–32.

34 Webb G, Copeman C. *The Nutrition of Older Adults*. London: Arnold; 1996.

35 *Staged Dysphagia Diet*. Department of Nutrition and Dietetics, North West Wales Trust. Bangor: Ysbyty Gwynedd; 1998.

36 Curtis J, Langmore S. Respiratory function and complications related to deglutition. In: Perlman A, Schulze-Delrieu K, editors. *Deglutition and its Disorders: anatomy, physiology, clinical diagnosis and management*. San Diego, CA: Singular Publishing; 1997: Chapter 4.

37 Clifford T, Finnerty J. The dental awareness and needs of a Parkinson's disease population. *Gerodontology*. 1995; **12**: 99–103.

38 Clifford TJ, Warsi MJ, Burnett CA, *et al*. Burning mouth in Parkinson's disease sufferers. *Gerodontology*. 1998; **15**: 73–8.

39 Persson M, Sterberg T, Granrus A-K, *et al*. The influence of Parkinson's disease on oral health. *Acta Odontol Scand*. 1992; **50**: 37–42.

40 Fiske J, Davis D, Frances C, *et al*. The emotional effects of tooth loss in edentulous people. *Br Dent J*. 1998; **184**: 90–3.

41 Samaranayake LP. *Essential Microbiology for Dentistry*. London: Churchill Livingstone; 1996.

42 Jolly DE, Paulson RB, Paulson GW, *et al*. Parkinson's disease: a review and recommendations for dental management. *Special Care in Dentistry*. 1989; **9**: 74–8.

43 Finnerty J. *Parkinson's and Dental Health*. Parkinson's Disease Society, code B45; 1996.

9

Sleep dysfunction in Parkinson's disease

K RAY CHAUDHURI

Introduction

The earliest description of sleep problems of Parkinson's disease (PD) dates back to the original description of PD by James Parkinson. He describes in his original monograph, *The Shaking Palsy*, a patient in whom 'his attendants observed, that of late the trembling would sometimes begin in his sleep, and increase until it awakened him: when he always was in a state of agitation and alarm'.[1] This may have been the first description of nocturnal akinesia and tremor and also, perhaps, rapid eye movement behaviour disorder (RBD) that complicate sleep of people with PD. In spite of sleep dysfunction being a key aspect of the non-motor symptom complex (NMS) of PD, it is only recently that sleep disturbances related to PD have received diagnostic and therapeutic attention, with emergence of some relevant reviews and research-based publications.[2–8] The issue of sleep dysfunction and its treatment has also become relevant as evidence suggests that sleep problems are a key determinant of quality of life of patients and effective treatment may improve overall health-related quality of life.[9,10] 'Poor nights' for people with PD may occur not only in advanced PD, but also in early untreated PD or may even precede the motor symptoms. Such morbidity may have significant adverse effects on day-time functioning and functional capacity (such as driving) of the patient, as well as on quality of life.[9–12] Certain sleep disorders may provide useful diagnostic information in differentiating between parkinsonian syndromes and may be important prognostic indicators of neuropsychiatric disturbance and dementia.[13]

Epidemiology

Sleep dysfunction in PD is multifactorial and as many as 98% of patients with PD may suffer at some time from nocturnal symptoms that can disturb their sleep.[2] Overall prevalence figures range from 25% to 98% (*see* Table 9.1). A community-based study reported 60% of patients with PD (144 of 239) with sleep problems, compared with 33% of healthy controls (33 of 100) with the same age and sex distribution,[4] while others[5] reported that 64% of patients with PD had a sleep disorder, compared with 33% of controls. More recently, the NMSQuest study in 123 PD patients across all age groups and 96 age-matched controls, using a validated non-motor symptoms questionnaire in an international multicentre setting, identified high rates for a range of sleep-related disorders.[14] While some, such as nocturia (67%) are common in controls, other complaints such as insomnia (41%), intense/vivid dreams (31%), acting out during dreams (33%), restless legs (37%) and day-time sleepiness (28%) are more prevalent in PD and may reflect more fundamental dysfunction of sleep-related mechanisms (*see* Figure 9.1). Another observational study evaluated PD patients followed for a period of 15–18 years after being recruited to a bromocriptine versus levodopa trial.[15] One-third of the original cohort were evaluated and most had significant NMS, including sleep disorders which were more troublesome and disabling than the motor symptoms or levodopa-induced dyskinesias. Despite these figures, such disorders are frequently overlooked, even in specialist centres.[16]

TABLE 9.1 Prevalence of sleep problems in Parkinson's disease

Nausieda, *et al*, 1982[32]		74%
Lees, *et al*, 1988[3]		98%
Factor, *et al*, 1990[31]		89%
Smith, *et al*, 1997[33]	M	25%
	F	41%
Tandberg, *et al*, 1998[4]		60%
Stocchi, 2001[34]		72%

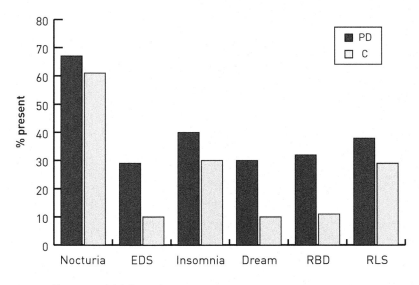

Dream = vivid dreaming
EDS = excessive day-time sleepiness
RBD = REM behaviour disorder
RLS = restless legs syndrome

FIGURE 9.1 Sleep dysfunction in PD compared with age matched controls. NMSQuest study. Source: Chaudhuri *et al.*[14]

Sleep disturbances of PD may be grouped into four broad categories: insomnia; motor-function related; urinary difficulties, and neuropsychiatric or parasomnias (*see* Table 9.2). Day-time somnolence or excessive day-time sleepiness (EDS) is also an important issue. Sleep architecture studies in PD show variable results, but on the whole a common feature is reduced total sleep time and sleep efficiency, multiple sleep arousals and fragmentation of sleep.[7,8,17,18] A circadian variation of symptoms has been identified and in terms of this, patients can be classified into a 'morning better', 'morning worse' and a non-affected group.[7] EDS is an important aspect of sleep-related morbidity of PD and may be caused by the underlying dopaminergic denervation, or may be due to poor nocturnal sleep.[17] In the following section we will review some key aspects of pathophysiology of sleep dysfunction in PD and related individual sleep disorders.

Pathophysiology

Sleep disorders related to PD are multifactorial and for this reason, attributing causation is complex. The pathophysiology of much of sleep disturbance in PD is complex and largely unknown. Degeneration of central sleep regulatory neurones, either directly due to dopaminergic cell loss, or due to an indirect effect of dopaminergic cell loss in the brainstem and related thalamocortical pathways, is implicated.[17,19,20] A preclinical

TABLE 9.2 Causes of night-time sleep disruption and day-time sleepiness in Parkinson's disease

Disease-related	
Insomnia	Fragmentation of sleep (sleep maintenance insomnia)
	Sleep-onset insomnia
Motor function-related	Akinesia (difficulty turning)
	Restless legs/Akathisia
	Periodic limb movements of sleep
	Sensory problems (pain, paraesthesia)
Urinary difficulties	Nocturia
	Nocturia with secondary postural hypotension
Neuropsychiatric/ parasomnias	Depression-related insomnia
	Vivid dreams
	Nightmares
	Sleep talking
	Nocturnal vocalisations
	Somnambulism
	Hallucinations
	Panic attacks
	REM behaviour disorder
	Confusional awakenings
Treatment-related	
Motor	Nocturnal 'off'-period-related tremor
	Dystonia
	Dyskinesias
	'Off'-period-related pain/paraesthesia/muscle cramps
Urinary	'Off'-period-related incontinence of urine
Neuropsychiatric	Hallucinations
	Vivid dreaming
	? 'Off'-period-related panic attacks
	? REM behaviour disorder
	Akathisia
Sleep-altering medications	Alerting effect, nocturnal agitation

Source: Adapted from Chaudhuri[6]

pathological staging of PD has been proposed by Braak.[21] It has been believed traditionally that the pathological process of degeneration of dopaminergic neurones starts in the substantia nigra. Braak proposes an alternative and has introduced the concept of a six-stage pathological process, beginning at clearly designated 'induction sites'.[21] In Braak stage-1 of PD, there is degeneration of the olfactory bulb and the anterior olfactory nucleus and this may clinically manifest as olfactory dysfunction. Progression of the pathological process to the lower brainstem occurs in Braak stage-2 and these are key areas mediating NMS – such as olfaction, sleep homeostasis and other autonomic features. The brainstem areas, particularly the raphe nucleus (serotonin), locus caeruleus (norepinephrine) and pedunculopontine nucleus play a major role in the sleep–wake cycle and mediate the so-called flip-flop switch (*see* Figure 9.2) that mediates thalamocortical arousal.[22] The clinico-pathological correlates are becoming increasingly evident. There is strong evidence that symptoms such as olfactory dysfunction and sleep disturbances like RBD or excessive day-time sleepiness may indeed precede the development of motor symptoms of PD, thus correlating with Braak stages 1 and 2.[2,23,24,25]

Degeneration of brainstem nuclei (such as the locus caeruleus, raphe nuclei and the pedunculopontine nucleus) plays a critical role in thalamo-cortical arousal and the sleep–wake cycle and leads to dysregulation of basic rapid eye movement (REM) and non-REM sleep architecture.[19,20,26,27] Clinically the manifestations are insomnia, parasomnias and excessive day-time sleepiness. The latter may be dependent on dysfunction of the flip-flop switch (*see* Figure 9.2).[22,28] It is suggested that the brain can be either 'off' (promoting sleep by activating the ventrolateral preoptic area (VLPO) thought to be a sleep-promoting centre), or 'on' (promoting wakefulness by activation of the tuberomamillary nucleus (TMN)) which is the wake-promoting area along with the locus caeruleus and the raphe nuclei.[22] Regulation of the internal rhythm between the two switches is via the suprachiasmatic nucleus (SCN) and also possibly, hypocretin 1 (orexin), a hypothalamic peptide.[28,29] Hypocretin 1 is virtually undetectable in narcolepsy, and may have a complex relationship with the dopaminergic

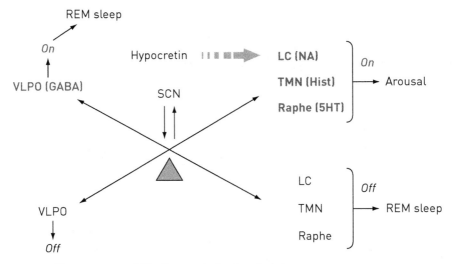

FIGURE 9.2 The concept of flip flop switch of wakefulness.
Source: Chaudhuri *et al.*[2] based on the concept of Saper *et al.*[22]

systems in the basal ganglia.[17] The hypocretin neurones, for instance, project to the dopaminergic neurones in the substantia nigra.[17] Hypocretin-1 could function as an external regulator of the flip-flop switch promoting wakefulness. Dopaminergic dysfunction caused by neuronal degeneration can destabilise this switch and its regulators, promoting rapid transitions to sleep intruding on wakefulness. Although hypocretin-1 insufficiency has not been confirmed by studies of cerebrospinal fluid in three patients with PD and excessive day-time sleepiness associated with dopamine agonist use, one study has reported low hypocretin-1 levels in ventricular fluid of advanced PD patients.[30,46]

Other nocturnal disabilities in PD arise from causes secondary to the progression of disease causing 'destructuring of sleep' and motor complications generated by dopaminergic treatment.[70] Examples of the latter include nocturnal akinesia, early-morning dystonia and excessive day-time sleepiness. The cause of RLS in PD is unknown. Sleep-disordered breathing is increasingly being recognised in PD and may reflect a combination of central and peripheral mechanisms.[7,18]

The symptoms
Nocturnal akinesia
Night-time akinesia is perhaps the clinically most relevant symptom that patients complain of. Nocturnal akinesia usually results from a relatively 'drug-free' period for PD as most regimes use the last dopaminergic treatment well before bedtime. Theoretically this would mean that a 'wearing off' period would occur after the medication half-life expires. There is some support of this observation in the fact that some studies have reported a significant reduction in symptoms of nocturnal akinesia such as pain, spasm and stiffness after nocturnal dosing use of a long-acting dopamine agonist such as cabergoline or sustained infusion of apomorphine through the night.[35,36] Nocturnal akinesia presents as a complex of symptoms which range from difficulty in turning in bed to emergence of tremor (*see* Tables 9.2 and 9.3).

TABLE 9.3 Symptoms and signs of nocturnal akinesia and night-time wearing off

- Difficulty in turning
- Spasm/cramps in muscle
- Pain
- Early morning dystonia
- Restless legs syndrome
- Periodic limb movements
- Nocturia
- Tremor
- Panic attacks

The parasomnias

REM sleep behaviour disorder (RBD)

RBD was first reported in 1986 and is a parasomnia which is typically characterised by vivid and usually frightening dreams or nightmares associated with a paradoxical simple or complex movement during REM sleep when usually muscles are atonic.[13,23] RBD is thought to have a population prevalence of 0.5% and during REM sleep patients enact their dreams, which can be vivid or unpleasant and partners report vocalisations (talking, shouting, vocal threats) and abnormal movements (arm/leg jerks, falling out of bed, violent assaults).[39–42] Typical clinical features are summarised in Table 9.4, while the criteria for diagnosis of RBD as suggested by the International Sleep Disorders Society is shown in Table 9.5.

TABLE 9.4 Clinical features characterising REM behaviour disorder

Predilection for male gender
Mean age of onset 50–65 yrs (wide age range reported varying from 20 to 80 yrs)
REM associated vocalisations, shouting, swearing, screaming, groaning (catathrenia)
Simple and complex motor movements:
• Muscle twitching
• Arm/leg jerking
• Kicking
• Fighting (boxing or trying to hit/strangulate partner)
• Falling out of bed
• Self and partner injury
Dreams associated with attacks by animals or humans or insects
Behaviours are indicative of content of dream
Occurs during the latter half of sleep period (early morning)

Source: Modified from Boeve et al.[13]

Although clinical history may suggest a diagnosis in some situations – such as when there is a high risk of physical injury or if loud snoring suggestive of obstructive sleep apnoea is observed – confirmation of diagnosis should be obtained by a single night of polysomnography (PSG) with video telemetry. PSG would show an increased EMG activity during REM sleep. Symptoms of RBD may predate the diagnosis of PD with reports that in 11 of 29 men (38%) 50 years or older in whom idiopathic RBD was diagnosed, a parkinsonian disorder was identified after a mean interval of 3.7 ± 1.4 (SD) years following the diagnosis of RBD, and 12.7 ± 7.3 years after the onset of RBD.[39] A recent study has suggested an increased risk of developing PD in individuals who have RBD and olfactory disturbance.[45] This concept is consistent with the recent hypothesis of Braak and colleagues who suggest that the preclinical stages 1 and 2 of PD start at the olfactory and medullary area of the brainstem.[21] Although the pathological basis of RBD is unknown, speculation is that RBD is related to degeneration of lower brainstem nuclei like the pedunculopontine and peri-caeruleal nucleus. Specifically based on studies in cats, several brainstem areas (such as latero-dorsal tegmental nucleus (LDTN), peri locus caeruleus region (peri-LC), nucleus reticularis magnocellularis and the ventrolateral reticulospinal tracts) in addition to the PPN have been implicated.[13] Lesions in the peri-LC regions lead to REM sleep without atonia and in one of the first cases of RBD to come to autopsy, there was a marked reduction in the number of neurones in LC while increase in neuronal numbers in PPN and LDTN were observed.[43] The authors suggested that RBD could have been caused by a decreased cholinergic activity of the LC and reduced disinhibition of PPN and LTDN. This is, however, controversial as others have noted depletion of neuro-melanin neurones in LC and depleted choline-acetyl transferase neurones in LDTN/PPN in multiple system atrophy cases.[44] Furthermore, why clonazepam remains the most effective drug for treatment of RBD cannot be explained by these possible pathophysiological mechanisms.

TABLE 9.5 The International Sleep Disorders Society criteria for diagnosis of RBD

A: The patient has a complaint of violent or injurious behaviour during sleep
B: Limb or body movement is associated with dream mentation
C: At least one of the following occurs: 1. Harmful or potentially harmful sleep behaviours 2. Dreams appear to be acted out 3. Sleep behaviours disrupt sleep continuity

D: Polysomnographic monitoring demonstrates at least one of the following electrophysiological measures during Rapid Eye Movement (REM) sleep:
1. Excessive augmentation of chin electromyographic (EMG) tone
2. Excessive chin or limb phasic EMG twitching, irrespective of chin EMG activity and one or more of the following:
   a. Excessive limb or body jerking
   b. Complex, vigorous or violent behaviours
   c. Absence of epileptic activity in association with the disorder

E: The symptoms are not associated with mental disorders but may be associated with neurological disorders
F: Other sleep disorders (e.g. sleep terrors or sleepwalking) can be present but are not the cause of the behaviour

Source: American Sleep Disorders Association[37] and Mahowald et al.[38]

RBD: differential diagnosis with other parasomnias

A list of differential diagnosis of RBD is provided in Table 9.6. Somnabulism usually complicates early non-REM sleep and exhibits purposeful movements, such as walking away from the bed, not necessarily associated with violent dreams; or abrupt movements such as kicking, fighting or jumping. Night terrors and confusional episodes occur early in sleep unlike in RBD and may involve screaming or incoherent speech but there is no recall of the dream. Nocturnal panic attacks in PD may complicate nocturnal akinesia with dysautonomic symptoms such as palpitations, hyperhidrosis and immediate full awareness without dream enactment while seizures may be associated with tonic-clonic posturing, tongue biting, incontinence of urine and post-ictal confusion.

TABLE 9.6 The possible differential diagnosis of RBD

Parasomnias of non-REM sleep:
• somnabulism
• confusional arousal
• night terrors
Nocturnal panic attacks
Nightmares
Nocturnal seizures
Severe periodic limb movements of sleep
Obstructive sleep apnoea

Excessive day-time somnolence (EDS) and sudden onset of sleep

EDS is a common complaint in PD and one study reported a prevalence of 15.5% of these patients compared with only 1% of healthy age-matched controls.[4] In another study the occurrence of EDS in 142 patients in 1993 and subsequently four years later was examined. While 7% had EDS in 1993, by 1997 the figure had risen to 29% and the authors concluded that EDS may occur at a rate of 6% new patients per year in PD.[63] The causation is complex and may represent a destabilisation of the flip-flop switch of wakefulness due to dopaminergic denervation.[22,28] In addition, the effect of poor nocturnal sleep and anti-parkinsonian or other drugs may be causative (*see* Table 9.7). EDS may manifest as a feeling of sleepiness and slowly drifting off to sleep, while other patients may experience fatigue. A controversial notion is the concept of sudden onset of sleep (SOS) without any preceding drowsiness, resembling narcolepsy in some patients.[17,47,48] Some had originally suggested the term 'sleep attacks' linked to use of non-ergot dopamine agonists.[49] However, recent reviews suggest that 'sleep attacks' are not drug-specific but rather a class effect of all dopamine agonists used to treat PD as well as of dopaminergic agents such as levodopa; and furthermore, use of the term 'sleep attack' is discouraged.[49,50,51]

Like RBD, EDS can occur early in PD and may predate the diagnosis in some cases.[52,53] However, based on a study in 15 untreated PD patients, there is no evidence of EDS in untreated PD based on PSG, multiple sleep latency test (MSLT) or Epworth Sleep Scale (ESS), but EDS occurs after treatment with dopaminergic agents.[68] One study was performed using PSG and MSLT in PD patients with and without hallucinations.[54] EDS was present in 50% of each group while sleep onset REM periods and sleep latency below 10 minutes characteristic of narcolepsy were present mainly in the hallucinating group.[54] This would suggest that a subset of PD patients may have an intrinsic susceptibility to sudden onset of sleep which may be unmasked by use of some dopaminergic drugs. Irresistible sleepiness not preceded by obvious somnolence or warning has been shown to be present in 14% of a Chinese PD population compared with its presence in fewer than 2% of controls.[55] Such subjects may, therefore, be susceptible to falling asleep while driving or operating machinery. EDS may need to be differentiated from fatigue, and also post-prandial hypotension in PD may unmask sleepiness and akinesia.[56] Fatigue may be present up to 43% of PD patients and is usually associated with sleepiness although tiredness is a key feature.[57]

TABLE 9.7 Possible causes of excessive day-time sleepiness in Parkinson's disease

Non-drug-therapy-related reasons:
• Advancing disease
• Nocturnal sleep disruption
• Parasomnias
• Depression
Drug-therapy-related reasons:
• Dopaminergic treatment in susceptible patients
• Antihistamines
• Hypnotics
• Anxiolytics
• Selective serotonin re-uptake inhibitors

Source: Adapted from Chaudhuri[6]

Driving, EDS and sudden onset of sleep

The combination of motor dysfunction of PD, the propensity to day-time sleepiness and fatigue may pose a particular problem in relation to driving. A questionnaire survey of 6620 patients with 361 phone interviews suggested that 60% of this population were still driving and that, of those holding a driving licence, 11% were implicated in the causation of at least one road traffic accident in the preceding five years.[69] The risk factors identified for accidents included: a high ESS score; moderately severe motor disability of PD, and a previous history of sudden onset of sleep while driving.

Restless legs syndrome (RLS) and periodic limb movements (PLM)

RLS and PLM commonly occur together and both can be effectively treated by dopaminergic drugs – raising speculation that there may be an underlying dopaminergic dysfunction and a link with PD. There are few studies addressing the prevalence of RLS in PD. One observational study reported RLS to occur in PD at a rate twice the normal prevalence of RLS in general population.[58] A recent comparative study suggested a prevalence rate of 24% RLS in PD.[59] RLS may occur across all stages of PD and even in untreated PD.[60] A study of sleep and periodic leg movement patterns (PLM) in untreated PD and multiple system atrophy using two nights' polysomnography[60] reported frequent problems with sleep disruption and increased PLM index in untreated PD. This observation is in agreement with recent clinical findings in a study of untreated PD versus controls and advanced PD using a bedside sleep scale of PD.[61] However, a confusing issue is that in some cases (more than 65% of PD patients in one study), RLS may emerge after the diagnosis of PD, when patients are already on dopaminergic therapy, which is thought to be first-line treatment for RLS. Furthermore, in PD, RLS may be confused with akathisia which may be related to dopaminergic dyskinesia. For a formal diagnosis of PLM, overnight PSG is useful (*see* Figure 9.3).

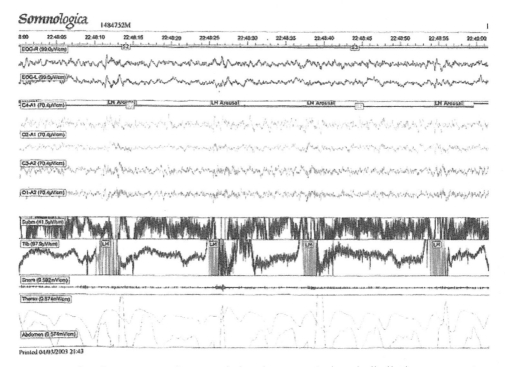

FIGURE 9.3 A polysomnography record showing repeated periodic limb movements (marked as LM) causing awakening in a PD patient. This was abolished by nocturnal dopamine agonist treatment.
Source: Courtesy of Dr A Williams. Lane–Fox Sleep Centre, St Thomas' Hospital, London, UK.

Sleep disordered breathing

EDS may overlap with day-time somnolence due to sleep disordered breathing. Obstructive sleep apnoea (OSA) causing sleep disordered breathing may be suggested by a history of loud crescendo snoring and irregular snoring with snorting and gasping and gaps, particularly in an overweight subject. Partner-corroborated history of observed apnoeic episodes and day-time fatigue and somnolence also suggests OSA. Formal polysomnography will identify sleep apnoea, and OSA may occur in up to 50% of patients with PD with resultant day-time sleepiness and tiredness.[18,62] Sleep apnoea may co-exist with RLS, PLM or RBD and it is important to diagnose it, since treatment for RBD with clonazepam, for instance, may aggravate OSA.

Nocturia

Nocturia has consistently been shown to be one of the commonest problems causing sleep disruption in PD. A rate of 43% nocturia among 200 PD patients has been reported,[34] with a suggested overall prevalence of 30–80% for nocturia in PD.[6,89] The validation study of the newly developed Parkinson's disease sleep scale (PDSS) and an independent study of Spanish validation of PDSS both reported nocturia as the most prevalent nocturnal symptom of PD.[71,72] The causation is unclear. Nocturia may reflect a symptom of nocturnal wearing off while an underlying striatal dopamine D1-receptor-related dysfunction has also been implicated.[64,65] Nocturia associated with nocturnal 'off' period may lead to incontinence of urine and bed soiling. Nocturia also appears to be problem of advancing PD rather than early or untreated PD as indicated in a study using PDSS in untreated and advanced PD compared with controls.[61]

Neuropsychiatric comorbidities complicating sleep in PD

Depression is common in PD and affects sleep quality, causing insomnia, usually sleep onset in type.[6,7] Dementia will also lead to sleep dysfunction with evidence of RBD, insomnia and nocturnal hallucinations. Hallucinations may complicate nocturnal sleep and some have suggested an overlap with RBD.[41,54] An eight-year follow-up study of cases with RBD and PD suggested a high rate of development of visual hallucinations in those with RBD.[66] RBD could be a risk factor for future development of hallucinations and cognitive failure.[67]

Drug-induced sleep disruption in PD

Insomnia and night-time agitation may be caused by late dosing of selegiline, probably as a result of its amphetamine metabolite, while other drugs (such as amantadine and anticholinergics) may also produce an alerting effect. The effect of rasagiline on sleep is unclear. Selective serotonin re-uptake inhibitors (SSRIs) may need to be avoided at bedtime, as they may impair sleep onset.[7] Dopamine agonists and levodopa have a variable and dose-dependent effect on sleep, either promoting or disrupting sleep, although studies suggest that overnight sustained dopaminergic stimulation improves sleep in PD by reducing nocturnal akinesia and RLS/PLM.[6,7]

Investigations for sleep disorders in PD

Until 2002 there were no specific instruments to clinically assess sleep problems of PD in a comprehensive and holistic fashion. Existing sleep scales for other disorders – such as the Pittsburgh Sleep Quality Index (PSQI), Stanford Sleepiness Scale or the Karolinska Sleepiness Scale – are not specific for PD and have problems when these are used in PD.[72–75] For instance, the Pittsburgh Sleep Quality Index, although quantifiable, does not specifically address sleep disturbances of PD such as restlessness of legs, painful posturing of arms or legs, tremors or fidgeting; while the Stanford

Sleepiness Scale and the Karolinska Sleepiness Scale appear to be too short for a comprehensive assessment of sleep problems. The gold standards for measurement of physiological aspects of sleep architecture are PSG and MSLT, although these are tests of sleep structure, need specialised sleep laboratories, and are expensive. In the UK, for instance, facilities for sleep studies are not readily available. Furthermore, these studies do not provide any information on aspects of sleep dysfunction in PD such as nocturnal tremor, akinesia, nocturia or hallucinations.

The Unified Parkinson's Disease Rating Scale (UPDRS) is used widely for motor examination and contains only one sleep-related inquiry: 'Does the patient have any sleep disturbances, for example, insomnia or hypersomnolence?'[79] This is inadequate for sleep assessment of PD and a proposed revision of the scale may have more sleep-related items incorporated.[79,80]

The Epworth Sleepiness Scale (ESS) is a self-administered questionnaire, and is aimed at assessment of excessive day-time somnolence in eight situations of daily life.[81] The ESS is used widely in relation to PD and correlates well with the relevant question (Question 15) on PDSS. A high ESS score in a patient with moderately advanced PD may predict a risk for sudden onset of sleep and road traffic accidents.[69] However, ESS does not quantify the types of sleep disturbance that occur in PD. Furthermore, the interpretation of the ESS suffers from cross-cultural differences and uncertain test–retest reliability.

TABLE 9.8 The items listed in the SCOPA sleep scale[78]

Night-time sleep	Day-time sleepiness	Other sleep parameters
• Difficulty falling asleep	• Falling asleep unexpectedly	• Using sleep medications, number (%)
• Being awake too often	• Falling asleep while sitting	• Sleep initiation time, minutes
• Lying awake too long	• Falling asleep watching TV	• Time awake per night, hours
• Waking too early	• Falling asleep while talking	• Actual sleep per night, hours
• Having too little sleep	• Difficulty staying awake	• Sleep in day-time, minutes
• Overall sleep quality (0–6)	• Sleepiness problematic	• Planned naps, number (%)
		• Unplanned naps, number (%)
		• Unexpected sleep, number (%)

The first bedside scale for a comprehensive assessment of sleep problems is the PDSS which has now been used across the world for a bedside assessment of clinical aspects of sleep disabilities of PD.[71,72] The PDSS is 15-question visual analog scale which can be administered easily at the bedside and has also undergone formal linguistic validation in Italy, Spain and Japan (see Figure 9.4 on p. 209).[72,88]

The PDSS has robust test–test reliability and good discriminatory power between patients with PD and healthy controls. Patients and caregivers respond to individual questions based on their experiences in the past week, and scores for each item range from 0 (symptom severe and always experienced) to 10 (free of symptoms). The maximum cumulative score for the PDSS is 150 (patient is free of all symptoms). The PDSS aims to distinguish between sleep-onset and sleep-maintenance insomnia (Questions 2 and 3 of the PDSS); nocturnal motor symptoms (Questions 10 to 13 of the PDSS); nocturnal restlessness, dystonia, and pain (Questions 4, 5, 10, and 11 of the PDSS); neuropsychiatric symptoms (Questions 6 and 7 of the PDSS); and nocturia (Questions 8 and 9 of the PDSS). Excessive day-time sleepiness is addressed by Question 15, while Question 14 addresses sleep refreshment. A total score below 90 or an individual item score below 6 is likely to indicate significant sleep disturbance. One criticism is that PDSS does not specifically address the issue of sleep disordered breathing and RBD and a modification has been suggested.[77]

As part of a program for development of scales to address various aspects of PD, a validated SCOPA-SLEEP scale has been developed (*see* Table 9.8).[78] This is a short, two-part scale that assesses nocturnal sleep and day-time sleepiness and contains non-disease-specific items. SCOPA-SLEEP has been validated in PD and is reliable. Unlike the PDSS, it is not a visual analog scale and does not address some problems specific to PD, such as nocturnal hallucinations, pain, dystonia, tremor, and nocturia which can be quantified in PDSS.

Sleep architecture can be studied using PSG and MSLT providing measures of alertness. These studies are not required routinely for assessment of sleep in PD. However, in cases where obstructive sleep apnoea or severe PLM is suspected, PSG is essential. In cases of severe RBD or other parasomnias, PSG is useful for confirmation of diagnosis. A pathological MSLT result (sleep latency < 10 minutes) in a PD patient may also suggest a propensity to sudden onset of sleep.

Treatment

There is a poor evidence base for treatment of sleep problems in PD and the issue is complicated by the fact that treatment of sleep problems needs to take into account the multi-factorial nature of sleep disturbance in PD. A recent review by the Movement Disorders Society Task Force reported that there were no robust trials of dopaminergic agents for treatment of non-motor symptoms in PD, including sleep.[82] Only modafinil (for EDS) and melatonin (for insomnia) have been studied in randomised double-blind trials in a small number of patients in PD (*see* Table 9.9). Other published evidence of drug treatment addressing sleep disorders in PD consists of a number of case-series-related observations and open-label trials with a limited and inadequate evidence base for treatment.

The use of PDSS enables the clinician to adopt a systematic and pragmatic approach to treatment of night-time symptoms. An example would be that patients with low scores (< 6) for Questions 10–13 in the PDSS (indicating nocturnal motor disabilities due to wearing off) might benefit from extending the action of levodopa by combining levodopa with entacapone, using Stavelo or a night-time cabergoline, a long-acting dopamine agonist. Low scores in response to Questions 6 and 7 (indicating hallucinations) might warrant withdrawal of night-time dopamine agonists or treatment with clonazepam if RBD is suspected. A summary of management strategies for sleep disturbances related to Parkinson's disease is outlined in Table 9.9.

TABLE 9.9 Management strategies for symptoms contributing to nocturnal disturbance in Parkinson's disease

Insomnia-related symptoms	Fragmented sleep with difficulty in sleep onset and sleep maintenance
Non-pharmacologic measures	Avoidance of night-time alcohol, caffeine, tobacco
	Increase in day-time physical activity and ensuring exposure to daylight
	Psychological therapies: relaxation training, cognitive therapies, biofeedback training
Pharmacologic strategies	Short-acting benzodiazepines: clonazepam, temazepam, diazepam
	Non-benzodiazepine hypnotics: zopiclone
	Tricyclic antidepressants: amitriptyline (may help nocturia but may aggravate RLS)
Motor symptoms	Fidgeting, painful cramps and posturing, tremor, sleep akinesia, RLS-type symptoms
Non-pharmacologic measures	Use of satin bed sheets and bed straps to help moving in bed
	Bed rails
Pharmacologic strategies (based on case series and open-label trials)	Sustained dopaminergic stimulation (night-time dosing of):
	• CR levodopa ± COMT inhibitor, Stalevo™
	• Long-acting dopamine agonists, e.g. cabergoline
	• Nocturnal apomorphine infusion (severe RLS/PLM/dystonia/cramps)
	• Combination of day-time apomorphine and evening cabergoline (dual agonist therapy)
Practical measures to aid bioavailability of dopaminergic medications	Avoidance of high-protein meals at night
	Domperidone if delayed gastric emptying
REM behaviour disorder	Clonazepam (usually first choice)
	Pramipexole
	Melatonin
	Carbamazepine
	Donepezil
	Levodopa

cont.

Neuropsychiatric symptoms	Distressing dreams, hallucinations, depression
Non-pharmacologic measures	Consider alternative diagnosis: MSA, LBD, PSP
Pharmacologic strategies	Hallucinations: • ? Drug-induced: optimise therapy • Atypical neuroleptics: quetiapine
	Depression: • Amitriptyline; noradrenaline reuptake inhibitors; dopamine agonists, e.g. pramipexole
	Panic attacks: • During 'on' periods: alprazolam, lorazepam • During 'off' periods: CR levodopa ± COMT inhibitor; cabergoline; apomorphine infusion • Any time: sertraline, fluoxetine, paroxetine
Urinary symptoms	Nocturia Incontinence of urine because of inability to move during 'off' phase
Non-pharmacologic measures	Reduction of evening fluid intake Emptying bladder before going to bed Use of condom catheters/bedside commode If associated with postural hypotension, head-up tilt of bed
Pharmacologic strategies	Low-dose amitriptyline Possible role for D1/D2 agonists, e.g. cabergoline, pergolide, apomorphine If associated with detrusor instability: oxybutinin, tolterodine If associated with morning hypotension: desmopressin nasal spray; avoidance of evening diuretics, antihypertensives, vasodilators

CR = controlled-release; COMT = catechol-*O*-methyl-transferase; MSA = multiple system atrophy; LBD = Lewy body dementia; PSP = progressive supranuclear gaze palsy; RLS = restless legs syndrome; PLM = periodic limb movement.

Source: Adapted from Chaudhuri[6] and Garcia-Borreguero, *et al.*[7]

Sleep benefit and sleep hygiene

Sleep benefit which implies improvement in mobility and motor state of variable duration, ranging from 30 minutes to 3 hours, after sleep is a common phenomenon in PD.[7] The mechanism of sleep benefit is unknown and possible causes include: (a) recovery of dopaminergic function and storage during sleep; (b) a circadian rhythm-related phenomenon, or (c) a pharmacological response to dopaminergic drugs.[7,30] Good sleep hygiene is useful and includes activities such as: taking a hot bath about two hours before bedtime; maximising day-time activity and ensuring bright light exposure; having a hot sweet drink or a light snack at bedtime; use of handrails in

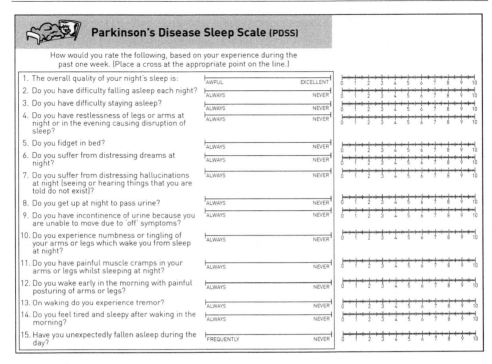

FIGURE 9.4 The Parkinson's Disease Sleep Scale (PDSS). The scale on the right is on a transparency, and it needs to be applied on the printed scale after the scale has been scored by placing a cross mark on each 10-cm line by patient/partner.

bed and/or satin sheets to make turning in bed easier; flexible bedtimes; the use of a reclining armchair for some, and avoiding stimulants such as tea or coffee at bedtime.[90] Nocturia remains one of the commonest causes of sleep disruption in PD and needs to be tackled by avoiding diuretics or tea/coffee at bedtime, and use of a nasal spray of desmopressin in some patients.[89] Some have suggested use of combined D2/D1-receptor dopamine agonists such as pergolide, but this has not been established in clinical trials.[91] In cases with risk of urinary incontinence, condom catheters or a bedside urinal is essential to ensure a good-quality sleep with minimal interruption.

Nocturnal akinesia

Nocturnal akinesia is usually caused by night-time wearing off and strategies promoting overnight dopaminergic stimulation may be helpful. Sustained-release levodopa/benserazide significantly improved night-time akinesia (ability to turn in bed) and reduced total time awake in a 12-month open-label, non-comparative trial including 15 patients with PD and distressing nocturnal symptoms.[84] Open-label comparative observational reports in PD patients with severe sleep disruption due to nocturnal motor symptoms suggest that cabergoline, the long-acting once-a-day dopamine agonist may be superior to levodopa or pergolide.[85,86] Overnight apomorphine infusion also has been reported to be beneficial for nocturnal motor and non-motor symptoms of

PD.[87] These studies were performed prior to the availability of the PDSS and currently studies investigating the efficacy of controlled-release formulations of agents (such as ropinirole and rotigotine transdermal patch) on nocturnal akinesia are under way.

Excessive day-time somnolence (EDS)

In PD, severe EDS needs treatment and first of all, concurrent medications that may be sedating should be eliminated or reduced (*see* Table 9.7). Modafinil (100–400 mg/day), a non-addictive sleep–wake cycle activator is non-stimulating and the only drug which has shown efficacy in improving EDS in double-blind placebo controlled trials (*see* Table 9.10).[92,93] A seven-week double-blind placebo crossover study of 200 mg modafinil followed by a four-week open-label extension (200 and 400 mg) study showed significant improvement in ESS with modafinil and improvement in clinical global impression scores for wakefulness in the open-label arm.[93] Those with high ESS scores and a history of sudden onset of sleep should be advised not to drive alone or long distances. Dopamine agonists, when started, should be titrated up slowly, especially in older patients.

Neuropsychiatric problems

Depression affects approximately 40% of patients with PD and may contribute to sleep disturbances, necessitating active treatment with sedating antidepressants (e.g. trazodone or mirtazepine) (*see* Table 9.9). Panic attacks can occur in both 'on' and 'off' periods and 'off'-related panic can be overcome by sustained dopaminergic stimulation. Successful treatment of the neuropsychiatric problems often leads to improvement of sleep quality in PD.

REM behaviour disorder and restless legs syndrome (RLS)

The treatment of choice for RBD is clonazepam, a benzodiazepine, although the mechanism is unknown and there are no controlled trials.[13] Other drugs thought to be helpful for RBD, should clonazepam fail, inlcude pramipexole, levodopa, carbamazepine, donepezil or melatonin.[89,94,95,98] Caution needs to be exercised with the use of clonazepam as in some cases RBD may be confused with OSA which can be worsened by clonazepam. Night-time dosing with drugs such as selegiline may aggravate RBD. There are reports of paradoxical worsening of RBD during deep-brain stimulation of the subthalamic nucleus (STN).[96]

RLS may complicate PD and may cause significant sleep disruption and there are no trials investigating treatment of RLS in PD. In some cases, targeted treatment with a long-acting dopamine agonist such as cabergoline, given at night-time, may be effective.[85,86] The role of drugs such as a rotigotine transdermal patch or a controlled-release version of ropinirole needs to be investigated. In severe cases, hospital admission with overnight apomorphine infusion may be required.[87]

Deep-brain stimulation of the subthalamic nucleus (STN-DBS)

Long-term STN-DBS may improve sleep quality through decreased nocturnal mobility and reduction of sleep fragmentation.[96,97] STN-DBS seems to be an effective therapeutic option for the treatment of advanced PD because it improves the cardinal symptoms and also seems to improve sleep architecture.

TABLE 9.10 List of trials of pharmacological and surgical interventions in sleep disorders in PD

	Drug/ intervention	Study design	Patient numbers and duration	Mean dose	Outcome
Akinesia and sleep time					
1	Levodopa + Benserazide	Open label	15/12 mths	CR levodopa (200 mg)	Improved total time awake (p = 0.046)
2	Cabergoline	Retrospective, comparative with levodopa CR	25(CBG) vs 15 (LD)/ 6 mths	Cbg = 4 mg od CR levodopa (200 mg)	Reduction of painful dyskinesias, early morning akinesia (p<0.05)
3	Melatonin	DBPC, Crossover	40	Melatonin (50 mg)	Improved total sleep time (10 min, p<0.05)
RBD					
1	Clonazepam	Open label	93/4½ yrs	Clonazepam (0.25–1 mg)	RBD treatment completely or partially successful in 87% of patients
3	Melatonin	Case series	13/14 mths	7 patients on clonazepam (0.5–1.0) + melatonin (3–12 mg) 12 patients on melatonin	8 patients reported continued benefit with melatonin for 1 yr
4	Pramipexole	Case series	8 (idiopathic RBD and periodic limb movements)	Pramipexole (1.5–4.5 mg)	5 patients reported reduction in REM sleep time (p = 0.09), and % of REM sleep (p = 0.07)
EDS					
1	Modafinil	DBPC crossover study	15/4 wks	Modafinil 100 mg 1st wk, 200 mg 2nd wk	ESS significantly improved in all pts (p= 0.011)
2	Modafinil	DBPC	21/6 wks	Modafinil 200 mg/day	Improvement in CGI for change (p = 0.07) on modafinil

cont.

Drug/ intervention	Study design	Patient numbers and duration	Mean dose	Outcome
Deep-brain stimulation				
1 Subthalamic nucleus stimulation (bilateral)	5 yrs prospective study	49/5 yrs	Patients assessed at 1, 3 & 5 yrs with and without levodopa	Improved sleep and activities of daily living (p<0.001)
2 Subthalamic nucleus stimulation (bilateral)	Observational study	386/3 mths	NA	Decreased day-time somnolence and improved sleep quality
3 Subthalamic nucleus stimulation (bilateral)	Case control	5/3 mths	NA	Significant improvement in total mean PDSS score

NA = Not applicable. DBPC = Double-blind placebo-controlled. ESS = Epworth sleepiness scale. PDSS = Parkinson's disease sleep scale.

The future

The natural history and much of pathophysiology of sleep disorders of PD remains unknown and treatment of several aspects of sleep disorders in PD lacks robust evidence base. These areas will need investigation and research in future. A key area of interest is likely to focus on unraveling the role of hypocretin and other hormones such neuronal activity related pentraxin (NARP) in the causation of sleep dysfunction (if any) in PD. Pathophysiological and observational studies will also help devise better treatment strategies for nocturnal parasomnias such as RBD, restless legs syndrome and sleep disordered breathing. Currently, some trials related to aspects of nocturnal akinesia using oral or non-oral formulations of dopamine agonists are already planned.

Conclusion

Sleep disorders in patients with PD are common; are a key component of the non-motor symptom complex of PD, and remain under-diagnosed and under-treated. Sleep problems may arise from uncontrolled motor symptoms, from degeneration of the neuro-anatomical substrates responsible for the sleep/wake cycle, or from unwanted medication side effects. Routine assessment of patients with PD should include inquiry regarding the quality of sleep and sleep-related symptoms. Use of validated bedside clinical tools such as the PDSS, SCOPA-SLEEP and ESS offer a robust way to assess the presence or absence of sleep disruption, and also to guide treatment. Uncontrolled nocturnal motor symptoms may be ameliorated by long-acting dopaminergic agents, while other sleep disruptions such as hallucinations or

RBD require a different approach. In resistant cases, patients may need to undergo polysomnography and/or multiple sleep latency tests (MSLT). Targeted night-time treatment should result in improved sleep for patients with PD.

REFERENCES

1 Parkinson J. An essay on the shaking palsy [reprint of monograph published by Sherwood, Neely, and Jones, London, 1817]. *J Neuropsychiatry Clin Neuro Sci.* 2002; **14**: 223–36.

2 Chaudhuri KR, Healy D, Schapira AHV. The non motor symptoms of Parkinson's disease: diagnosis and management. *Lancet Neurology.* 2006: **5**(3): 235–45.

3 Lees AJ, Blackburn NA, Campbell VL. The nighttime problems of Parkinson's disease. *Clin Neuropharmacol.* 1988; **11**: 512–9.

4 Tandberg E, Larsen JP, Karlsen K. Excessive daytime sleepiness and sleep benefit in Parkinson's disease: a community-based study. *Mov Disord.* 1999; **14**: 922–7.

5 Karlsen K, Larsen JP, Tandberg E, *et al.* Fatigue in patients with Parkinson's disease. *Mov Disord.* 1999; **14**: 237–41.

6 Chaudhuri KR. Nocturnal symptom complex in PD and its management. *Neurology.* 2003; **61** (Suppl. 3): S17–S23.

7 Garcia-Borreguero D, Larosa O, Bravo M. Parkinson's disease and sleep. *Sleep Med Rev.* 2003; **7**: 115–29.

8 Adler CH, Thorpy MJ. Sleep issues in Parkinson's disease. *Neurology.* 2005; **64** (12 Suppl. 3): S12–S20.

9 Karlsen KH, Larsen JP, Tandberg E, *et al.* Influence of clinical and demographic variables on quality of life in patients with Parkinson's disease. *J Neurol Neurosurg Psychiatry.* 1999; **66**: 431–5.

10 Aarsland D, Larsen JP, Tandberg E, *et al.* Predictors of nursing home placement in Parkinson's disease: a population-based, prospective study. *J Am Geriatr Soc.* 2000; **48**(8): 938–42.

11 Findley L, Aujla MA, Bain PG, *et al.* Direct economic impact of Parkinson's disease: a research survey in the United Kingdom. *Mov Disord.* 2003; **18**(10): 1139–45.

12 Bosanquet N, May J, Johnson N. Alzheimer's disease in the United Kingdom: burden of disease and future care. *Health Policy Review Paper* No. 12. London: Health Policy Unit, Imperial College School of Medicine; 1998.

13 Boeve BF, Silber MH, Ferman TJ, *et al.* Association of REM sleep behaviour disorder and neurodegenerative disease may reflect an underlying synucleinopathy. *Mov Disord.* 2001; **16**: 622–30.

14 Chaudhuri KR, Martinez-Martin P, Schapira AHV, *et al.* An international multicentre pilot study of the first comprehensive self-completed non motor symptoms questionnaire for Parkinson's disease: The NMSQuest study. *Mov Disord.* 2006; **22**(11): 916–23.

15 Hely MA, Morris JGL, Reid WGJ, *et al.* Sydney multicenter study of Parkinson's disease: non-L-dopa-responsive problems dominate at 15 years. *Mov Disord.* 2005; **20**: 190–9.

16 Shulman LM, Taback RL, Rabinstein AA, *et al.* Non-recognition of depression and other non-motor symptoms in Parkinson's disease. *Parkinsonism Relat Disord.* 2002; **8**(3): 193–7.

17 Rye DB, Jankovic J. Emerging views of dopamine in modulating sleep/wake state from an unlikely source: PD. *Neurology.* 2002; **58**: 341–6.

18 Arnulf I, Konofal E, Merino-Andreu M, *et al.* Parkinson's disease and sleepiness: an integral part of PD. *Neurology.* 2002; **58**: 1019–24.

19 Shouse MN, Siegel JM. Pontine regulation of REM sleep components in cats: integrity of the pedunculopontine tegmentum (PPT) is important for phasic events but unnecessary for atonia during REM sleep. *Brain Res.* 1992; **571**: 50–63.

20 Lai YY, Siegel J. Physiological and anatomical link between Parkinson-like disease and REM behaviour disorder. *Curr Treat Options Neurol.* 2003; **5**: 231–39.

21 Braak H, Del Tredici K, Rüb U, *et al.* Staging of brain pathology related to sporadic Parkinson's disease. *Neurobiol Aging.* 2003; **24**: 197–210.

22 Saper C, Chou TC, Scammell TE. The sleep switch: hypothalamic control of sleep and wakefulness. *Trends in Neurosci.* 2001; **24**: 726–31.

23 Schenck CH, Mahowald MW. REM sleep behavior disorder: clinical, developmental, and neuroscience perspectives 16 years after its formal identification in SLEEP. *Sleep.* 2002; **25**: 120–38.

24 Abbott RD, Ross GW, White LR, *et al.* Excessive daytime sleepiness and the future risk of Parkinson's disease. *Mov Disord.* 2005; **20** (Suppl. 10): S101 (P341).

25 Ross W, Petrovitch H, Abbott RD, *et al.* Association of olfactory dysfunction with risk of future Parkinson's disease. *Mov Disord.* 2005; **20** (Suppl. 10): P439 (Abstract).

26 Parent A, Hazrati LN. Functional anatomy of the basal ganglia. 1. The cortico-basal ganglia-thalamo-cortical loop. *Brain Res Review.* 1995; **20**: 91–127.

27 Karachi C, Yelnki J, Tande D, *et al.* The pallidosubthalamic projection: an anatomical substrate for non motor functions of the subthalamic nucleus in primates. *Mov Disord.* 2005; **20**: 172–80.

28 MacMahon D. Why excessive daytime sleepiness is an important issue in Parkinson's disease. *Adv Clin Neurol and Rehab.* 2005; **5**(2): 46–9.

29 Nishino S, Ripley B, Overseem S, *et al.* Hypocertin (orexin) deficiency in human narcolepsy. *Lancet.* 2000; **355**: 39–40.

30 Ripley B, Overseem S, Fujuki N, *et al.* CSF hypocretin/orexin levels in narcolepsy and other neurological conditions. *Neurology.* 2001; **57**: 2253–8.

31 Factor SA, McAlarney T, Sanchez Ramos JR, *et al.* Sleep disorders and sleep effect in Parkinson's disease. *Mov Disord.* 1990; **5**: 280–5.

32 Nausieda PA, Weiner WJ, Kaplan LR, *et al.* Sleep disruption in the course of chronic levodopa therapy: an early feature of levodopa psychosis. *Clin Neuropharmacol.* 1982; **5**: 183–94.

33 Smith MC, Ellgring H, Oertel WH. Sleep disturbances in Parkinson's patients and spouses. *J Am Geriatr Soc.* 1997; **45**: 194–9.

34 Stocchi F, Vacca L, Valente M, *et al.* Sleep disorders in Parkinson's disease. *Adv Neurol.* 2001; **86**: 289–93.

35 Chaudhuri KR, Bhattacharya K, Agapito C, *et al.* The use of cabergoline in nocturnal parkinsonian disabilities causing sleep disruption: a parallel study with controlled-release levodopa. *Eur J Neurol.* 1999; **6** (S 5): S11–S15.

36 Reuter I, Ellis CM, Chaudhuri KR. Nocturnal subcutaneous apomorphine infusion in Parkinson's disease and restless legs syndrome. *Acta Neurol Scand.* 1999; **100**: 163–7.

37 American Sleep Disorders Association. *International Classification of Sleep Disorders, Revised: diagnostic and coding manual.* Rochester, Minneapolis: American Sleep Disorders Association; 1997: 177–80.

38 Mahowald M, Schenck C. REM sleep behaviour disorder. In: Kryger M, Roth T, Dement W, editors. *Principles and Practice of Sleep Medicine*, 3rd ed. Philadelphia: WB Saunders; 2000: 724–41.

39 Schenck CH, Bundlie SR, Mahowald MW. Delayed emergence of a parkinsonian disorder in 38% of 29 older men initially diagnosed with idiopathic rapid eye movement sleep behavior disorder. *Neurology.* 1996; **46**: 388–93.

40 Olson EJ, Boeve BF, Silber MH. Rapid eye movement sleep behaviour disorder: demographic, clinical and laboratory findings in 93 cases. *Brain.* 2000; **123**: 331–9.

41 Fantini ML, Ferini-Strambi L, Montplaisir J. Idiopathic REM sleep behavior disorder: toward a better nosologic definition. *Neurology.* 2005; **64**(5): 780–6.

42 Comella CL, Nardine TM, Diederich NJ, *et al.* Sleep-related violence, injury, and REM sleep behavior disorder in Parkinson's disease. *Neurology.* 1998; **51**(2): 526–9.

43 Schenck CH, Garcia-Rill E, Skinner RD, *et al.* A case of REM sleep behaviour disorder with autopsy confirmed Alzheimer's disease: post-mortem brain-stem histochemical analyses. *Biol Psychiatry.* 1996; **40**: 422–5.

44 Benarroch EE, Schmeichel AM. Depletion of cholinergic mesopontine neurons in multiple system atrophy: a substrate for REM behaviour disorder? *Neurology*. 2002; **58** (Suppl. 3): A345.

45 Stiasny-Kolster K, Doerr Y, Moller JC, *et al.* Combination of 'idiopathic' REM sleep behaviour disorder and olfactory dysfunction as possible indicator for alpha-synucleinopathy demonstrated by dopamine transporter FP-CIT-SPECT. *Brain*. 2005; **128** (Part 1): 126–37.

46 Drout X, Moutereau S, Nguyen J, *et al.* Low levels of ventricular orexin/hypocretin in advanced PD. *Neurology*. 2003; **61**: 540–3.

47 Ondo WG, Dat Vuong K, Khan H, *et al.* Daytime sleepiness and other sleep disorders in Parkinson's disease. *Neurology*. 2001; **57**: 1392–6.

48 Olanow CW, Schapira AH, Roth T. Waking up to sleep episodes in Parkinson's disease. *Mov Disord*. 2000; **15**: 212–5.

49 Frucht S, Rogers JD, Greene PE, *et al.* Falling asleep at the wheel: motor vehicle mishaps in persons taking pramipexole and ropinirole. *Neurology*. 1999; **52**: 1908–10.

50 Andreu N, Chale J-J, Senard J-M, *et al.* L-dopa-induced sedation: a double-blind cross-over controlled study versus triazolam and placebo in healthy volunteers. *Clin Neuropharmacol*. 1999; **22**: 15–23.

51 Ferreira JJ, Galitzky M, Montastruc JL, *et al.* Sleep attacks in Parkinson's disease. *Lancet*. 2000; **355**: 1333–4.

52 Fabbrini G, Barbanti P, Aurilia C, *et al.* Excessive daytime sleepiness in de novo and treated Parkinson's disease. *Mov Disord*. 2002; **17**(5): 1026–30.

53 Abbott RD, Ross GW, White LR, *et al.* Excessive daytime sleepiness and the future risk of Parkinson's disease. *Mov Disord*. 2005; **20** (Suppl. 10): S101 (P341).

54 Arnulf I, Bonnet AM, Damier P, *et al.* Hallucinations, REM sleep and Parkinson's disease: a medical hypothesis. *Neurology*. 2000; **55**: 281–8.

55 Tan EK, Lum SY, Fook-Chong SMC, *et al.* Evaluation of somnolence in Parkinson's disease: comparison with age and sex matched controls. *Neurology*. 2002; **58**: 465–8.

56 Chaudhuri KR, Ellis C, Love-Jones S, *et al.* Postprandial hypotension and parkinsonian state in Parkinson's disease. *Mov Disord*. 1997; **12**(6): 877–84.

57 van Hilten JJ, Weggeman M, van der Welde EA, *et al.* Sleep, excessive daytime sleepiness and fatigue in Parkinson's disease. *J Neural Transm*. [P-D Sect] 1993; **5**: 235–44.

58 Ondo WG, Dat Vuong K, Khan H, *et al.* Daytime sleepiness and other sleep disorders in Parkinson's disease. *Neurology*. 2001; **57**(8): 1392–6.

59 Lussi F, Peralta C, Wolf E, *et al.* Restless legs in idiopathic Parkinson's disease. *Parkinsonism Relat Disord*. 2005; **11** (Suppl. 2): 207 (Abstract PT029-10).

60 Wetter TC, Collado-Seidel V, Pollmacher T, *et al.* Sleep and periodic leg movement patterns in drug free patients with Parkinson's disease and multiple system atrophy. *Sleep*. 2000; **23**(3): 361–7.

61 Dhawan V, Dhoat S, Williams A, *et al.* The range and nature of sleep dysfunction in untreated Parkinson's disease. A comparative clinical study using the Parkinson's disease sleep scale and selective polysomnography. *J Neurol Sci*. 2006; **248**(1–2): 158–62.

62 Diederich NJ, Vaillant M, Leischen M, *et al.* Sleep apnoea syndrome in Parkinson's disease: a case-control study in 49 patients. *Mov Disord*. 2005; **20**(11): 1413–18.

63 Gjerstad MD, Aarsland D, Larsen JP. Development of daytime somnolence over time in Parkinson's disease. *Neurology*. 2003; **58**: 1544–6.

64 Jenner PG. Is stimulation of D1 and D2 dopamine receptors important for optimal motor functioning in Parkinson's disease? *Eur J Neurol*. 1997; **4** (Suppl. 3): S3–S11.

65 Yoshimura N, Sass M, Yoshida O, *et al.* Dopamine D1 receptor-mediated inhibition of micturition reflex by central dopamine from the substantia nigra. *Neurourol Urodyn*. 1992; **11**: 535–45.

66 Onofrj M, Thomas A, D'Andreamatteo G, *et al.* Incidence of RBD and hallucinations in patients affected by Parkinson's disease: 8 year follow up. *Neurol Sci*. 2002; **23**: S91–S94.

67 Sinforiani E, Zangaglia R, Manni R, *et al*. REM sleep behaviour disorder, hallucinations and cognitive impairment in Parkinson's disease. *Mov Disord.* 2006; **21**(4): 426–6.

68 Kaynak D, Kinziltan G, Kaynak H, *et al*. Sleep and sleepiness in patients with Parkinson's disease before and after dopaminergic treatment. *Eur J Neurol.* 2005; **12**(3): 199–207.

69 Meinorfner C, Korner Y, Moller JC, *et al*. Driving in Parkinson's disease: mobility, accidents, and sudden onset of sleep at the wheel. *Mov Disord.* 2005; **20**(7): 832–42.

70 Diederich NJ, Vaillant M, Lyen P, *et al*. Progressive 'sleep destructuring' in Parkinson's disease: a polysomnographic study in 46 patients. *Sleep Med.* 2005; **6**(4): 313–8.

71 Chaudhuri KR, Pal S, Di Marco A, *et al*. The Parkinson's disease sleep scale: a new instrument for assessing sleep and nocturnal disability in Parkinson's disease. *J Neurol Neurosurg Psychiatry.* 2002; **73**: 629–35.

72 Martinez-Martin P, Salvador C, Menendez-Guisasola L, *et al*. Parkinson's disease sleep scale: validation study of a Spanish version. *Mov Disord.* 2004; **19**(10): 1226–32.

73 Chaudhuri KR, Martinez-Martin P. Clinical assessment of nocturnal disability in Parkinson's disease: the Parkinson's disease sleep scale. *Neurology.* 2004; **63** (Suppl. 3): S17–S20.

74 Buysse DJ, Reynolds CF III, Monk TH, *et al*. The Pittsburgh Sleep Quality Index: a new instrument for psychiatric practice and research. *Psychiatry Res.* 1989; **28**: 193–213.

75 Hoddes E, Zarcone V, Smythe H, *et al*. Quantification of sleepiness: a new approach. *Psychophysiology.* 1973; **10**: 431–6.

76 Gillberg M, Kecklund G, Akerstedt T. Relations between performance and subjective ratings of sleepiness during a night awake. *Sleep.* 1994; **17**: 236–41.

77 Tse W, Liu Y, Barthlen GM, *et al*. Clinical usefulness of the Parkinson's disease sleep scale. *Parkinsonism Relat Disord.* 2005; **11**(5): 317–21.

78 Marinus J, Visser M, van Hilten JJ, *et al*. Assessment of sleep and sleepiness in Parkinson disease. *Sleep.* 2003; **26**: 1049–54.

79 Movement Disorder Society Task Force on Rating Scales for Parkinson's Disease. The Unified Parkinson's Disease Rating Scale (UPDRS): status and recommendations. *Mov Disord.* 2003; **18**(7): 738–50.

80 Dodel RC, Dubois B, Fahn S, *et al*. Addressing non-motor impairments in Parkinson's disease: the new version of the UPDRS. *Mov Disord.* 2005; **20** (Suppl. 10): S83 (P 277).

81 Johns MW. A new method for measuring daytime sleepiness: the Epworth Sleepiness Scale. *Sleep.* 1991; **14**: 540–5.

82 Goetz CG, Poewe W, Rascol O, *et al*. Evidence-based medical review update: pharmacological and surgical treatments of Parkinson's disease: 2001–2004. *Mov Disord.* 2005; **20**(5): 523–39.

83 Comella CL, Stebbins GT, Bohmer J. Sleep benefit in Parkinson's disease. [Abstract]. *Neurology.* 1995; **45**(S4): A286.

84 Van Den Kerchove M, Jacquy J, Gonce M, *et al*. Sustained-release levodopa in parkinsonian patients with nocturnal disabilities. *Acta Neurol Belg.* 1993; **93**(1): 32–9.

85 Chaudhuri KR, Bhattacharya K, Agapito C, *et al*. The use of cabergoline in nocturnal parkinsonian disabilities causing sleep disruption: a parallel study with controlled-release levodopa. *Eur J Neurol.* 1999; **6**(S5): S11–S15.

86 Ghatani T, Agapito C, Bhattacharya K, *et al*. Comparative audit of pergolide and cabergoline therapy in the treatment of nocturnal 'off' periods causing sleep disruption in Parkinson's disease. *Eur J Neurol.* 2001; **8** (Suppl. 1): 8–11.

87 Reuter I, Ellis CM, Chaudhuri KR. Nocturnal subcutaneous apomorphine infusion in Parkinson's disease and restless legs syndrome. *Acta Neurol Scand.* 1999; **100**: 163–7.

88 Abe K, Hikita T, Sakoda S. Sleep disturbances in Japanese patients with Parkinson's disease – comparing with patients in the UK. *J Neurol Sci.* 2005: **234**(1–2): 73–8.

89 Grandas F, Iranzo A. Nocturnal problems occurring in PD. *Neurology.* 2004; **63**: S8–S11.

90 Schapira AH. Present and future drug treatment for Parkinson's disease. *J Neurol Neurosurg Psychiatry.* 2005; **76**(11): 147–8.

91 Yoshimura N, Mizuta E, Kuno S, *et al*. The dopamine D1 receptor agonist SKF 38393 suppresses detrusor hyperreflexia in the monkey with parkinsonism induced by MPTP. *Neuropharmacology*. 1993; **32**: 315–21.
92 Hogl B, Saletu B, Brandauer E, *et al*. Modafinil for the treatment of daytime sleepiness in Parkinson's disease: a double blind, randomised, crossover, placebo controlled, polygraphic trial. *Sleep*. 2002; **25**(8): 905–9.
93 Adler CH, Caviness JN, Hentz JG, *et al*. Randomised trial of modafinil for treating subjective daytime sleepiness in patients with Parkinson's disease. *Mov Disord*. 2003; **18**: 287–93.
94 Fantini ML, Gagnon J-F, Filipini D, *et al*. The effects of paramipexole in REM sleep behavior disorder. *Neurology*. 2003; **61**: 1418–20.
95 Tan A, Salgado M, Fahn S. Rapid eye movement sleep behavior disorder preceding Parkinson's disease with therapeutic response to levodopa. *Mov Disord*. 1996; **11**: 214–6.
96 Krack P, Van Blercom N, Chabardes S, *et al*. Five-year follow-up of bilateral stimulation of the subthalamic nucleus in advanced Parkinson's disease. *N Eng J Med*. 2003; **349**: 1925–34.
97 Hjort N, Ostergaard K, Dupont E. Improvement of sleep quality in patients with advanced Parkinson's disease treated with deep-brain stimulation of the subthalamic nucleus. *Mov Disord*. 2004; **19**: 196–9.
98 Dowling GA, Mastick J, Colling E, *et al*. Melatonin for sleep disturbances in Parkinson's disease. *Sleep Med*. 2005; **6**(5): 459–66.

PART 4

Motor dysfunction

10

Motor problems in Parkinson's disease: fluctuations, gait, balance and falls

HELEN ROBERTS AND PETER OVERSTALL

Introduction

Postural instability, causing unsteadiness when standing and walking, is a cardinal feature of Parkinson's disease (PD), and is particularly associated with disease onset after the age of 70 years. Older patients are more likely to have balance impairment, both at onset and after five years of treatment, and its presence as the major criterion for Hoehn and Yahr stage 3 marks a significant shift from mild to more disabling disease. Mobility and independence are threatened, and the risk of serious injury from a fall increases. Patients with imbalance appear to have a more rapidly progressive form of the disease, and the presence of a gait disorder in a parkinsonian patient doubles the relative risk of death.[1,2] Whether or not these patients have a different underlying pathology is still unclear, although co-morbidity – in particular cerebrovascular disease – is likely to be the explanation in at least some of these patients.

The challenge for clinicians is therefore twofold: first, to decide whether the patient with the all-too-common presentation of falls and 'off his/her legs' really does have idiopathic PD; and second – having made the diagnosis – to determine the best form of treatment. Unfortunately, gait continues to deteriorate despite levodopa treatment.[3] However, modern gait laboratories, which can measure balance using force platforms and surface electromyography (EMG), both during quiet standing and following perturbations and when walking using three-dimensional (3D) motion analysing systems, have provided important information on the kinetics and kinematics of PD and possible physical therapies.

Normal standing balance

During normal quiet standing, balance is maintained when the vertical projection of the centre of mass (COM) on the ground (often called the centre of gravity, COG) is kept within the support base provided by the feet. Maintenance of this upright position is associated with body sway mainly in the anterior/posterior (A/P) direction, and this sway may be measured either as degrees of angular movement or using force platforms as the excursions of the centre of pressure (COP). The COP is independent of the COM and represents the pressure over the surface of the feet in contact with the ground. There is a separate COP under each foot, and when both feet are in contact with the ground, the net COP lies somewhere between the two feet, depending on the relative weight taken by each foot.[4] Both A/P sway velocity and area increase in normal elderly subjects (i.e. those who report that their balance is normal and are functionally independent), and this difference is more obvious if the difficulty of the test is increased by using a moving platform or when the eyes are closed.[5] Further increases in A/P sway have been correlated with spontaneous falls, but a better predictor of falls is medio-lateral sway.[6]

In contrast to this increased sway that is seen in normal elderly subjects, PD patients have an unusually small sway area – about half that seen in elderly controls. They do not appear to have any difficulty using visual, somatosensory or vestibular information, and the sway areas remain small even under challenging sensory conditions.[7] This reduced sway may be due to higher intrinsic musculoskeletal stiffness, or it may be compensation for inadequate postural control when the COM is displaced. The result is an overall increase in stiffness, which offers a certain advantage in resisting minor displacements. However, because postural responses to perturbations are impaired, the PD patient is like a tin soldier in that, although there is increased stability during quiet standing, stable equilibrium can be maintained only over a very small area, and loss of balance follows even modest displacements. Interestingly, an increase in medio-lateral sway has been noted in PD patients – especially those who have fallen – and this may be a response to the postural inflexibility seen in the A/P direction. PD patients are unable to achieve extremes of forward or backward leaning, and this has been blamed on their reduced sway: the increased sway seen in these extreme positions in controls reflects not instability but rather a deliberate action aimed at reducing further displacement. The increased medio-lateral sway may thus be a compensatory strategy, which introduces the necessary slight shifts and postural adjustments to counteract the restricted A/P movement.[8,9]

Senile gait

There has been a long-running debate on what constitutes a normal gait in old age, and the cause of the senile gait (idiopathic gait disorder). There are undoubtedly some elderly people who maintain a normal gait with a speed greater than 1 m/s.[10] A normal gait has been observed in 18% of a community living sample aged between 88 and 96 years.[11] However, gait laboratory studies show subtle changes even in carefully screened healthy elderly subjects. Gait slowing is due to a decreased stride length, and cadence (steps per minute) remains unaltered. Stance time and double support time increase, and there is a less vigorous push-off. Whether this represents an early degeneration of the balance control system or an adaptation to make the gait safer is unclear.[12] Recently the importance of executive function in performing dual task has been recognised.[13]

It is now apparent that the senile gait disorder, which is characterised by caution and shorter and more frequent strides (for which there is no apparent cause) and is said to occur in 15–24% of the elderly, is not due to age but to underlying neurodegenerative syndromes and stroke. These patients have a twofold increased risk of cardiovascular death compared with age-matched subjects with a normal gait, further supporting the view that senile gait is caused by subclinical cerebrovascular disease.[14] The considerable confusion over the aetiology of different gait disorders in the elderly can been clarified by the their classification into three broad categories of gait disorder: (i) the lowest level due to peripheral skeletomuscular or sensory problems; (ii) a middle level causing distortion of appropriate postural and locomotor synergies (early Parkinsonism could be included in this category); and (iii) highest-level disorders, which are those most commonly seen by geriatricians.[15] The last category includes five gait types of which subcortical dysequilibrium, frontal dysequilibrium and frontal gait disorder are the most relevant, since all of these gaits may include an element of parkinsonism.

In deciding whether or not a patient with impaired balance and gait has PD, it should be remembered that for postural instability to be regarded as a cardinal sign of PD it must be unrelated to primary visual, cerebellar, vestibular or proprioceptive dysfunction. In practical terms, the important diagnoses to exclude are a frontal gait disorder due to cerebrovascular disease or normal pressure hydrocephalus, and a cervical myelopathy. For further discussion of the differential diagnosis, see Chapter 4.

Differential diagnosis
Arteriosclerotic parkinsonism
This is also called lower-half parkinsonism, and the gait is sometimes described as *marche à petits pas*. It is characteristically a frontal gait disorder. The gait tends to be wider than in idiopathic PD, the steps are short and shuffling, and there is start and turn hesitation.[15] Disequilibrium can be more marked than in idiopathic PD, and in both conditions there is increased reliance on visual cues. A possible explanation is that the multiple vascular lesions produce a disconnection of cortical modulation rather than an impairment of the functions of the basal ganglia. If the periventricular lesions affect the afferent loop between the basal ganglia and the supplementary motor area, there will be a loss of internally triggered movements and increased reliance on visually triggered external movements.[16] Other clues that distinguish it from idiopathic PD are the upright trunk and leg posture and the preservation of arm swing. Pyramidal tract signs and pseudobulbar palsy are common in arteriosclerotic parkinsonism, but not in PD. Although it is sometimes said that the upper limbs are normal in arteriosclerotic parkinsonism, it is not uncommon in elderly patients to find both bradykinesia and rigidity (and even occasionally tremor), although the limb rigidity is more likely to be symmetrical than in idiopathic PD. A good response to levodopa would make one question the diagnosis of arteriosclerotic parkinsonism, but a modest improvement in symptoms (up to 50%) is occasionally seen.[17]

Computed tomography (CT) scanning of patients with arteriosclerotic parkinsonism and gait abnormalities shows leuko-araiosis and ventricular enlargement in 90% of cases.[18] Lacunar strokes and white matter lesions on CT are better predictors of the development of parkinsonism than territorial strokes. White matter lesions are more likely to be found in patients with idiopathic PD than in healthy subjects, and are a marker for more severe disease, particularly bradykinesia, postural instability and gait difficulties. These patients have shorter disease duration and their bradykinesia responds less well to levodopa.[19]

Cervical myelopathy
This is a common cause of gait disorder in the elderly, and is due to degenerative arthritis of the cervical spine. In advanced cases there is spasticity and hyper-reflexia in the legs, with dorsal column signs and urinary urgency. The patient has a spastic gait and often there are lower motor neurone signs in the upper limbs, with reduced neck movements. However, before these patients develop the typical stiff-legged para-spastic gait there is impairment of balance apparent to the patient, who compensates by

producing a protective gait pattern. Gait velocity, step length and cadence are reduced, and step width is increased. Improvement may follow decompressive surgery.[20]

Alzheimer's disease

Parkinsonian signs are more likely to occur in Alzheimer's disease (AD) patients than in the general population. There are similarities (but also differences) between AD with parkinsonism and dementia with Lewy bodies (DLB). In both, the parkinsonism is typically symmetrical, and rest tremor is uncommon. However, in DLB there is a male predominance and the parkinsonian signs – and particularly the gait abnormalities – occur early, whereas in AD dementia is the presenting feature and the parkinsonian signs occur late. The neuropathological findings in patients with AD and parkinsonism are variable, but most cases are associated with subcortical Lewy bodies.[21]

Normal gait initiation

In order to understand what is happening in start hesitation, it is helpful to recall normal gait initiation. This begins with anticipatory postural adjustments (APA), the first of which is inhibition of the swing limb gastrocnemius-soleus, causing the COP to move posteriorly. Simultaneously, the tensor fascia lata is inhibited on the stance limb and activated on the swing limb, resulting in the COP moving towards the swing limb with loading of the swing limb and unloading of the stance limb. There is then rapid unloading of the swing limb and loading of the stance limb as the COP shifts to the stance limb. The COM accelerates forwards and towards the stance limb and, at the point of toe-off of the swing limb, the entire body weight is over the stance limb. The body falls forwards, and the COM moves towards the point where the heel of the swing foot will land.[4] The APA are programmed in advance of the intended voluntary movement, and shifting the COM allows a step to be taken.

Gait initiation in Parkinson's disease

In 1961, Purdon Martin conducted a famous study of 130 post-encephalitic parkinsonian patients cared for at Highlands Hospital in north London. He observed that some patients, although able to stand, were unable to walk either forwards or backwards, but if they were tilted slightly forwards and rocked from side to side, they could walk more or less normally. He concluded that the stepping mechanism as such is not disordered, and that the fault lies in disturbance of the APA, essential for the initiation and continuation of regular stepping.[22] This observation has remained at the heart of PD gait research ever since. In essence, in PD patients the APA and the forward velocity of the COM at heel-off are significantly reduced, but are improved by levodopa.[23] The APA show several changes, the initial standing posture is abnormal with increased likelihood of activation of quadriceps, hamstrings and tibialis anterior. This change in the postural set appears to prolong the time interval between gastrocnemius-soleus inhibition and heel-off of the swing limb. Even when standing EMG activity is normal, the APA may be slowed by prolonged recruitment of tibialis anterior before heel-off, but the most common abnormality is a loss of effectiveness of the APA. The initial inhibition of gastrocnemius-soleus may either be repeated several times, or be incomplete or even completely absent. Activation of tibialis anterior is desynchronised or absent and where soleus inhibition is present, there can be marked delay before activation of tibialis anterior. The defective APA means that the initial posterior shift of the COP is reduced (proportional to the degree of disability of the patient), and this in turn reduces the force of forward propulsion.[24,25,26]

Stepping in response to an external stimulus improves both force and velocity of the APA,[23] and is consistent with the observation that visual and auditory cues assist gait initiation. Although the precise function of the basal ganglia is unclear, it has been suggested that one important role is to provide an internal non-specific cue to trigger switching from one sequential movement to the next. Automatic predictable movement sequences appear to be particularly impaired in PD.[27]

Motor fluctuations

These eventually trouble most patients, and appear to be related to the length of time that the patient has been on levodopa. The pathophysiology of the development of motor complications is thought to be related to pulsatile delivery of levodopa, and long-acting forms of levodopa (e.g. Duodopa™) and dopamine agonists (e.g. apomorphine infusions) have been shown to improve motor fluctuations. This has led to the concept of continuous dopamine stimulation as a means of reducing these complications.[28]

The fluctuations can be divided into fluctuations of short duration (which last seconds to minutes and consist of sudden, transient freezing episodes), of medium duration and diurnal (minutes to hours) and of long duration (days).[29]

Medium-duration fluctuation begins as gradual end-of-dose deterioration. The patient's increasing awareness of this reflects an increased amplitude of the 'on/off' difference. Eventually, the development of sudden dramatic fluctuations indicates that a threshold level of dopaminergic stimulation has been reached, where the patient is either 'on' or 'off', with very little useful time in between. Frequent small doses may mean that the patient does not turn on at all, or has unpredictable fluctuations, and there is a more predictable response with larger, less frequent doses. Although this may improve the quality of the 'on' time, the 'off' time is subsequently worse. Diurnal variations are often noted, with, typically, the patient being better in the morning than in the afternoon and evening.

Freezing

Freezing tends to be a later feature of PD, but analysis of the DATATOP study reveals that it may occur in the early stages of idiopathic PD.[30] It can occur in both the 'on' and 'off' states, and even in the absence of levodopa treatment. Freezing is not pathognomonic of PD, and indeed it occurs more commonly in progressive supra-nuclear palsy (PSP), arteriosclerotic parkinsonism and normal-pressure hydrocephalus. It is very rare in drug-induced parkinsonism, and was thought to be rare in multiple system atrophy. However recent clinico-pathological studies have found freezing in patients with MSA with parkinsonian features.[31] Early severe freezing is unusual in PD, and would suggest a diagnosis of PSP.

The most common type of freezing is start hesitation (gait ignition failure). The patient attempts to start walking, but the feet remain stuck to the ground. Several short incomplete steps may be made before the patient is able to move forwards. Patients may freeze when passing through doorways[30] and turning hesitation is common and often noted to be worse in one direction than in another. Freezing is also observed in speech, the eyelids, when writing, and when performing tasks such as shaving.

The most important predictor for freezing is not disease duration, but progression of disease as measured by the Hoehn and Yahr scale. Duration of levodopa treatment is the second most significant factor, followed by duration of treatment with agonists. Treatment with selegiline reduced the development of freezing in the DATATOP trial, but is less effective once symptoms have developed.[32] There is a significant association between freezing and the presence of dyskinesia, early morning foot dystonia, postural instability and dementia.[33]

Deficient force production during gait initiation does not explain freezing.[23] It appears that during freezing the 'gain', i.e. velocity of the forward movement, reduces to zero[4] and is associated with a total absence of any APA. Freezing is notoriously resistant to treatment with levodopa, and yet both the delayed APA and the reduced force production for a self-generated step can be improved with levodopa. In other words, gait initiation – but not freezing – improves with levodopa, suggesting that in freezing either the levodopa fails to produce a normal response or else other non-dopaminergic pathways are involved. Impaired serotonin (5HT) neurotransmission has been suggested as a possible candidate.[34]

Pathophysiology

The pathophysiology underlying freezing remains unclear. Frontal lobe disease and, more specifically, frontal white matter lesions, have been suggested.[15,17] However, patients with severe freezing due either to idiopathic PD or to isolated gait ignition failure have not been shown to have significant frontal hypoperfusion (using single photon emission computed tomography, SPECT), although hypoperfusion can be demonstrated in patients with PSP. Interestingly, only 5% of this PSP group had freezing, so the frontal lobe hypoperfusion that was observed may be related to other deficits, such as cognitive impairment, rather than to gait ignition failure.[35]

Another hypothesis centres on basal ganglia malfunction leading to motor set deficits (hypokinesia) while altered motor cue production leads to a sequence deficit with progressively smaller movements as seen in festination. A recent study found that visual cues improved sequencing, while the hypokinesia improved with medication, attentional strategies and visual cues.[36] Again dual task studies have indicated that patients who freeze are more dependent on attention when walking than those who don't experience freezing.[37]

Recent studies have demonstrated increased variability in stride length while walking without freezing, in patients who freeze compared with those who don't, leading to the hypothesis that freezing may be due to a loss of locomotion rhythm.[38]

Treatment

Treatment of freezing depends crucially on distinguishing between episodes occurring when the patient is 'off' or is starting to develop end-of-dose deterioration, and the episodes of those patients whose episodes are unpredictable and unrelated to their 'on' or 'off' state. 'Off' freezing improves with levodopa, apomorphine or stimulation of the sub-thalamic nucleus. A small open-label trial of botulinum injections into the calf muscles improved freezing in one study[39] and botulinum toxin injected into the calf muscles can be particularly helpful for patients with dystonic posturing. Up to five injections may be required. Improvement may not be noticed for a week, but the benefit lasts for about six weeks. 'On' freezing is rare and improves with a reduced dose. Patients with unpredictable freezing, who are taking frequent small doses of levodopa may be helped by a change to less frequent, larger doses. Physical measures to overcome freezing include advice from the physiotherapist on how to turn, various trick manoeuvres such as marching on the spot to command or stepping over an object, a small electronic metronome worn on the belt and strips of white tape on the floor in parts of the house such as the WC where freezing tends to occur.

Dyskinesias

About 10% of PD patients on levodopa treatment develop dyskinesias each year, and eventually virtually all patients are affected. They can be particularly problematical in younger patients[40] but do not appear to impact on quality of life so much in older patients.[41] The most common type is peak-dose dyskinesia, which appears earlier in patients with more severe disease. Typically, it is choreiform and painless and appears first on the most affected side, although in the elderly the lips, mouth or head are frequently involved. High doses of levodopa and long duration of treatment increase the risk, whereas agonist monotherapy reduces it. These dyskinesias can significantly interfere with the patient's gait and balance and, if the legs are severely affected, the dyskinesias must be controlled by reducing the levodopa dosage before the physiotherapist can start work on the patient. Unfortunately, for many patients, turning 'on' becomes synonymous with dyskinesias. A variety of strategies can be tried, including controlled-release preparations of levodopa, agonists, apomorphine and amantadine. Apomorphine can remain effective for at least five years[42] and some patients can be weaned off levodopa altogether, provided that the dosage reduction is very gradual (50 mg per week). Patients with severe dyskinesias who have had PD for at least four years and are under 75 years of age are increasingly being considered for surgery. Stimulation or lesioning of globus pallidus interna or the subthalamic nucleus are the most promising operations at present.

'Off'-period dystonias may occur at the beginning or end of dose, during 'off' periods, or in the early morning.[29] Typically, the patient wakes in the morning with the foot distorted and painful, usually on the least affected side. The patient can be advised to stay in bed until the first dose of levodopa starts to work. Apomorphine or an injection of botulinum toxin can also be effective.

Biphasic dyskinesias (occurring at the onset and end of levodopa action) are more common in young-onset patients and are best managed by larger and less frequent doses of levodopa and, if this is unsuccessful, by neurosurgery.

Gait

In most patients, PD first becomes apparent in the arms and trunk, and it may be months (or even years) before any abnormality is noted in the legs. Initial symptoms affecting only the legs are unusual.

Usually the first sign of gait impairment is a reduction in step length and changes in the swing phase. A reduction both in knee flexion and heel elevation causes the heel to scuff as the foot moves forwards. Further progression of the disease is shown by slowing of walking speed; a tendency to take smaller steps and to slow down when turning; and increasing flexion of arms, neck and trunk. PD patients typically walk at 40–60 m/min compared with 75–90 m/min in age-matched control subjects, with a reduced stride length of 1 m or less, compared with 1.2 to 1.5 m in healthy older people.[43] In advanced disease the patient is severely flexed forwards and there is complete loss of the normal toe raise at the end of leg swing, so that the patient takes short quick steps by sliding his/her toes along the floor.

Gait analysis shows that PD patients have increased stride-to-stride variability, and they walk slowly because they are unable automatically to regulate their stride length. If asked to walk faster, they normally increase cadence (steps per minute) but not step length unless trained to do so.[43] Why patients can maintain or increase their cadence yet are unable accurately to regulate stride-to-stride gait is unknown, but it may represent a loss of automaticity in smoothly maintaining sequential movements so that walking becomes a matter of separate steps rather than a continuous flowing motion. Inability to generate adequate muscle force at foot 'push-off' may also be a factor.[23] Additionally, stride width increases early in PD, possibly to compensate for altered posture, then narrows in later disease with an associated risk of falls.[44]

Current views on the role of the basal ganglia suggest two main functions. First, they contribute to cortical motor set (i.e. the tonic discharge in motor cortical neurones that keeps the motor plans in a state of readiness). Motor set allows initiation of the motor plan and enables it to run with the correct amplitude, to completion and without attention. The second function is to provide internal cues to ensure that the motor plans, which are thought to be a predetermined set of submovements, run precisely and accurately with correct timing between the submovements. The basal ganglia, supplementary motor area and motor cortex form a loop and it is thought that the basal ganglia provides internal cues to the supplementary motor area that allows the correct submovement, in well-learned automatic movement sequences, to occur smoothly. Abnormal internal cues would impair submovement preparation and interrupt habitual movements such as walking. Another possibility is that the gait disturbance could be due to a disorder of motor set for the entire movement sequence. A series of experiments has shown that PD patients are able to generate normal stride length, not only with visual cues – e.g. light coloured strips placed on the floor at appropriate step length for the individual – but also with attentional strategies where the patient is asked to form a mental picture of the correct step size or mentally rehearse the step.[43] Furthermore, patients maintain the ability to produce rhythmic steps in response to a metronome cue, suggesting that it is not a loss of movement timing that causes the reduced stride length, but rather a defective scaling of stride size. Cerebral blood flow studies have demonstrated that activity in the pre-motor cortex and supplementary motor area is increased in PD patients when external cues or attentional strategies are used.[45] Peak speed and stride length respond to levodopa, whereas temporal variables such as cadence, swing and stance duration are dopa resistant.[46] The variability seen in walking performance in patients with PD is attributed to variability in medication levels over time rather than being an inherent feature of the disease.[47]

Similarly, people with PD may walk in a straight line relatively easily but find more difficulty performing complex tasks such as turning, or performing dual motor and cognitive tasks, or attempting to walk in complex community settings like crowded shops.[43]

Axial movements

Rigidity of the shoulder, neck and trunk can be detected early in the course of PD. The arms swing less when the trunk is rotated by the examiner. Increased neck rigidity is felt when the head is passively flexed and extended. The head and shoulders are thrust slightly forwards, the trunk appears stiff when walking, and when the patient turns, the body is seen to turn en bloc instead of displaying the normal smooth sequential movement of pelvis, lumbar and thoracic spine.

Most common tasks require frequent turns, and turning while walking is a potent source of akinetic blocks, leading to freezing episodes and falls. Disordered axial movement also shows up as difficulty in turning over in bed, and its presence appears to be related more to the duration of disease than the age of onset.[48] Although difficulty in turning in bed is regarded as a characteristic feature of PD it is not diagnostic, as it can be found in 9% of healthy elderly subjects and in 38% of elderly patients without neurological disease attending a geriatric day hospital.[49] Difficulty in turning over in bed is not an apraxia, but is due to bradykinesia and disruption of the normal limb and trunk synergies. Thus it can be regarded, along with disordered gait and loss of arm swing when walking, as another example of basal ganglia disease causing loss of sequencing of a well-practised, automatic movement. Difficulty in turning in bed is associated significantly with disturbed gait, postural instability, difficulty in rising from a chair, whole-body bradykinesia and axial rigidity. All of these axial motor impairments respond to levodopa.[48]

Falls

Falls are not usually a presenting feature of idiopathic PD, and their presence within the first year raises the possibility of one of the 'Parkinson's plus' syndromes, such as PSP. Two recent prospective studies of older people with PD found an annual incidence of falls of around 68%, with 50% describing recurrent falls.[50,51] Up to 90% of patients will eventually fall, but the fall frequency probably declines in late-stage disease because of the patient's immobility. [52]

Falls correlate with previous falls, increasing PD duration, the patient's age, severity of disease, rigidity, bradykinesia, motor complications, and cognitive impairment.[50] However, the main determinant of whether or not a PD patient will fall is postural instability, particularly impairment in the response to perturbations and in the anticipatory postural adjustments. Although the increased stiffness of the PD patient improves standing balance, the loss of flexibility increases the risk of falls. Other important factors are the reduced height of the foot from the ground during the swing phase; this increases the risk of tripping. The tendency to walk on the balls of the feet also reduces postural stability.

Many falls occur on turning or on transferring from a chair or bed; falls due to trips or slips are relatively rare. Patients also describe falling when they freeze; their feet remain rooted to the ground while their upper body continues to move. PD patients tend to fall forwards (45% of all falls) or laterally (20%), presumably due to the forward shift of the centre of gravity provided by the stooped posture. In contrast, patients with PSP tend to fall backwards, and often spontaneously.[52]

The fall rates in PD undoubtedly depend very much on the age of the group studied, since in the normal elderly population falls increase linearly with age, reaching 50% in those aged 85 years and over. Thus, postural instability due to PD may not be the only explanation for falls in older patients. Other relevant factors include the presence of small-vessel disease,[19] visual impairment, vestibular disease, cutaneous and proprioceptive loss in the feet, cervical spondylosis, muscle weakness and a general slowing of central information processing.[53,54,55]

Most PD patients fall indoors, and the fracture rate is unclear, although one study found 25% of participants to have sustained a hip fracture within ten years of diagnosis.[56] Patients with recurrent falls have an increased mortality risk, with average survival reduced to approximately seven years from the onset of falling.[57] Additionally the loss of confidence and effect on quality of life and mood is considerable, and falls may cause patients to move into rest or nursing homes.

Response to perturbation

Laboratory studies of PD patients who are deliberately thrown off balance by a sudden movement of the platform on which they are standing has shown that the main deficit is an inability to produce a postural response, both quickly enough and of sufficient force.[52]

Responses to an external perturbation consist of corrective responses, such as the ankle and hip strategies, muscle stiffening and co-contraction, which do not require any change in the base of support provided by the feet, and protective responses where one or more steps are taken or an arm is thrown out to grab hold of an external support.[58] Although the timing of the onset of corrective responses in PD has variously been described as normal or delayed, the main abnormalities in addition to inadequate force are an inappropriate sequencing of postural strategies. These result in co-contraction and joint stiffness, which interferes with the rapid corrective movements needed to prevent a fall, e.g. arms are adducted against the trunk during a fall, possibly explaining the low incidence of wrist fractures in PD. There are also changes in reflex amplitude, with an increased medium latency reflex and decreased long latency reflexes. As a result, PD patients sway further backwards than controls following toe-up tilt of the platform, and this cannot be corrected by levodopa. Furthermore, the inappropriately large medium latency reflexes to the stretched gastrocnemius soleus muscles – which destabilises the response to the toe-up perturbation – is unresponsive to levodopa. This suggests that non-dopaminergic lesions contribute to the postural instability seen in PD.[59]

The protective responses are characterised by change in support strategies (CIS), and involve stepping and grasping reactions. These are not reactions of last resort and are often initiated very early after the onset of an unexpected perturbation. Indeed, these CIS reactions are much more rapid than even the fastest voluntary limb movements. In contrast to a voluntary step, which is invariably preceded by a large APA, the APA is small or even absent during CIS reactions. The lack of APA shortens the time to unload the limb, but at the cost of increasing medio–lateral instability.[60] The typical CIS strategy of a young subject is a single step, but older subjects take more steps and the second step is often a lateral one, suggesting that they have difficulty controlling the tendency of the COM to fall to the unsupported side during stepping. Rather than using a cross-over step, elderly subjects take a sequence of small side steps.[61] Why there is this change in strategy is not clear, but it is probably related to reductions in muscle strength, especially of the quadriceps, slowing in psychomotor speed and reduced plantar sensation due to loss of pressure receptors in the sole of the foot. In the control of compensatory stepping there appears to be a trade-off between speed and stability. A single-step reaction offers maximum stability, but where stability is already compromised, additional steps will be required.[62]

In PD, the compensatory step made in response to a platform perturbation produces perseveration of the APA. Instead of one weight shift over the stance foot before foot-off, the weight shifts between left and right foot several times with gradually increasing force until the last one is larger than in controls. As a result, the time to foot-off is significantly prolonged. This perseveration may be due to an inability either to trigger a step or to sequence stepping and posture quickly enough to maintain balance. Patients with PD fall frequently during these perturbations, especially when off levodopa and when distracted by a cognitive task. Levodopa improves both voluntary and compensatory stepping and reduces perseveration of the APAs.[63]

Some aspects of the APA are actually impaired by levodopa. The normal baseline tone particularly in tibialis anterior and quadriceps in PD patients is reduced by levodopa, so there is a reduction in the normal stiffness that resists perturbation and patients are unable to produce adequate bursts of muscle activity to correct the displacement.

Testing postural control is an important part of the clinical examination, but the usual retropulsion test – where the examiner stands behind the patient and gives a gentle tug on the shoulders – is a poor predictor of falls[51] and variability leads to inadequate evaluation of postural instability.[64] The first time the test is done is usually the most reliable, as patients learn what is expected. For research purposes a battery of four tests – tandem stance, single limb stance, functional reach, and external perturbation – distinguishes between fallers and non-fallers.

Effect of attention on posture

Postural control, even during quiet standing, is not entirely automatic and requires cognitive input. Patients with PD are at particular risk of falling when their balance is threatened if at the same time they are distracted by a cognitive task, especially when off levodopa.[65] Additional motor and particularly cognitive tasks have also been to shown to reduce gait speed and mean step length in PD patients.[66] It is postulated that competition for attention in these patients, who have an over-reliance on cortically-mediated attentional mechanisms, leads to the reduction in mobility. This may explain why studies of the use of cues in complex environments resulted in increased mobility, possibly by enhancing the attention.[67] The role of attentional strategies is clearly important in the rehabilitation of PD patients. Both rhythmic auditory and visual cueing have been shown to manipulate the speed of walking in patients with PD.[68,69] Developing a mental picture of an ideal stride size is as effective as asking patients to walk over lines on the floor in improving gait, and when distracted by cognitive tasks the deterioration in gait is proportional to the complexity of the task.

Effect of surgery on motor function

Motor problems in PD are associated with altered activity in the cortico-basal ganglia-thalamo-cortical loop, thus surgical manipulation at various sites within this closed loop can affect the clinical state. Neurosurgery is usually reserved for patients with advanced disease suffering from motor fluctuations and dyskinesias, or those with isolated severe tremor. Most surgery aims to reduce abnormally increased neuronal activity through thermo-ablation, deep-brain stimulation (DBS), or – less commonly – gamma knife radiation (associated with difficulty with lesion size and accuracy and radiation necrosis). The main target sites are the following.

1. Thalamus: thalamotomy and DBS are particularly good for tremor control (90% improvement in the contralateral side). Some studies report improvement in dyskinesias with lesioning of the posterior nuclei. There is no effect on bradykinesia.
2. Globus pallidus: pallidotomy is particularly effective in controlling contra-lateral dyskinesias, but a lesser improvement in ipsi-lateral dyskinesia has been reported up to two years after surgery.[70] There is an increase in dyskinesia-free 'on' time, and reduction in 'off' time and generally improvement in contralateral bradykinesia, rigidity and tremor. However, balance, freezing and bulbar problems are not helped. Pallidotomy may be more effective at reducing dyskinesia than globus pallidus interna (GPi) DBS. Bilateral pallidotomy is rarely performed due to an

increased incidence of worsening speech, swallowing, falling or cognition.
3. Sub-thalamic nucleus (STN): the surgery of choice is usually DBS rather than ablation. Tremor and bradykinesia can be markedly improved. Dyskinesia improves in most patients, and gait freezing in about one-half. Surgery on the STN has the advantage of a greater reduction in levodopa dosage than following pallidotomy/ GPi stimulation, and the requirement for lower stimulation parameters prolongs the battery life. A randomised controlled trial of DBS of the GPi versus the STN found that both improved 'off' motor scores, but STN stimulation improved bradykinesia more and allowed greater reduction in L-Dopa dose, but was less effective against dyskinesias and was associated with cognitive and behavioural complications.[71] Depression, hypomania, euphoria, mirth and hyper-sexuality have all been described after DBS, but permanent cognitive complications appear rare.[72] Gait laboratory studies on patient who have undergone DBS in either STN or GPi show that DBS improves step initiation: the force of lateral COP shift before a self-initiated step is increased, and the latencies of foot-off are reduced, this improvement being more marked with DBS than with levodopa. DBS also improves the scaling of automatic postural responses following a backwards platform perturbation, and this is not seen with levodopa.

Recent surgical strategies to augment the dopaminergic tone of the striatum and the substantia nigra have largely been disappointing. Transplants of human foetal mesencephalic tissue to the putamen produced little if any motor improvement, and many patients developed dyskinesias despite reduction/elimination of dopamine medication.[73] Similarly, infusions of glial cell line–derived neurotrophic factor (GDNF) to the putamen have been disappointing in phase 2 studies.[74] Intra-striatal implantation of human retinal pigment epithelial cells (which produce L-Dopa, and can be grown in culture and attached to micro-carriers) improved motor symptoms in one small study, and are now undergoing further evaluation.[75] Finally, a phase-1 human gene therapy trial is under way, based on the inhibitory neuro-transmitter GABA in the STN.

Conclusions

Patients usually find that their most significant motor problem is impaired balance control. Falls occurring as a result of this have a major effect on quality of life, and only when patients become chair-or bed-bound is there a reduction in fall risk. Levodopa appears to have little effect on preventing falls, but physiotherapy can be helpful in teaching patients to use visual/auditory cues and attentional strategies. Recent advances in surgery promise considerable improvement for patients with advanced disease and gait and balance impairment. The question of which non-dopaminergic pathways are involved in the control of balance still remains unanswered, and standardised, reliable functional balance tests, which can be used in the clinic, need to be developed.

REFERENCES

1 Hely MA, Morris JGL, Reid WGJ, *et al.* Age at onset: the major determinant of outcome in Parkinson's disease. *Acta Neurol Scand.* 1995; **92**: 455–63.

2 Bennett DA, Beckett LA, Murray AM, *et al.* Prevalence of Parkinsonian signs and associated mortality in a community population. *N Eng J Med.* 1996; **334**: 71–6.

3 Klawans HL. Individual manifestations of Parkinson's disease after ten or more years of levodopa. *Mov Disord.* 1986; **1**: 187–92.

4 Winter DA. *ABC of Balance During Standing and Walking.* Waterloo, Ontario: Waterloo Biomechanics; 1995.

5 Baloh RW, Fife TD, Zwerling L, *et al.* Comparison of static and dynamic posturography in young and older normal people. *J Am Geriatr Soc.* 1994; **42**: 405–12.

6 Lord SR, Rogers MW, Howland A, *et al.* Lateral stability, sensorimotor function and falls in older people. *J Am Geriatr Soc.* 1999; **47**: 1077–81.

7 Horak FB, Nutt JG, Nashner LM. Postural inflexibility in parkinsonian subjects. *J Neurol Sci.* 1992; **111**: 46–58.

8 Mitchell SL, Collins JJ, DeLuca CJ, *et al.* Open-loop and closed-loop postural control mechanism in Parkinson's disease: increased mediolateral activity during quiet standing. *Neurosci Lett.* 1995; **197**: 133–6.

9 Schieppati M, Hugon M, Grasso M, *et al.* The limits of equilibrium in young and elderly normal subjects and in parkinsonians. *Electroencephalogr Clin Neurophysiol.* 1994; **93**: 286–97.

10 Imms FJ, Edholm OG. Studies of gait and mobility in the elderly. *Age Ageing.* 1981; **10**: 147–56.

11 Bloem BR, Haan J, Lagaay AM, *et al.* Investigation of gait in elderly subjects over 88 years of age. *J Geriatr Psychiatry Neurol.* 1992; **5**: 78–84.

12 Winter DA. *The Biomechanics and Motor Control of Human Gait,* 2nd ed. Waterloo, Ontario: Waterloo Biomechanics; 1991.

13 Springer S, Giladi N, Peretz C, *et al.* Dual-tasking effects on gait variability: the role of aging, falls, and executive function. *Mov Disord.* 2006; **21**(7): 950–7.

14 Bloem BR, Gussekloo J, Lagaay AM, *et al.* Idiopathic senile gait disorders are signs of subclinical disease. *J Am Geriatr Soc.* 2000; **48**: 1098–101.

15 Nutt JG, Marsden CD, Thompson PD. Human walking and higher-level gait disorders particularly in the elderly. *Neurology.* 1993; **43**: 268–79.

16 Trenkwalder C, Paulus W, Krafezyk S, *et al.* Postural stability differentiates 'lower body' from idiopathic parkinsonism. *Acta Neurol Scand.* 1995; **91**: 444–52.

17 Yamanouchi H, Nagura H. Neurological signs and frontal white matter lesions in vascular Parkinsonism. *Stroke.* 1997; **28**: 965–9.

18 van Zagten M, Lodder J, Kessels F. Gait disorders and Parkinsonian signs in patients with stroke related to small deep infarcts and white matter lesions. *Mov Disord.* 1998; **13**: 89–95.

19 Piccini P, Pavese N, Canapicchi R, *et al.* White matter hyperintensities in Parkinson's disease. *Arch Neurol.* 1995; **952**: 191.

20 Kuhtz-Buschbeck JP, Jöhnk K, Mäder S, *et al.* Analysis of gait in cervical myelopathy. *Gait Posture.* 1999; **9**: 184–9.

21 Mitchell SL. Extrapyramidal features in Alzheimer's disease. *Age Ageing.* 1999; **28**: 401–9.

22 Martin JP. *The Basal Ganglia and Posture.* London: Pitman Medical; 1967.

23 Morris ME, McGinley J, Huxham F, *et al.* Constraints on the kinetic, kinematic and spatiotemporal parameters of gait in Parkinson's disease. *J Hum Movement Sci.* 1999; **18**: 461–83.

24 Crenna P, Frigo C, Giovannini P, *et al.* The initiation of gait in Parkinson's disease. *Motor Disturbances.* 1990; **II**: 161–73.

25 Lee RG, Tonolli I, Viallet F, *et al.* Preparatory postural adjustments in Parkinsonian patients with postural instability. *Can J Neurol Sci.* 1995; **22**: 126–35.

26 Halliday SE, Winter DA, Frank JS, *et al.* The initiation of gait in young elderly and Parkinson's disease subjects. *Gait Posture.* 1998; **8**: 8–14.

27 Georgiou N, Iansek R, Bradshaw JL, *et al.* An evaluation of the role of internal cues in the pathogenesis of Parkinsonian hypokinesia. *Brain.* 1993; **116**: 1575–87.

28 Olanow W, Schapira AH, Rascol O. Continuous dopamine-receptor stimulation in early Parkinson's disease. *Trends Neurosci.* 2000; **23** (Suppl.): S117–S126.

29 Quinn NP. Classification of fluctuations in patients with Parkinson's disease. *Neurology.* 1998; **51** (Suppl. 2): S25–S29.

30 Giladi N, McDermott MP, Fahn S, *et al.* Freezing of gait in PD: prospective assessment in the DATATOP cohort. *Neurology.* 2001; **56**(12): 1712–21.

31 Gurevich T, Giladi N. Freezing of gait in multiple system atrophy (MSA). *Parkinsonism Relat Disord.* 2003; **9**(3): 169–74.

32 Shoulson I, Oakes D, Fahn S, *et al.* Impact of sustained deprenyl (selegiline) in levodopa-treated Parkinson's disease: a randomized placebo-controlled extension of the deprenyl and tocopherol antioxidative therapy of parkinsonism trial. *Ann Neurol.* 2002; **51**: 604.

33 Shabtai H, Treves TA, Korczyn AD, *et al.* Freezing of gait in patients with advanced Parkinson's disease. Poster, International Symposium on Gait Disorders; 1999; Prague.

34 Sandyk R. Freezing of gait in Parkinson's disease is improved by treatment with weak electromagnetic fields. *Int J Neurosci.* 1996; **85**: 111–24.

35 Fabre N, Brefel C, Sabatini U, *et al.* Normal frontal perfusion in patients with frozen gait. *Mov Disord.* 1998; **13**: 677–83.

36 Iansek R, Huxman F, McGinley J. The sequence effect and gait festination in Parkinson disease: contributors to freezing of gait? *Mov Disord.* 2006; **21**(9): 1419–24.

37 Bond JM, Morris M. Goal-directed secondary motor tasks: their effects on gait in subjects with Parkinson disease. *Arch Phys Med Rehabil.* 2000; **81**(1): 110–6.

38 Nieuwboer A, Dom R, De Weerdt W, *et al.* Abnormalities of the spatiotemporal characteristics of gait at the onset of freezing in Parkinson's disease. *Mov Disord.* 2001; **16**(6): 1066–75.

39 Giladi N, Gurevich T, Shabtai H, *et al.* The effect of botulinum toxin injections to the calf muscles on freezing of gait in parkinsonism: a pilot study. *J Neurol.* 2001; **248**(7): 572–6.

40 Shrag A, Quinn N. Dyskinesias and motor fluctuations in Parkinson's disease: a community-based study. *Brain.* 2000; **123** (Part 11): 2297–305.

41 Marras C, Lang A, Krahn M, *et al.* Parkinson Study Group. Quality of life in early Parkinson's disease: impact of dyskinesias and motor fluctuations. *Mov Disord.* 2004; **19**(1): 22–8.

42 Manson AJ, Turner K, Lees AJ. Apomorphine monotherapy in the treatment of refractory motor complications of Parkinson's disease: long-term follow-up study of 64 patients. *Mov Disord.* 2002; **17**(6): 1235–41.

43 Morris ME, Huxham F, McGinley J, *et al.* The biomechanics and motor control of gait in Parkinson's disease. *Clin Biomechanics.* 2001; **16**(6): 459–70.

44 Charlett A, Weller C. Breadth of base whilst walking: effect of ageing and parkinsonism. *Age Ageing.* 1998; **27**: 49–54.

45 Jueptner M, Weiller C. A review of differences between basal ganglia and cerebellar control of movements as revealed by functional imaging studies. *Brain.* 1998; **121**: 1437–49.

46 Bowes SG, Dobbs RJ, Henley M, *et al.* Objective evidence for tolerance, against a background of improvement, during maintenance therapy with controlled release levodopa/carbidopa. *Eur J Clin Pharmacol.* 1992; **43**(5): 483–9.

47 Ebersbach G, Sojer M, Valldeoriola F, *et al.* Comparative analysis of gait in Parkinson's disease, cerebellar ataxia and sub-cortical arteriosclerotic encephalopathy. *Brain.* 1999; **122**: 1349–55.

48 Steiger MJ, Thompson PD, Marsden CD. Disordered axial movement in Parkinson's disease. *J Neurol Neurosurg Psychiatry.* 1996; **61**: 645–8.

49 Duncan G, Wilson JA. Extrapyramidal signs in dementia of Alzheimer type. *Lancet.* 1989; **ii**: 1392.

50 Wood BH, Bilclough JA, Bowron A, *et al.* Incidence and prediction of falls in Parkinson's disease: a prospective multidisciplinary study. *J Neurol Neurosurg Psychiatry.* 2002; **72**: 721–5.

51 Ashburn A, Stack E, Pickering RP, *et al.* Predicting fallers in a community-based sample of people with Parkinson's disease. *Gerontology.* 2001; **47**: 277–81.

52 Bloem BR, Hausdorff JM, Visser JE, *et al.* Falls and freezing of gait in Parkinson's disease: a review of two interconnected, episodic phenomena. *Mov Disord.* 2004; **19**(8): 871–84.

53 Maki BE, McIlroy WE. Postural control in the older adult. *Clin Geriatric Med.* 1996; **12**: 635–58.

54 Overstall PW. Falls. *Rev Clin Gerontol.* 1992; **2**: 31–8.

55 Colledge N. Falls. *Rev Clin Gerontol.* 1997; **7**: 309–15.

56 Johnell O, Melton ILJ, Atkinson EJ, *et al.* Fracture risk in patients with parkinsonism: a population based study in Olmsted County, Minnesota. *Age Ageing.* 1992; **21**: 32–8.

57 Hely MA, Morris JGL, Traficante R, *et al.* The Sydney multicentre study of Parkinson's disease: progression and mortality at 10 years. *J Neurol Neurosurg Psychiatry.* 1999; **67**: 300–7.

58 Rogers MW. Disorders of posture, balance and gait in Parkinson's disease. *Clin Geriatric Med.* 1996; **12**: 825–45.

59 Bloem BR, Beckley DJ, van Dijk JG, *et al.* Influence of dopaminergic medication on automatic postural responses and balance impairment in Parkinson's disease. *Mov Disord.* 1996; **11**: 509–21.

60 McIlroy WE, Maki BE. Controlling change-in-support reactions. *Gait Posture.* 1999; **9** (Suppl. 1): S10.

61 Maki BE, McIlroy WE, Perry SD, *et al.* Control of change-in-support reactions to whole body instability. *Gait Posture.* 1999; **9** (Suppl. 1): S10.

62 Maki BE, McIlroy WE. Control of foot placement during compensatory stepping. *Gait Posture.* 1999; **9** (Suppl. 1): S6.

63 Horak FB, Jones C, Nutt J. Patients with Parkinson's disease perseverate postural adjustments for compensatory stepping. *Gait Posture.* 1999; **9** (Suppl. 1): S9.

64 Munhoz RP, Li JY, Kurtinecz M, *et al.* Evaluation of the pull test technique in assessing postural instability in Parkinson's disease. *Neurology.* 2004; **62**(1): 125–7.

65 Rochester L, Hetherington V, Jones D, *et al.* Attending to the task: interference effects of functional tasks on walking in Parkinson's disease and the roles of cognition, depression, fatigue and balance. *Arch Phys Med Rehab.* 2004; **85**(10): 1578–85.

66 O'Shea S, Morris ME, Iansek R. Dual task interference during gait in people with Parkinson's disease: effects of motor versus cognitive secondary tasks. *Phys Ther.* 2002; **82**: 888–97.

67 The Rescue project. www.rescueproject.org (accessed 9 June 2006).

68 Willems AM, Nieuwboer A, Chavret F, *et al.* The use of rhythmic auditory cues to influence gait in patients with Parkinson's disease: the differential effect for freezers and non-freezers, an exploratory study. *Disabil Rehabil.* 2006; **28**(11): 721–8.

69 Van Wegen E, Lim I, de Goede C, *et al.* The effects of visual rhythms and optic flow on stride patterns of patients with Parkinson's disease. *Parkinsonism Relat Disord.* 2006; **12**(1): 21–7.

70 Metman LV, O'Leary ST. Role of surgery in the treatment of motor complications. *Mov Disord.* 2005; **20**(11): S45–S56.

71 Anderson VC, Burchiel KJ, Hogarth P, *et al.* Pallidal vs subthalamic nucleus deep-brain stimulation in Parkinson disease. *Arch Neurol.* 2005; **62**(4): 554–60.

72 Burn DJ, Troster AI. Neuropsychiatric complications of medical and surgical therapies for Parkinson's disease. *J Geriatr Psychiatry.* 2004; **17**(3): 172–80.

73 Olanow CW, Goetz CG, Kordower JH, *et al.* A double-blind controlled trial of bilateral fetal nigral transplantation in Parkinson's disease. *Ann Neurol.* 2003; **54**(3): 403–14.

74 Lang AE, Gill S, Patel NK, *et al.* Randomized controlled trial of intraputamenal glial cell line-derived neurotrophic factor infusion in Parkinson disease. *Ann Neurol.* 2006; **59**(3): 459–66.

75 Stover NP, Bakay RA, Subramanian T, *et al.* Intrastriatal implantation of human retinal pigment epithelial cells attached to microcarriers in advanced Parkinson disease. *Arch Neurol.* 2005; **62**(12): 1833–7.

11

Driving and safe mobility in Parkinson's disease

DESMOND O'NEILL

The importance of safe mobility

The irresistible rise of the internal combustion engine has had a profound effect on our society. In a little over one hundred years there has been a revolution in our expectations of safe and accessible transportation. Never in history have personal and public transportation been so widely available. This mobility is important at all ages and is particularly so in later life. At the White House Conference on Ageing in 1971, transportation was rated as third in importance in older people's lives, after health and finance.[1] This high ranking persists in the 2005 White House Conference on Ageing, with access to transportation ranked ahead of Medicaid and Medicare.[2]

There is also a negative cost to this ease of mobility, in terms of pollution, land use and injuries and deaths due to crashes. Deaths from road crashes are set to rise from ninth to sixth place in the Global Burden of Disability.[3] Society has accepted a certain toll from car crashes, and safety is not the overriding concern in transportation policies: if it were, speed limits would be fixed at 25 km/hr (20 mph) and car engines would be fitted with governors to limit their speed at this level. Convenience, financial efficiency, and other factors shape policy with equal force. A consciousness of this unstated but accepted level of risk should form the background to any discussion of transportation policies, particularly in the context of neurodegenerative illness. Medical approaches to illness and safe mobility are relatively under-developed, and in automotive terms are still at the stage of the man with the red flag walking in front of the car. Much of the medical and regulatory literature is couched in terminology which is negative. It seems more concerned with limiting personal mobility than with providing solutions to the question of how people with disease and disability can participate fully in society. Those sections which deal with fitness to drive concentrate on detecting those who cannot drive rather than enabling them to drive more safely and with ease.[4]

Enabling or policing?

Although the literature on enabling drivers is embryonic, the underlying philosophy is all-important. Patients attend their physician in the expectation of achieving health and social gain. Safe mobility, increasingly but not exclusively by means of driving, is a key function which needs to be safeguarded just as we attempt to do for continence, mobility and balance. The handful of empirical studies on driving in PD between 1999 and 2006 have also shown this bias, with an emphasis on risk rather than on mobility.[5-9] Although it is early to state yet, it is likely that even the perceived risk may be an overstatement of actual risk, representing selected populations and not taking into account restrictions on driving practices and mileage by the patients,[10] their carers and physicians. For these reasons, studies on driving in Alzheimer's disease seem to show this pattern: in public health terms, no clear increased risk for the group, but in clinical terms, a proportion of patients will present a dilemma for clinicians. As PD is an age-related illness, it is important to appreciate the changes in how older people fulfil their mobility needs. In developed countries, this is increasingly done by using cars. In the US, less than 3% of trips by older people are made using public transport. While the European experience is somewhat different, in the UK the car accounts for over half of trips of less than 100 km made by those aged 65–74. Older people are in general safe drivers: an oft-quoted statistic is that older drivers are involved in more crashes per kilometre travelled than younger people. However, not only do they drive considerably fewer kilometres than their younger peers, but at least two studies have shown that this finding is an artifact of low mileage – if low mileage is controlled for in comparisons with younger drivers, the difference in crash rate disappears.[11,12] Health is a major determinant of older driver ease and eventual cessation.[13] One estimate suggests that women will not drive for the last ten years of their lives, and men for the last seven years of their lives.[14] There is some concern that older drivers may quit driving without appropriate assessment and remediation of age-related disease. Older people who stop driving seem to have difficulty with adapting to public transportation: even when it is provided cost-free, they use it with a lesser intensity than those who have never driven, and loss of driving has been associated with entry to nursing home care.[15]

Models of driving behaviour

While the geriatrician is aided in the assessment and rehabilitation of problems with balance and gait by an understanding of the underlying mechanisms, driving is an even more complex task, and there has been a marked lack of progress in developing a comprehensive model of driving behaviour. At least five main types of model have been explored: psychometric, motivational, hierarchical controls, information processing, and error theory.[16] Because of the relative ease of measuring cognitive function, clinicians may look to psychometric measures as a means of assessing older drivers. A preliminary emphasis on psychometric measures relating to accident-causing behaviour has been faulted for having been conducted without the benefit of a process model of driving; for focusing primarily on accident-causing behaviours and not on everyday driving, and for relying heavily on post-hoc explanations. Motivational models which distinguish between drivers' performance limits and on-road driving offer a different perspective. For example, a pioneering Swedish study showed that when drivers are asked to remember road signs, the accuracy ranged from 17–78%, depending on the subjective importance of the sign, i.e. the amount of risk involved in ignoring the sign.[17] Early models assume risk to be a primary motivating factor; second-generation motivational models have given emphasis to motives other than risk, i.e. pleasure in driving, traffic risks, driving time and expense.[18] They also factor in concurrent activity at operational, manoeuvring and strategic levels and portray the driver as an active decision maker rather than as a passive responder, as was implicit in early information-processing models. The driver's allocation of attention depends on the immediate driving situation and the driver's motives which include the level of risk and other motives relating to the purpose of the trip. The main research interest is in identifying factors that influence the driver's allocation of attention among the tasks of the different control levels.

TABLE 11.1 A combined model of a control hierarchy and a automaticity/controlled processing scheme

	Strategic	Tactical/manoeuvring	Operational/control
Knowledge	Navigating in unfamiliar area	Controlling skid	Novice on first lesson
Rule	Choice between familiar routes	Passing other vehicles	Driving unfamiliar vehicle
Skill	Route used for intersection	Negotiating familiar curves	Vehicle handling on daily commute

Much of routine driving is done automatically. Automaticity, which is fast, effortless cognitive processing, can occur at all three levels of control and contrasts with control processing which is demanding of attention and resources. This automaticity can develop as a response to several types of stimuli and underlies much of experienced driving behaviour until knowledge-based problem solving is required. A combined model of a control hierarchy and an automaticity/controlled processing scheme is illustrated in Table 11.1.

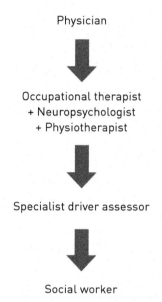

FIGURE 11.1 Assessment cascade.

A practical hierarchical approach

One practical scheme has been outlined, with an emphasis on a hierarchy of strategic, tactical and operational factors.[19] Strategic performance includes the planning of choice of route, time of day (avoiding rush hour), or even the decision not to drive and to take public transport. Tactical decisions are those aspects of the driving style which are characteristic of the driver and are consciously or unconsciously adopted for a great range of reasons. Examples are decisions on whether or not to overtake, whether or not to go through amber lights, or decisions to signal in good time before turning. Operational performance is the response to specific traffic situations, such as speed control, braking and signalling. Driving a car requires organisation of action at and between all three levels, and this model should be considered in assessments of fitness to drive.[20] Clinical assessment up to now has tended to dwell on deficiencies on the operational level, i.e. whether an illness affects the subject's appreciation of distracting stimuli or the reaction time to a hazardous situation. This emphasis is misguided: reaction time (a measure which is an integral part of operational tasks) is shortest in the 15–25 year age-group, the group with the highest accident rate.

This places the delayed reaction time noted in PD[21,22] in context. It is very likely that decisions at a strategic and a tactical level are much more important in causing accidents. Older drivers are known to use strategic and tactical measures widely to avoid delay, stress and risk by driving less at night and during bad weather, avoiding rush hours and unfamiliar routes. Drivers with PD also limit their mileage and their speed,[23] both of which are safety-enhancing manoeuvres.

The application of these three levels of function can be of practical help in decision making. This is illustrated by studies of drivers with acquired brain damage, particularly stroke.[24] Evidence for impairment at all levels may be collected by discussion with patient and relatives as well as by clinical observation. At a strategic level we would look for evidence of inappropriate planning of trips or lack of selective use of cars. Poor planning, poor judgement, lack of insight, and impulsivity affect both strategic and tactical levels. Impulsivity is attributed to disinhibition and/or cognitive impairment. Factors which interfere with the operational level include inadequate visual scanning of the environment, poor visual tracking, slowness in acting, and confusion when more complex acts have to be carried out.

Assessment

The methodology for assessment of, and intervention in, driving mobility is beginning to appear in the geriatric and rehabilitation literature, with chapters on driving assessment in two of the three main textbooks in geriatric medicine. This has paralleled the appearance of papers which show positive effects of interventions to improve driver ease and safety in the case of illnesses such as cataract and arthritis. The first step is the recognition of transportation needs as a relevant part of assessment of those with Parkinson's disease. This is not as clearly recognised as it might be: studies of patients with dementia,[25] stroke,[26] syncope[27] and arthritis[28] show a poor appreciation by healthcare providers of the interaction between disease and driving.

PD is of particular interest as it represents the most complex of all illnesses in terms of multiple influences on driving skills. The illness may involve the following:
➤ problems of motor function, including fluctuations, on/off syndrome
➤ depression
➤ impaired cognitive function
➤ tendency to sleepiness[29]
➤ impact of medications (both positive – enabling driving – and negative, including dyskinesia, neuropsychiatric effects or precipitation of sudden disabling sleepiness[30]).

Rather than stating that Parkinson's disease is dangerous for driving, it is vital to take a balanced approach, emphasising lost mobility as well as compromise in driving ability. The author can only find one study on Parkinson's disease and transport mobility (sometimes termed 'automobility'), suggesting that 20% of those with the illness were confined to home, compared with 1.5% of controls.[31] Clinically, a phenomenological approach is indicated. The depression and the motor function must be treated, psychoactive medications minimised, sudden onset of sleep and cognitive function assessed and managed before any decisions are made about the most appropriate approach to mobility, whether this involves using public transport or driving.

Assessment strategy

The schedule for the assessment of a driver with PD is akin to that of geriatric assessment of older people, a process which is marked by the following qualities: medical and functional assessment; detection and prioritisation of diseases; interdisciplinary assessment and remediation (*see* Table 11.2). Functional assessments, such as a comprehensive test of visual processing, a falls history, and a review of current medications may be of greater relevance than specific medical aspects in the identification of older at-risk drivers.[32] Early specialist referral may prove beneficial for the primary care physician who does not have access to an interdisciplinary team.

TABLE 11.2 Assessment process

History
• Patient, family/informant
• Driving history
Examination
Functional status
Other illnesses and drugs
Vision
Mental status testing
Diagnostic formulation and prioritization
Disease severity and fluctuations
Remediation
Re-assess
In-depth cognitive/perceptual testing
± On-road assessment
Overall evaluation of hazard
• Strategic
• Tactical
• Operational
Advice to patient/carer ± DMV
If driving too hazardous, consider alternative mobility strategies

A cascade system for interdisciplinary assessment is probably the most cost-effective way to approach the patient (*see* Figure 11.1). For example, if the physician detects visual acuity below the standard for the jurisdiction, referral to an ophthalmologist and maximal remediation of vision should occur before returning to the assessment cascade. Similarily, should a patient in the European Union have a homonymous hemianopia (one of the few absolute medical contra-indications to driving), then referral to the social worker for developing strategies for alternative transportation is the next step in the cascade.

Decision making

It is worth remembering that many dementia clinics do not use the same neuro psychological batteries. Their utility depends on the care that clinicians take in developing a liaison and familiarity with local occupational therapists and neuropsychologists, so that results can be taken in context. It is likely that the same approach is critical to good assessment practice in driving competency in PD.

To most clinicians, it is relatively easy to detect those patients who represent a low risk and those who represent a high risk for driving. A caveat to this is that one study showed that a single neurologist tended to overrate the driving performance of drivers with PD.[7] It is those in between who represent the greatest challenge. Using the meagre literature on PD as well as that of the dementias, we can glean some interesting information from various components of the assessment and treatment processes outlined above.

Disease severity scales

It is unclear whether there is a correlation between disease severity scales and driver performance. Although some report more crashes in the case of patients with a more advanced PD stage (Hoehn and Yahr stage 3), they conclude that disability scales do not reliably predict ability to drive.[33] Others found a similar link to disease stage (Hoehn and Yahr) but not to severity (UPDRS).[34] On simulator performance, there is again a confusing picture, with one study showing a correlation between performance and disease severity (Webster scale),[35] one showing a correlation with one measure of severity (UPDRS) but not with another (Webster scale),[36] and a further study suggesting correlation between both the severity (UPDRS) and the disease stage (Hoehn and Yahr).[37]

A Finnish on-road study showed no correlation with disease severity,[7] while an Australian study found a significant correlation with disease duration but not with motor severity scores (UPDRS) or stage (Hoehn and Yahr).[8] It is likely that in estimating safety to drive, disease severity scales and staging are secondary in importance to multidisciplinary assessment and occupational therapy/neuropsychology testing: however, they are clearly important as targets for remediation, and also as a focus in car choice and adaptation.

Sudden onset of sleepiness (SOS)

Although it was a study originally in the context of medication which triggered an interest in SOS and driving,[30] it has been long recognised that disorders of sleep and vigilance are part of the spectrum of parkinsonism.[38] Although estimates vary, the largest study so far suggests that 8% of drivers have experienced SOS at the wheel, but unfortunately this was carried out without a control group,[29] and sleepiness at the wheel is recognised as a risk factor for crashes for the general population, accounting for up to 10% of accidents.[39] It is possible that SOS may be associated with certain medications, but in reality it may occur whilst on any dopaminergic medication for parkinsonism. Although the makers of some synthetic dopamine agonists have stated on medication inserts that those on these medications should not drive, in reality a more considered position (as adopted in the UK) is to to advise patients taking all antiparkinsonian agents, especially ropinirole and pramipexole, that they may be prone to excessive drowsiness.[40] This may be compounded by the use of other sedative drugs and alcohol. Where SOS occurs, patients should cease driving until reviewed by a specialist, and medications should be altered until drowsiness and SOS are alleviated. If SOS cannot be alleviated, then alternative transportation options to personal driving should be sought.

Medication review

The potential and actual effect of drugs on driving may be an important factor in the safe mobility of older people,[41] and no journal article makes the point that good medication control helps transportation and driving. It is a complex area and very difficult to separate the effects of the disease from those of the medications. One complicated area is the use of the synthetic dopamine agonists, ropinirole and pramipexole. These have been associated with sudden, disabling and unheralded attacks of sleepiness. Eight cases have been reported with subsequent crashes: in five of these there was no warning.[30] Some of these patients were subsequently treated with other agents with no recurrence of these attacks. If driving is of importance to patients with PD, these agents should not be prescribed. Conversely, if a physician feels that this class of medication is important, patients should be counselled about driving and warned of the possibility that sleepiness will prevent them from driving.

The effect of other medications for PD is not well quantified. Overt neuropsychological side effects, such as drowsiness or psychotic phenomena, should be an indicator for driving cessation until the symptoms have resolved.

Mental status testing

Cognitive impairment or slowing has been found to correlate with an increased crash rate in PD.[5] There are no clear guidelines although there may be some guidance from studies of dementia and driving. Although a correlation has been established in numerous studies between various cognitive tests and driving skills in dementia – i.e. the MMSE[42,43,44] – this is not sufficiently well delineated to provide a useful screening measure. A consensus statement in 1994 could only state that at an MMSE of 17, drivers should have a further evaluation.[45] In view of the complex nature of the driving model, it is not likely that this approach offers much above its utility in the generic assessment of cognitive function.

Occupational therapy assessment

Although some good reviews on occupational therapy assessment in driving exist,[46,47] there is little yet by way of consensus for tests which are clearly superior in determining those who are and those who are not unfit to drive. It is likely that the opinion of an interested and experienced therapist, backed up by a standard test of cognition and perception is the most useful approach. Specific tests aimed at driving have as yet been disappointing.[48] A particularly interesting role for occupational therapy arises in countries where they are deeply embedded in the driving assessment process.

Neuropsychology tests

No specific battery has yet been established as being intrinsically helpful in the assessment of driving skills in PD. A thorough cognitive assessment is important. It has been suggested that the test battery should include the following measures: vigilance and concentration; visual perception; choice reaction times, and information processing in a complex situation. A battery including these measures correlated with an on-road assessment of driving ability.[7] More recent studies on those driving with PD suggest some additional insights from neuropsychological testing,[9,34] but the studies are small and it is difficult to truly blind experienced driving assessors or occupational therapists during assessments.

On-road tests

All patients, except the most severely affected, should have the right of access to a road test. A very large number of 'standardised' road tests have been described, some of which have been developed with healthcare professionals. Examples include the Washington University Driving test[49] and the Alberta Driving Test.[50] The results from the latter indicated that hazardous errors were the single best indicator of membership in a group of older drivers with early dementia. A regression analysis showed that five classes of driving errors accounted for over 57% of the variance associated with global ratings provided by expert driving instructors. Specialist driving assessors are available at a number of centres throughout North America. The discipline is achieving academic recognition, with university-level courses developing, e.g. Greenwich University in the UK, and addresses of centres for specialist on-road testing are available, i.e. from the Forum of Mobility Centres in the UK (*see* Appendix 2). A course of lessons may be prescribed to help the patient to adapt to any deficits uncovered during the assessment. The on-road test may also be invaluable for advising on car adaptation or choice if the patient is changing cars. Large door apertures, high chassis, built-up keys, mirrors and controls as well as power steering and automatic gears may help certain patients.

Advising the patient

All assessments and advice should be documented in the patient's file. The driver should be advised to consult the documentation from both their insurance companies and driving licensing authorities with regard to disclosure. The patient should be advised to re-attend for review at six- to twelve-month intervals – or sooner, should they or their carer detect any deterioration in driving habits. There is some early data to suggest that restrictions to driving locally, and by day, may be associated with fewer accidents in drivers with medical impairments.[51]

When driving is no longer possible

When driving cessation is indicated, it is important to explore alternatives with the patient. Intervention by a sympathetic social worker may be helpful, and he or she can work though the various options available to the patient. Public transport, even if free, is often irrelevant to older, compromised adults. Older drivers who stop driving have been shown to use public transport less frequently than those who have never driven.[52] Family members may be able to provide some driving input. The ideal situation is to provide a system of 'paratransit': affordable, tailored individual transportation. Various models have been developed (an excellent example is the service in Portland, Maine), but the funding remains problematic.[53]

Dangerous driving: reporting to driver licensing authorities

The breaking of medical confidence by physician is not to be undertaken lightly. It is likely that there will be wide-ranging differences in the cultural acceptance of reporting, and only some indication of the issues can be given. In the United Kingdom and Ireland, standard practice is that confidentiality cannot be broken unless (i) there is evidence of hazardous driving, (ii) the patients has been informed of the risk but fails to stop driving, (iii) the family has been informed but cannot stop the driving. There is concern that reporting over and above this may deter patients from seeking treatment for treatable illnesses if they perceive their physician as an agent for the authorities. In Canada, the licensing authority seems to promote reporting, whether or not it is mandatory in the province. This pre-supposes a trust in the assessment procedures, as well as faith that patients with severe dementia will stop driving if their driving licences are removed. Clinical experience does not necessarily support the latter outcome, and working with the patient and the family seems more ethical and also more practical.[54,55]

The future

It will be important to develop specialist assessment centres which build on the expertise already developed. Already geriatricians on both sides of the Atlantic have produced guides for clinicians,[56,57] and this philosophy has also informed the recent excellent guide from the American Medical Association guide on assessing older drivers.[58] One emerging research trend further strengthens the role of the geriatrician in the process. Several epidemiological studies have shown a strong association between falls and crashes[32,59] and it is tempting to speculate that the assessment and interventions strategies for falls (an area of expertise for geriatricians) may be developed to aid in assessing and intervening in compromised driving ability in later life. Another area of interest is be the possibility of cognitive training, and studies are under way using the Useful Field of View, a dynamic measure of the functionally useful field of view.[60] Information technology may also be of help but the technology is at a pre-testing phase. The preservation of safe mobility will also require some adequate substitute for the car for those who can no longer drive. Patterns of usage are developed at an earlier age and in health: this will require careful education of transportation planners in order not only to include those with mental and physical disability in the development of transportation but also to make the integration of public and private transport seamless and to encourage usage of a variety of transport measures at all ages.

REFERENCES

1 Carp FM, Byerts T, Gertman J, *et al.* Transportation. *Gerontologist.* 1980; **12**: 11–6.
2 *Proceedings of the White House Conference on Aging*; 2005; Washington DC, USA.
3 Lopez AD, Murray CC. The global burden of disease, 1990–2020. *Nat Med.* 1998; **4**(11): 1241–3.
4 White S, O'Neill D. Health and relicencing policies for older drivers in the European Union. *Gerontology.* 2000; **46**(3): 146–52.
5 Dubinsky RM, Gray C, Husted D, *et al.* Driving in Parkinson's disease. *Neurology.* 1991; **41**(4): 517–20.
6 Lings S, Dupont E. Driving with Parkinson's disease: a controlled laboratory investigation. *Acta Neurol Scand.* 1992; **86**(1): 33–9.
7 Heikkila VM, Turkka J, Korpelainen J, *et al.* Decreased driving ability in people with Parkinson's disease. *J Neurol Neurosurg Psychiatry.* 1998; **64**(3): 325–30.
8 Wood JM, Worringham C, Kerr G, *et al.* Quantitative assessment of driving performance in Parkinson's disease. *J Neurol Neurosurg Psychiatry.* 2005; **76**(2): 176–80.
9 Stolwyk RJ, Charlton JL, Triggs TJ, *et al.* Neuropsychological function and driving ability in people with Parkinson's disease. *J Clin Exp Neuropsychol.* 2006; **28**(6): 898–913.
10 Campbell MK, Bush TL, Hale WE. Medical conditions associated with driving cessation in community-dwelling, ambulatory elders. *J Gerontol.* 1993; **48**(4): S230–4.
11 Hakamies-Blomqvist L, Ukkonen T, O'Neill D. Driver ageing does not cause higher accident rates per mile. *Transportation Research Part F, Traffic Psychology and Behaviour.* 2002; **5**: 271–4.
12 Langford J, Methorst R, Hakamies-Blomqvist L. Older drivers do not have a high crash risk: a replication of low mileage bias. *Accid Anal Prev.* 2006; **38**(3): 574–8.
13 Anstey KJ, Windsor TD, Luszcz MA, *et al.* Predicting driving cessation over 5 years in older adults: psychological well-being and cognitive competence are stronger predictors than physical health. *J Am Geriatr Soc.* 2006; **54**(1): 121–6.
14 Foley DJ, Heimovitz HK, Guralnik JM, *et al.* Driving life expectancy of persons aged 70 years and older in the United States. *Am J Public Health.* 2002; **92**(8): 1284–9.
15 Freeman EE, Gange SJ, Munoz B, *et al.* Driving status and risk of entry into long-term care in older adults. *Am J Public Health.* 2006; **96**(7): 1254–9.
16 Ranney TA. Models of driving behaviour: a review of their evolution. *Accid Anal and Prev.* 1994; **26**(6): 733–50.
17 Johansson G, Backlund F. Drivers and road signs. *Ergonomics.* 1970; **13**(6): 749–59.
18 Rothengatter T, de Bruin R. Risk and the absence of pleasure: a motivational approach to modelling road user behaviour. *Ergonomics.* 1988; **31**: 599–607.
19 Michon JA. A critical review of driver behaviour models: what do we know, what should we do? In: Evans L, Schwing RC, editors. *Human Behaviour and Traffic Safety.* New York: Plenum; 1985: 487–525.
20 De Raedt R, Ponjaert-Kristoffersen I. Can strategic and tactical compensation reduce crash risk in older drivers? *Age Ageing.* 2000; **29**(6): 517–21.
21 Bloxham CA, Dick DJ, Moore M. Reaction times and attention in Parkinson's disease. *J Neurol Neurosurg Psychiatry.* 1987; **50**: 1178–83.

22 Jahanshani M, Brown RG, Marsden CD. Simple and choice reaction time and use of advance information for motor preparation in Parkinson's disease. *Brain.* 1992; **115**: 539–64.

23 Gimenez-Roldan S, Dobato JL, Mateo D. Vehicle drivers with Parkinson disease: behavior schedules of a patient sample from the Community of Madrid. *Neurologia.* 1998; **13**(1): 13–21.

24 van Zomeren AH, Brouwer WH, Minderhoud JM. Acquired brain damage and driving: a review. *Arch Phys Med Rehabil.* 1987; **68**: 697–705.

25 O'Neill D, Neubauer K, Boyle M, *et al.* Dementia and driving. *J R Soc Med.* 1992; **85**(4): 199–202.

26 Fisk GD, Owsley C, Pulley LV. Driving after stroke: driving exposure, advice, and evaluations. *Arch Phys Med Rehabil.* 1997; **78**(12): 1338–45.

27 MacMahon M, O'Neill D, Kenny RA. Syncope: driving advice is frequently overlooked. *Postgrad Med J.* 1996; **72**(851): 561–3.

28 Thevenon A, Grimbert P, Dudenko P, *et al.* Polarthrite rhumatoïde et conduite automobile. *Rev Rhum Mal Osteoartic.* 1989; **56**(1): 101–3.

29 Meindorfner C, Korner Y, Moller JC, *et al.* Driving in Parkinson's disease: mobility, accidents, and sudden onset of sleep at the wheel. *Mov Disord.* 2005; **20**(7): 832–42.

30 Frucht S, Rogers JD, Greene PE, *et al.* Falling asleep at the wheel: motor vehicle mishaps in persons taking pramipexole and ropinirole. *Neurology.* 1999; **52**(9): 1908–10.

31 Tison F, Barberger-Gateau P, Dubroca B, *et al.* Dependency in Parkinson's disease: a population-based survey in nondemented elderly subjects. *Mov Disord.* 1997; **12**(6): 910–5.

32 Sims RV, Owsley C, Allman RM, *et al.* A preliminary assessment of the medical and functional factors associated with vehicle crashes by older adults [see comments]. *J Am Geriatr Soc.* 1998; **46**(5): 556–61.

33 Dubinsky RM, Williamson A, Gray CS, *et al.* Driving in Alzheimer's disease [see comments]. *J Am Geriatr Soc.* 1992; **40**(11): 1112–6.

34 Grace J, Amick MM, D'Abreu A, *et al.* Neuropsychological deficits associated with driving performance in Parkinson's and Alzheimer's disease. *J Int Neuropsychol Soc.* 2005; **11**(6): 766–75.

35 Madeley P, Hulley JL, Wildgust H, *et al.* Parkinson's disease and driving ability. *J Neurol Neurosurg Psychiatry.* 1990; **53**(7): 580–2.

36 Lings S, Dupont E. Driving with Parkinson's disease: a controlled laboratory investigation [see comments]. *Acta Neurol Scand.* 1992; **86**(1): 33–9.

37 Zesiewicz TA, Cimino CR, Malek AR, *et al.* Driving safety in Parkinson's disease. *Neurology.* 2002; **59**(11): 1787–8.

38 Dhawan V, Healy DG, Pal S, *et al.* Sleep-related problems of Parkinson's disease. *Age Ageing.* 2006; **35**(3): 220–8.

39 Radun I, Summala H. Sleep-related fatal vehicle accidents: characteristics of decisions made by multidisciplinary investigation teams. *Sleep.* 2004; **27**(2): 224–7.

40 Parkinson's Disease Society. *Parkinson's and Driving.* London: Parkinson's Disease Society; 2002.

41 Alvarez FJ, Del Rio MC. Drugs and driving. *Lancet.* 1994; **344**: 282.

42 Fitten LJ, Perryman K, Ganzell S, *et al.* Driving ability and Alzheimer's disease: a prospective field and laboratory study. *Gerontologist.* 1991; **31** (special issue II): 88–9.

43 Fox GK, Bowden SC, Bashford GM, *et al.* Alzheimer's disease and driving: prediction and assessment of driving performance. *J Am Geriatr Soc.* 1997; **45**(8): 949–53.

44 Odenheimer GL, Beaudet M, Jette AM, *et al.* Performance-based driving evaluation of the elderly driver: safety, reliability, and validity. *J Gerontol.* 1994; **49**(4): M153–9.

45 Lundberg C, Johansson K, Ball K, *et al.* Dementia and driving: an attempt at consensus. *Alzheimer Dis Assoc Disord.* 1997; **11**(1): 28–37.

46 Quigley FL, DeLisa JA. Assessing the driving potential of cerebral vascular patients. *Am J Occupational Therapy.* 1983; **37**: 474–8.

47 Taira ED, editor. *Assessing the Driving Ability of the Elderly*. Binghampton, NY: Haworth Press; 1989.

48 Mitchell RK, Castledent CM, Fanthome YC. Driving, Alzheimer's disease and ageing: a potential cognitive screening device for all elderly drivers. *International Journal of Geriatric Psychiatry*. 1995; **10**: 865–9.

49 Hunt LA, Murphy CF, Carr D, *et al.* Environmental cueing may affect performance on a road test for drivers with dementia of the Alzheimer type. *Alzheimer Dis Assoc Disord*. 1997; **11** (Suppl. 1): 13–6.

50 Dobbs AR, Heller RB, Schopflocher D. A comparative approach to identify unsafe older drivers. *Accid Anal Prev*. 1998; **30**(3): 363–70.

51 Vernon DD, Diller EM, Cook LJ, *et al.* Evaluating the crash and citation rates of Utah drivers licensed with medical conditions, 1992–1996. *Accid Anal Prev*. 2002; **34**: 237–46.

52 O'Neill D, Bruce I, Kirby M, *et al.* Older drivers, driving practices and health issues. *Clin Gerontology*. 2000; **10**: 181–91.

53 Freund K. Independent Transportation Network: alternative transportation for the elderly. *TR News*. 2000; **206**: 3–12.

54 Bahro M, Silber E, Box P, *et al.* Giving up driving in Alzheimer's disease: an integrative therapeutic approach. *Int J Geriatr Psychiatry*. 1995; **10**: 871–4.

55 Donnelly RE, Karlinsky H. The impact of Alzheimer's disease on driving ability: a review. *J Geriatr Psychiatry Neurol*. 1990; **3**(2): 67–72.

56 Carr DB. Assessing older drivers for physical and cognitive impairment. *Geriatrics*. 1993; **48**(5): 46–8, 51.

57 O'Neill D. The older driver. *Rev Clin Gerontology*. 1996; **6**: 295–302.

58 American Medical Association. *Assessing Fitness to Drive in Older People*. Chicago: AMA; 2003.

59 Marottoli RA, Cooney LM Jr, Wagner R, *et al.* Predictors of automobile crashes and moving violations among elderly drivers [see comments]. *Ann Intern Med*. 1994; **121**(11): 842–6.

60 Ball K, Owsley C. Predicting vehicle crashes in the elderly: who is at risk? In: Johansson K, Lundberg C, editors. *Aging and Driving*. Stockholm: Karolinska Institutet; 1994: 1–2.

PART 5

Therapy and management

12

Organisation of services and health economics

DOUG MACMAHON AND SUE THOMAS

Introduction

Parkinson's disease (PD) has a considerable impact upon the mental, emotional and physical well-being of those affected. Not only does it impinge on the patient's lifestyle, but also that of their family and other carers. Both patients and carers are likely to require access to a wide range of services throughout the duration of the disease, as direct or indirect consequences of the condition or of its complications. While this may be true at all ages, elderly patients in particular, because of other co-morbidities, have need of a wide range of services that must be planned, co-ordinated, and well managed, in order to be accessible for people with impairment and disability. There is accumulating evidence that properly planned, accessible and integrated multidisciplinary services delivered by skilled, multidisciplinary teams can improve not only the care given to these patients, but also the quality of their lives and that of their carers – and in a cost-effective manner. This chapter investigates models of care, and introduces some of the current concepts of disease management applied to PD. It will also explore the context of the economics of providing this care and treatment, and the concept that appropriate team-working and disease management from diagnosis onwards can deliver better care by preventing or solving many of the problems that this disease may cause.

Services and structures

In the UK healthcare system, it is necessary to consider primary, secondary and tertiary healthcare; the role of the independent sector and social enterprise; local government and social services; self-care; volunteers (charities and voluntary societies such as the Parkinson's Disease Society UK), and – most importantly – carers. Devolution of government to the four UK countries – England, Northern Ireland, Scotland and Wales – has brought about a differing health and social care structure. The English system of health and social care will be referred to in this chapter but it should be recognised that, whilst there is not specific policy relating to PD in Wales, Scotland and Northern Ireland, policy for long-term conditions (which will include PD) exists. In Wales the NICE Guidelines for Parkinson's were commissioned jointly by the Welsh Assembly Government and thus also apply to health services in Wales. *Designed for Life* (Welsh Assembly) also outlines a future vision for chronic disease management services in Wales with an emphasis on early assessment, accurate and timely diagnosis and appropriate specialist service provision by a multidisciplinary team and support for self-management which is applicable to PD.

In Scotland systematic support for people with long-term conditions is a key requirement of *Delivering for Health*, the Scottish Executive's vision for the NHS. The overall direction of this policy is moving towards early interventional, community-based health services with multidisciplinary teams delivering patient-centred care. This contrasts with the traditional model of doctor-led hospital-focused services with high levels of unplanned admissions.

Primary care

All patients have access to a general practitioner, working in primary care with a host of community-provided health services. It has been suggested that with appropriate training and effective teamwork, primary care teams could manage complex chronic illnesses effectively. This model draws upon learning from other organisations and initiatives, such as the Expert Patients Programme, the Evercare model,[1] the American Kaiser Permanente approach and Supported Self Care. It is generally recognised that patients with long-term conditions such as PD need high-quality care which is personalised in order to meet their individual requirements and which will reduce the reliance on acute and secondary care services. However, it is also clear that they need education and support to make healthy choices about their lifestyle, diet and physical activity. A range of policy is influencing current delivery of health and social care:

➤ *Creating a Patient-led NHS*[2]
➤ *Your Health, Your Care, Your Say*[3]
➤ *Health and Social Care Green Paper*[4]
➤ *The National Service Framework for Older People*[5]
➤ *The National Service Framework for Long-term Conditions*[6]
➤ *The National Service Framework for Mental Health*[7].

These emerging policy drivers in the NHS outline three tiers of care for patients, similar to the model used by Kaiser Permanente in the USA. Each tier of patients will require a range of services and approaches which are adaptive yet specific to identified need:

➤ Level 1 – self-supported care and support for self-management for the 70% of people living with long-term conditions whose symptoms are fairly stable
➤ Level 2 – disease-specific care management from multidisciplinary teams to provide ongoing monitoring and review of patients with less severe clinical symptoms but who may be at high risk
➤ Level 3 – case management to provide intensive support for those with severe, complex problems, who are most at risk of hospitalisation.

Although the management of long-term conditions like PD has moved towards community-based systems of healthcare, referral to specialists – principally secondary-care-based neurologists and geriatricians – is required for their expertise and is the preferred model for diagnosis and ongoing care management in recently published guidelines.[8]

Secondary care

The delivery of care by a co-ordinated team of individuals has been assumed by many specialists (geriatricians and neurologists) to be a good thing, even though objective evidence has not been widely available. Patients are thought to benefit from the deployment of more staff, bringing the insights of different bodies of knowledge and a wider range of skills.

TABLE 12.1 The essential components of effective management of chronic disease

Treatment plans for each patient	Formal written plans help to organise the work of teams and help patients navigate the complexities of multidisciplinary care. Those that include patients' treatment preferences are more likely to result in satisfied, compliant patients.
Evidence-based clinical management	The identification or addition of team members to achieve greater concordance with complex treatment protocols by providers and patients has significantly improved outcomes in several chronic conditions.
Self-management support	Educational and supportive interventions directed at helping patients to change behaviour and become better self-managers have been shown to improve outcomes across a range of chronic illnesses.
	Effective interventions tend to emphasise the acquisition of skills rather than just knowledge, and systematically try to bolster patients' motivation and their confidence in managing their condition rather than encouraging dependency.
	The advantages of the team having a nurse or other professionals trained in behavioural counselling have been demonstrated in several studies.
More effective consultations	The limitations of a brief consultation with a chronically ill patient, who will have multiple needs, are obvious. Group consultations may provide a particularly efficient vehicle for the complementary functions of team care.
Sustained follow-up	Close follow-up ensures early detection of adverse effects, problems in compliance, failure to respond to treatment, and recrudescence of symptoms. It affords opportunities to solve problems and demonstrate the concern of the care team. Randomised trials have shown the effectiveness of telephone follow-up by other staff (including nurses) in chronic care.

During the past decade, intervention studies have begun to show clear advantages to people with long-term conditions when they are cared for by a team, within protocols designed to make best use of the particular team members' roles and functions (*see* Table 12.1). Consistently these have been associated with better outcomes. The involvement of – or even leadership by – appropriately trained nurses or other staff who complement the doctor in critical care functions (such as assessment, treatment, management, self-management support, and follow-up) has been demonstrated to improve adherence to guidelines. This can free the doctor to attend to those areas that only they have the training to complete; for example, diagnosis and medical treatment. The other elements – best performed by skilled nurses – include population management, protocol-based regulation of medication, support for self-management, and intensive follow-up (face-to-face, or by telephone). The participation of medical specialists in consultative and educational roles outside conventional referrals may also be beneficial. It is therefore apparent that sharing care between primary and secondary care would have significant advantages, and a specialist nurse can be in a pivotal position to facilitate these arrangements.

Self-care

Self-care is increasingly recognised as an important component of the management of all chronic illnesses, and has been highlighted as a government health priority in England and Wales. Patients are known to obtain information from a wide range of sources, although little systematic research has been carried out on the factors which inform healthcare-seeking decisions.

Concepts that have been developed for patient empowerment include telephone triage (e.g. NHS Direct); Expert Patient programmes, and the Working in Partnership Programme of self-care (www.wipp.nhs.uk/self-care). The concordance model of doctor–patient interaction may help understanding and implementation of self-care. The apparently insatiable demand of more traditional media (television and tabloid journalism particularly) for stories with medical interest demonstrates that the quality of this information may range between extremes of technical accuracy and nonsensical misinformation. Whether the spreading accessibility of the internet and other electronic media will improve the quality of this information or compound the distribution of inaccurate myths remains to be seen.

It is widely agreed that healthcare professionals need to understand patients' constructions of symptoms and illnesses better, and also their needs and expectations of healthcare – particularly in different cultural contexts. There is also a need to have a better understanding of the best ways of providing information in order to enable people to deal with their health concerns themselves. A better understanding of ways in which to help them use services most effectively and efficiently is equally important. This must be particularly true for conditions, such as PD,[9] with known cognitive elements.

Drawing on experience in asthma, partnerships with patients are central to effective disease control. Those teaching doctors and other healthcare professionals need to be aware of this and of the methodologies that can facilitate this approach.[10] Commercial disease-management partnerships may not be the most appropriate solution, for a variety of reasons – including professional and lay suspicion of commercial motives, and the results seen so far from such partnerships.[11]

Needs assessment

The needs of individuals with PD are frequently overlooked, and several surveys have shown under-recognition of cases in the community. Even once recognised, individuals often have a multiplicity of problems that change as the disease evolves, but that are often not recognised by the primary healthcare team.[12,13] Many problems (such as constipation) are easily dealt with once identified. However, many patients are only seen as result of a crisis occurring and therefore at a time when management is rendered much more difficult. Evidence is accruing that well-planned interventions can avoid such crises, with their attendant distress to both the patient and their family, and can not only improve quality of life but also reduce wastage of healthcare and social care budgets.[14,15]

Additionally, it needs to be emphasised throughout that the impact of this disease falls on a similar number of carers.[16] Carers typically perceive problems at and around the making of the diagnosis (when they may realise that this role may later be assumed by themselves), and also later in the complex and palliative phases when they perceive themselves as no longer able to cope. Referrals for residential and nursing-home care (with attendant cost implications) may be necessary – initially for respite care, and ultimately for long-term placement – and particularly when cognitive problems complicate the picture.

Services need to be designed to address each population group, recognising cultural, ethnic, and social issues as well as those related to the differing needs and wishes of patients at different stages of the disease. Information technology should be capable of informing and supporting disease-management packages. In addition to electronic communication, the value of a database – which could act as a disease register – has obvious potential. There remain issues of confidentiality, ownership of information (especially between different agencies) and also of commercial confidence. However, it is hoped that none of these is insurmountable and they are being addressed in the current discussion around electronic patient records and the National IT programme.

To make comprehensive plans for the whole of this population in one group is exceedingly difficult. This chapter will examine the issues involved in planning and delivering these services, and offer some solutions to the challenges raised. Owing to the complexity and scale of the problem, the chapter has been structured around the four-stage clinical scale developed to simplify the management of this disease (*see* Figure 12.1).[17] The average duration of each stage for patients with typical and atypical PD is given in Table 12.2.

TABLE 12.2 Audit of 'Pathways paradigm': duration of stages

Stage	Years (idiopathic)	Years (atypical)
Diagnosis	1.6 ± 1.5	1.8 ± 2.9
Maintenance	5.9 ± 4.8	3.0 ± 2.0
Complex	4.9 ± 4.4	3.5 ± 3.5
Palliative	2.2 ± 2.2	1.5 ± 1.2
TOTAL	14.6	9.8

Diagnosis

Idiopathic PD is a common, age-related, disabling neurodegenerative disorder. *Parkinsonism* is a term used to describe movement disorders characterised by similar symptoms to those of idiopathic PD. Idiopathic PD represents the cause of approximately three-quarters of cases of parkinsonism, the others being either similar neurodegenerative diseases with other features (Parkinson's–plus syndromes such as multiple system atrophy and progressive supranuclear palsy), cerebrovascular disease, and drug or toxic cases. In this chapter, the principles discussed refer to all causes

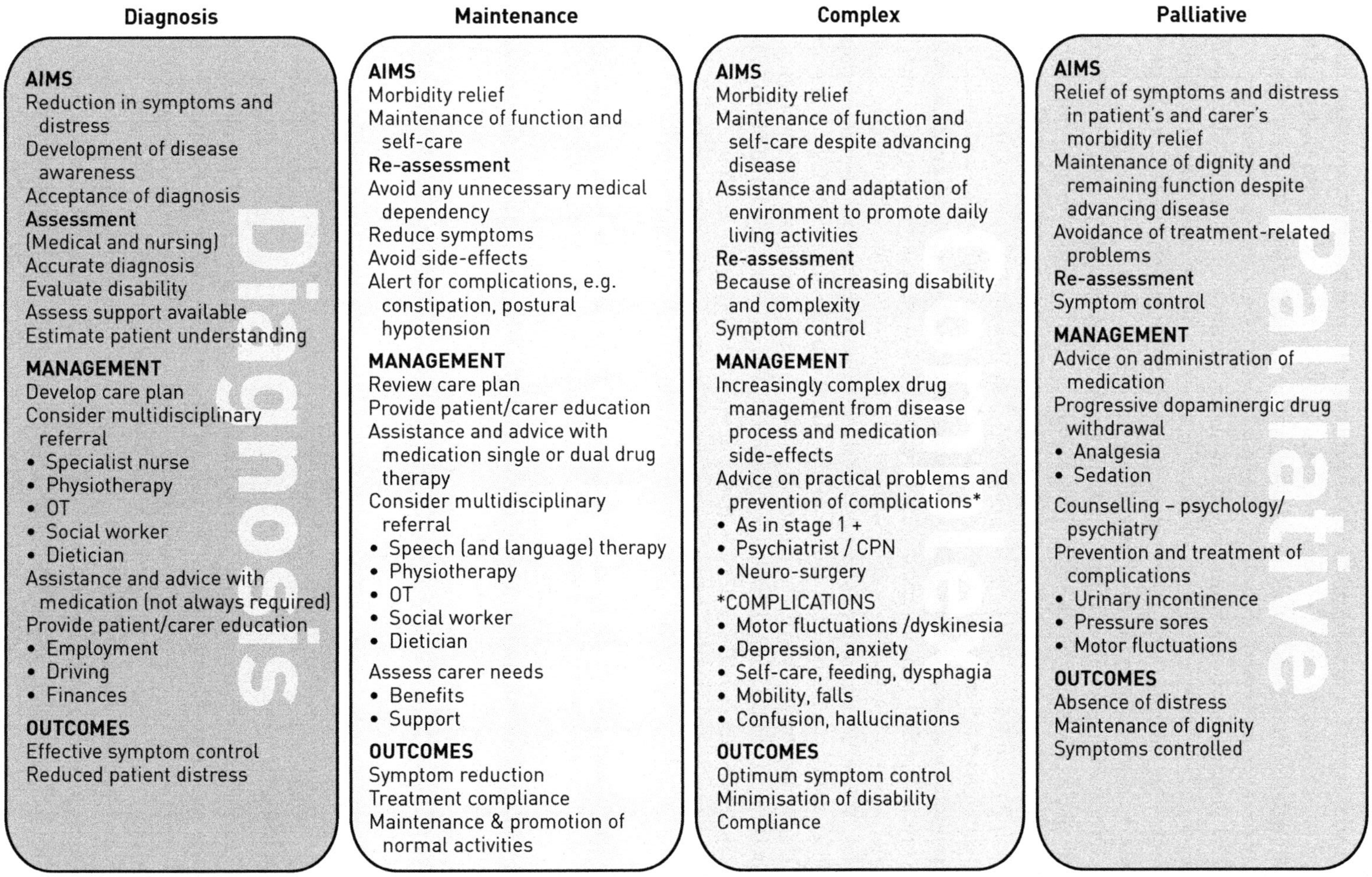

Diagnosis

AIMS
Reduction in symptoms and distress
Development of disease awareness
Acceptance of diagnosis

Assessment
(Medical and nursing)
Accurate diagnosis
Evaluate disability
Assess support available
Estimate patient understanding

MANAGEMENT
Develop care plan
Consider multidisciplinary referral
- Specialist nurse
- Physiotherapy
- OT
- Social worker
- Dietician
Assistance and advice with medication (not always required)
Provide patient/carer education
- Employment
- Driving
- Finances

OUTCOMES
Effective symptom control
Reduced patient distress

Maintenance

AIMS
Morbidity relief
Maintenance of function and self-care

Re-assessment
Avoid any unnecessary medical dependency
Reduce symptoms
Avoid side-effects
Alert for complications, e.g. constipation, postural hypotension

MANAGEMENT
Review care plan
Provide patient/carer education
Assistance and advice with medication single or dual drug therapy
Consider multidisciplinary referral
- Speech (and language) therapy
- Physiotherapy
- OT
- Social worker
- Dietician
Assess carer needs
- Benefits
- Support

OUTCOMES
Symptom reduction
Treatment compliance
Maintenance & promotion of normal activities

Complex

AIMS
Morbidity relief
Maintenance of function and self-care despite advancing disease
Assistance and adaptation of environment to promote daily living activities

Re-assessment
Because of increasing disability and complexity
Symptom control

MANAGEMENT
Increasingly complex drug management from disease process and medication side-effects
Advice on practical problems and prevention of complications*
- As in stage 1 +
- Psychiatrist / CPN
- Neuro-surgery

*COMPLICATIONS
- Motor fluctuations / dyskinesia
- Depression, anxiety
- Self-care, feeding, dysphagia
- Mobility, falls
- Confusion, hallucinations

OUTCOMES
Optimum symptom control
Minimisation of disability
Compliance

Palliative

AIMS
Relief of symptoms and distress in patient's and carer's morbidity relief
Maintenance of dignity and remaining function despite advancing disease
Avoidance of treatment-related problems

Re-assessment
Symptom control

MANAGEMENT
Advice on administration of medication
Progressive dopaminergic drug withdrawal
- Analgesia
- Sedation
Counselling – psychology/ psychiatry
Prevention and treatment of complications
- Urinary incontinence
- Pressure sores
- Motor fluctuations

OUTCOMES
Absence of distress
Maintenance of dignity
Symptoms controlled

FIGURE 12.1 A paradigm for disease management in Parkinson's disease.

of parkinsonism, since the problems of patients with parkinsonism are often similar to those of patients with PD, and the patients will often present with that diagnosis although their prognosis and response to treatment differs. Some units are organised to manage all movement disorders, of which PD is by far the most common.

To plan a service, it is sensible to quantify the number of cases that may need to access it. It is known that PD can occur at any age, but becomes very much more common in older age groups, with peak incidence in the seventh decade, and a prevalence of at least 2% in the ninth decade.

Other chapters will emphasise the fact that the diagnosis of PD can often be difficult, as each case is different and in some patients it may be quite difficult to distinguish PD from normal ageing or a number of similar conditions (parkinsonism) which have different, often worse prognoses. For this reason, referral to a specialist with an interest in this condition is recommended in all recently published guidelines.[8] Although most cases can be diagnosed sufficiently well on clinical grounds, NICE recommends that computerised tomography (CT) or magnetic resonance imaging (MRI) scans can be used by specialists to help with the differential diagnosis in atypical cases. While the definitive imaging is derived from positron emission tomography (PET) scans, single photon emission computed tomography (SPECT) scans are a cheaper alternative. Similarly, most cases will not require many haematological or biochemical tests, although in younger patients Wilson's disease should be excluded. On occasion, there is also a need to perform serological tests for syphilis.

For some patients, the time of diagnosis can be quite traumatic, and this distress needs to be handled carefully by an experienced multidisciplinary team. Depression can frequently coexist with anxiety at this time, and has a major impact on the patient's quality of life.

While the majority of patients will be able to cope at home for many years with the illness, older patients are more likely to suffer cognitive problems, and carry a higher risk of admission to residential or nursing-home care as a result of both physical and mental morbidity. PD carries a high mortality in such institutions, and evidence suggests that few patients admitted because of PD survive more than one year from admission.[18] While PD is a common cause of admission to institutional care,[19,20,22] it should be remembered that the condition can also develop in nursing-home residents.

Incidence

PD is estimated to affect 100–180 per 100 000 of the population (6–11 people per 6000 of the general population in the UK) and has an annual incidence of 4–20 per 100 000. There is a higher prevalence and incidence of PD in males, with a rising prevalence with age in both sexes.[8] One three-year prospective study showed that the average incidence of PD was estimated at 13 new cases per 100 000 population per annum. The mean age at onset is typically in the seventh decade, but in 1 in 7 cases the onset is below the age of 60 years, while 1 in 50 cases occurs below the age of 40 years.

Prevalence

Since PD is a chronic disease, it is not simply the incidence but also the prevalence that is an important factor in commissioning and providing services. World-wide age-adjusted prevalence ratios vary between 30 and 180 per 100 000, with a commonly accepted estimate in Western populations of 100–180, depending on demographic factors, especially weighting for age.[21] The prevalence rises to 2% of the population over the age of 80 years.[22] The prevalence of features of parkinsonism in the normal population is even higher (*see* Table 12.3).[23]

TABLE 12.3 Prevalence of parkinsonism

Age group (years)	Prevalence (%)
65–74	14.9
75–84	29.5
85+	52.4

Parkinsonism is not a benign condition, but has a mortality adjusted for age and sex which is double that of the control population (95% confidence interval, 1.6–2.6).[23] This difference was strongly related to the presence of gait disorders, and suggests that falls prevention strategies should be targeted on this group. There are also clear public health implications in this respect.

Thus, a health economy in the UK commissioning and providing care for a population of 500 000 can expect to have 800 adults with PD, and another 65 who will develop it each year. These will need to be distinguished from considerably more who will have features of parkinsonism.

Medical care

Most patients will have an established professional relationship with their general (primary care) practitioner. On suspicion of a problem, this is usually the first person to be consulted, and hence it is the general practitioner who starts the process of identification, diagnosis, and referral. Most GPs would concur with the UK guidelines and wish to refer a suspected case for confirmation of their diagnosis, and for the establishment of a plan for the patient's future treatment and care. Medical referral differs around the country, with younger patients almost universally being referred to a neurologist, while many older patients (and those with complex needs) are referred to geriatricians, the varied referral patterns depending on local expertise and resources. The UK differs from many other countries in that it has fewer neurologists, and a relatively well-established geriatric service. Since the majority of patients with disease are relatively elderly, geriatricians care for most. As most departments have established multidisciplinary teams, this has the advantage of facilitating access to therapy staff, particularly for more advanced cases.

While most cases will be cared for in primary and secondary care facilities, a few patients will need to access tertiary care centres, either because they have atypical features or because of difficulties with their treatment. The former category would include juveniles or PD appearing in relatively youthful persons, or suspected variants such as multiple system atrophy. These cases may require complex investigations (e.g. PET scans and/or chromosomal analysis) that are not normally required in the more typical, older cases. As far as the latter situation is concerned, neurosurgery is dealt with elsewhere in this book. In many other countries, neurologists take full medical responsibility for patients, irrespective of their age or circumstances. Whether 'managed care' or 'shared care' can improve the medical care arrangements remains to be seen.

The role of the PD nurse specialist (PDNS)

The value of the PDNS has been recognised and NICE guidelines[8] now suggest each person with PD should be referred to a PDNS. In the medical literature, most successful interventions in chronic diseases have utilised a nurse who has additional experience or training in the treatment of such conditions. The nurses may be nurse practitioners, advanced practice nurses or nurses with additional experience and qualifications in a particular chronic disease. The nurses personally case-manage patients by using local protocols, and adding clinical and self-management skills as well as a greater intensity of care than would be considered standard. In the UK, PD nurse specialists are now well established, and well-validated research has demonstrated their value.[15]

TABLE 12.4 PD core competencies (PDS, RCN PDNSA 2006)

1 Case management
2 Assessment
3 Symptom management
4 Medicines management
5 Referral to a multidisciplinary team (MDT)
6 Management through four stages
7 Assessing and managing complications
• Psychological problems
• Promoting independence
• Motor and non-motor fluctuations (including mobility and falls)
8 Providing support and advice to people with PD and carers
9 Accountability
10 Education and professional/personal development
11 Research and audit
• Surgery: Developing expert practice in functional surgical management

These nurses work in a variety of settings at the interface of primary and secondary care, including in geriatric and neurology units, and also in the community alongside general practice. Differing models have evolved according to local need and a suite of competencies for the role have been developed (*see* Table 12.4),[24] the main areas of their work being specifically around disease management and education of patients, carers and other professionals. Patient education is an important part of their role together with support and early identification of problems. This can ensure an improved quality of life for the PD patient and the prevention of complications. The breakdown of care in the community may be precipitated by ignorance of self-management strategies.

Lay health workers

The importance of lay health workers has often been underestimated by healthcare professionals. Community health workers have been shown to have important roles in bridging language and cultural gaps, especially between middle-class health professionals and culturally or ethnically different patient populations. Lay volunteers who have experience of certain illnesses have also been used to support and coach patients facing similar challenges. The effectiveness of self-management programmes led by lay workers has been shown for patients with arthritis and for those with chronic illness in general. The Expert Patient programme has, in a small number of locations, utilised lay workers in the management of PD, but this disease-specific programme is an area that requires evaluation.

Treatment

Treatment for PD has advanced in spectacular fashion since 1969, when *Brain's Diseases of the Nervous System*[25] gave standard therapy advice as: 'The sufferer should be encouraged to lead an active life as long as possible, but should avoid fatigue. A "zip" fastener on the trousers is a convenience.' As an afterthought, the sub-editor (presumably) inserted 'L-Dopa in doses up to 5 grams looks promising', heralding the new therapeutic age for PD.

Treatment strategies now include the following components:
➤ information and education
➤ health maintenance/promotion
➤ diet, exercise, and activity
➤ neurorehabilitative education and training strategies (occupational therapist and physiotherapist)
➤ drugs
➤ surgery.

It is generally agreed that there is no single way to treat and manage PD.[8] Controversies exist concerning initial treatment, and also the supplementary regimens required when initial treatment proves insufficient. To some extent therapy algorithms can provide graphical aids to assist decision making, and also suggest options. However, ultimately, decisions are individual, pragmatic, and require negotiation between the patient and their doctor, often assisted and informed by carers and other health professionals such as specialist nurses.

Early treatment: maintenance stage

The disabling effects of the disease can be reduced or limited with drug therapy, but when this should be initiated – and with which drug – remain individual decisions. Most specialists advocate that drug treatment be reserved until symptoms cause significant problems, or if there is difficulty in maintaining independence, employment or social activities. Essentially, the choice of initial treatment lies between levodopa preparations and other drugs (such as direct agonists or mono-amine-oxidase inhibitors, and in younger patients anticholinergics or amantadine), but this will be discussed elsewhere in this volume. To encourage the provision of some uniformity of care, algorithms and the NICE Guidelines have been published,[8] a further awareness document[13] expands on the care options for primary care, and a Scottish algorithm based on this awareness document is also available: www.pathways.scot.nhs.uk/Neurology/Neurol%20PD%2023Sep05.htm

Education, education, education

Many patients are hungry for information in the early stages, though others may be frightened or in a state of denial. This requires an individual assessment to be made of their wishes and needs, and such an assessment often involves both the doctor (usually a specialist) and specialist nurse and the provision of sufficiently detailed, but not exhaustive, information in an appropriate format. Often a carer will ask for written information, or a relative may seek information on the internet – and a list of appropriate sites is often willingly received (with advice to avoid the less stringently edited sites).

In addition, the potential of a highly effective clinical service may not be realised in practice because of a lack of appropriate education and knowledge among other healthcare and social care professionals. This is clearly a matter for those responsible for the design of undergraduate and postgraduate continuing medical education (CME), continuing professional development (CPD), vocational training schemes (VTS) and other educational programmes for the full range of healthcare professionals, including those who commission services or education. The British Geriatrics Society (BGS) PD Section has been instrumental in developing a masterclass for clinicians to provide a structured educational programme in PD management. (This is available via www.pdsection.org.uk.)

Maintenance therapy

The aims in this phase are for morbidity relief, prevention of complications, and the promotion and maintenance of good health. The main primary care team priorities are to be available for patients and their carers, and to be alert for complications. In order to care further for patients in primary care, the relationship and access to secondary care needs to be explicit and the primary care team may need to consider whether further referrals (or re-referrals) are indicated.

Many patients in this stage will access their hospital consultant occasionally (e.g. six- or twelve-monthly), but the availability of telephone contact has been shown to be highly beneficial in general terms, and specifically in PD. As far as possible, patients should be encouraged to avoid untoward admissions to hospital, and to develop coping strategies that minimise the impact of the disease. At this stage, specialist nurses and lay workers might provide valuable inputs, and tertiary care should have no role.

Complex care

In this phase, increasingly complex arrays of potentially toxic drugs will be deployed to counteract the advancing effects not only of the disease, but also of its complications – many of which are, at least in part, iatrogenic. Ultimately, surgical options may be required, usually delivered from tertiary care (specialist neurosurgical units – typically in regional centres). In addition, throughout the care phase, a range of ancillary therapies will be required, including physiotherapy, occupational therapy, speech and language therapy, dietetics, chiropody, and also social care, advocacy and advice. Management in this stage should seek to avoid hospital admission for anything other than re-assessment and review and Community Matrons or district nurse team leaders may be utilised to case-manage patients in partnership with the PD specialist team.

Tertiary care includes specialist neurological and neurosurgical treatments that will be covered elsewhere in this volume. It will require specialist commissioning for the small numbers of patients currently requiring surgical treatment – unless research shows that better outcomes are obtained with earlier surgical approaches.

Palliative care

As Parkinson's disease has no cure it could be argued that palliative care is required from the point of diagnosis; indeed, recent thinking advocates this.[8] The main aims of palliative care are to relieve symptoms and distress for both patient and carers; retention of dignity is also paramount. The needs of patients in the final, palliative care stage are often underestimated.[26,27] At the time when their needs are at a maximal level, it may be difficult for them to visit a hospital (or even a community-based) specialist because of immobility and it may also be difficult to assess their needs in a typical outpatient environment. For these reasons, day-hospital attendance or domiciliary-based services – in which the specialists, including Community Matrons visit the home – may be easier. This has the additional advantages of not only facilitating a better assessment of the domestic circumstances and current problems, but also providing a platform to allow the diffusion of practical advice and guidance. This is especially true where the patient is in institutional care. To achieve these aims, often there is a need to progressively reduce and eventually even to withdraw dopaminergic drugs. There may be needs for other palliative measures such as analgesia or sedation, and for other therapies such as physiotherapy. However, the delivery of these modalities of care will usually be a function of residence – that is, the patient's own home, residential, or nursing home and, for a few, long-term hospitalisation. The services may be from community and/or secondary care, depending on circumstances and may include both health and social care.

Dementia is the major concern, and some longitudinal studies make concerning reading. The cumulative proportion of patients with PD who developed dementia in several longitudinal series have exceeded 50% at ten years.[28] An earlier paper published on this cohort (up to five years) suggested that age of onset, duration of PD and disability all correlated with the development of dementia. In addition, those who became demented had minor intellectual changes at inclusion, suggesting that even slight reduction in a generic mental test score (in this case a Folstein mini-mental test score of 25–29) may be significantly associated with the later development of dementia.[29]

The prevalence of PD in nursing homes has been variously estimated as between 5% and 10% of residents. While some may have developed PD since entering care, we know from American figures[18] that PD is a common cause of admission, and predictors of admission include hallucinations and the combination of both mental and physical disability. Those PD patients admitted to nursing homes showed a mean survival of less than one year, and all had died within two years.[19]

End-of-life care should take account of:
➤ Liverpool Care Pathway
➤ Gold Standards Framework
➤ preferred place of care.

Whilst the majority of palliative care can be given by the PD specialist team, liaison with palliative care services is useful for advice and support in difficult cases.

Specific roles of a palliative care service
Specialist palliative care services can provide the following support for people with PD:
➤ management of distressing symptoms, particularly pain, nausea and vomiting, breathlessness, anxiety/depression, insomnia
➤ support for end-of life decisions and planning
➤ support of the dying person and their family
➤ spiritual support, bereavement counselling
➤ advisory/liaison service; links to local palliative care resources and teams
➤ education of other professionals in how to provide palliative care and support
➤ description of service style: enabling patients and carers to understand how to access care and support.

Health economics: costs and 'burden'
Parkinson's disease has a major socio-economic impact on society that has not been extensively quantified, because of difficulties in estimating the prevalence, and in identifying and measuring costs.

It is the sum total of these factors that contributes to the 'economic burden' of this disease. The direct health costs reflect expenditure on drugs, primary and secondary care services, and are matched by direct social costs of domiciliary support, and residential or nursing-home care. Indirect costs consist of lost earnings, both of the individual patient with PD, and also of any carer. In addition, if an economic value were to be placed on time spent by carers in the processes of caring (including lost work and costing domestic and caring inputs at an economic rate), the sum total economic burden is vast.

NICE estimates the direct cost burden of PD to the NHS to be approximately £2298 (in terms of GB pounds in 1998)[30] per patient per year. Significant cost drivers include the onset of motor fluctuations and dyskinesias.[31] In addition, since the condition is a frequent cause of falls, and thus fractures, the costs may be rising as the population ages. The total annual cost of care including NHS, social services and private expenditure per patient in the UK has been estimated at approximately £5993 (GB pounds in 1998).[31] This results in direct costs of approximately £599 300 000 per year in the UK for 100 000 individuals with PD. Costs to the NHS were approximately 38% of the total costs. Total costs of care increase with age and disease severity.[30] The pharmaceutical industry estimated the cost of PD drugs in 1999 as £46 million. In addition, there has been an increasing range of drug and other therapeutic measures, including high-technology electrical functional stimulation and stereotactic surgery. UK estimates are typically lower than others for a variety of reasons, reflecting local practice. If the German costs were extrapolated to the UK scenario, this would increase the total cost of drugs to £140.5 million. Therapy and nursing costs are typically low, largely because of low referral rates in direct contrast to both professional and lay opinion.[32] Considerable sums are also expended on other issues, including the treatment of constipation, incontinence, or of erectile dysfunction which increase the hidden costs of this disease.

In terms of the 'burden of disease' the costs are even greater, when the impact on the individual, the family and society are considered. Work done by Professor Sir Brian Jarman investigating the value of nurse interventions has shown specialist nurses not only to be well received by patients and their carers, but also to be both effective (reduced mortality and fewer falls and fractures) and cost saving (approximately £300 per patient per annum).[15]

A British study[30] was conducted to evaluate a sample of patients with PD to calculate the true economic impact (direct and indirect costs) of PD. The mean direct annual costs per patient were found to increase from around £4000 at age 65 years to £9400 at age 85 years, and to over £19 000 in the highest-cost cases in nursing care. Total costs increased both with age and with advancing disease stage. In younger patients, the greatest single costs were drugs (11%) and lost earnings. In older patients, long-term institutional care was the greatest cost. An interesting phenomenon was that drug cost was inversely proportional to age, with drugs accounting for only 6% of total costs in older patients. Secondary health services account for an increasing proportion of costs with advancing disease (27% in Hoehn and Yahr stages 0–1; 62% in Hoehn and Yahr stage 5). The direct costs of patients cared for at home were found to be only 22% of those in long-term institutional care. A move to long-term care implies a net annual increase of almost £12 000 per annum, much of which is a cost falling upon individuals and their families in the present funding systems. These figures confirmed earlier predictions[32] that PD is an expensive disease, but quantified a much higher expenditure than the earlier study, with costs falling on patients, their carers, and both healthcare and social care agencies.[33]

Estimated direct costs of PD were:[34]
- ➤ £3500 to £10 000 per patient
- ➤ £7000 to £20 000 per GP
- ➤ £560 000 to £1.6 million per Primary Care Group (PCG).

Value is now being placed on audit data within local health economies, because of the need to meet Public Service Agreement targets. Meeting quality requirements within the National Service Framework for Long Term Neurological Conditions through use of specialist practitioners could keep patients within community settings and reduce care costs and hospital re-admission rates.

Expert opinion estimates that PDNS care can reduce admission for PD by 50%. Hospital in-patient and outpatient figures obtained from Hospital Episodic Statistics (HES) data in England showed 6313 admissions for PD in 2004/5. Using cost data of £1220 per admission (2006/7 Payment by Results (PbR) tariff), a PDNS could prevent admission for 3157 patients with a cost saving of £3 851 540.

Expert opinion suggests PDNS can potentially reduce outpatient care by 40% by taking over clinical monitoring and medication adjustment. Outpatient attendance for PD is estimated at 62 569 which is 14% neurology follow-up OP attendance (reference costs 2005). Based on HES data (2004/5), PD represents 14% of all finished consultant episodes (FCE) which has been used as the basis for estimating the proportion of OP attendance. Cost data of £103 per attendance was obtained from the 2006/7 PbR tariff. The above assumptions lead to an estimated saving of £6 million when providing this service by a PDNS.[8]

There are also costs savings associated with patient access to physiotherapy, occupational therapy and speech and language therapy. Although there will be cost implications in employment of extra nurses and therapists to meet quality requirements, overall cost savings should result (NICE Costing Schedule).

Further research has shown the cost neutrality of employing a PDNS.[15] A 2002 study demonstrated qualitatively the value of MS specialist nursing to patients and quantitatively to the NHS: a cost saving of £64 611.45p net per annum in bed days and unplanned admissions comparing a year pre- and a year post-nursing appointment.

Commissioning services in the new NHS

Chronic illness is increasingly recognised as the dominant feature of healthcare expenditure. Its impact on health services will grow with increased focus on disability, the move towards managed healthcare, lay expectations about the benefits from health-care, and the anticipated growth of the elderly population in all societies. As a relatively common chronic disabling disease, PD has a widespread impact upon patients, carers, social services, and primary and secondary health services, and is a common cause of admissions to institutional care. However, there is evidence that these services are currently often poorly structured and unco-ordinated. In a number of studies, and even more anecdotes, it has been demonstrated that the health and well-being of patients with chronic progressive neurological diseases can be significantly improved through a well-developed service.

There is mounting evidence that a properly planned and commissioned service would better deliver these services; in addition, there are also data to suggest that this approach would deliver more effective care more cost-effectively.

It is vitally important that services for people with PD are commissioned in an appropriate way, as prior development has largely been ad hoc with responsive, specialist services developing through local 'champions' spearheading services rather than as a result of a needs-based approach to care. There is now a drive towards primary care-led commissioning which is likely to be led by primary healthcare clinicians, particularly GPs using their knowledge of patients' needs and services combined with a requirement to meet government-led targets and exert budgetary control over resources. Primary care-led commissioning will involve the devolution of resources, decision-making power over the use of these resources and accountability for their use – either to individual practices or to groups of practices – with general practitioners (GPs) driving the commissioning process, in part through the leverage that budgetary control brings.

Primary care-led commissioning is also a part of the trend visible in NHS policy intended to challenge specialist and hospital providers and to bring about a shift in the balance of power within the system so that a primary care perspective and community-based alternatives to hospitals are given greater consideration when resource allocation decisions are made. One of the key requirements identified in managing PD effectively, however, is referral to a specialist clinician in PD for diagnosis and onward referral to the specialist PD team which, to date, has largely been secondary-care based. Changes in the specification and configuration of services will, in future, see services commissioned through practice-based commissioning (PbC) and payment by results (PbR).

Demands for the service

Evidence about consumers' perspectives on PD services is growing. International interest has also been focused on the neurodegenerative diseases, and in 1997 the World Health Organization made PD a public health priority. With an increasingly ageing population and greater public awareness, demands for comprehensive PD services are predicted to increase further during the next few decades.

Sustained improvements in managing chronic diseases require better practice systems, improvement in doctors' skills, and more effective use of non-physician providers. Practice system changes that have shown the greatest promise of success integrate self-management support programmes, guideline-based treatment plans, nurse case management, more intensive follow-up, and registries that provide reminders and feedback.[35]

In summary, planned services are required for the following reasons.
- ➤ PD is a devastating disease.
- ➤ PD is costly, to all health and social agencies, as well as to individuals.
- ➤ Early detection is important to prevent falls and other costly morbidity, to avoid complications, and to delay the onset of the complex care stage.
- ➤ Treatment has advanced remarkably during the 30 years since the advent of

levodopa, but remains palliative (directed at overcoming functional difficulties, symptoms and signs) rather than curative.

➤ Each GP will have experience of a few (typically two or three) patients, but insufficient experience to handle them alone through the course of the disease, which can span several decades.

➤ Ongoing support for this chronic disease is required intermittently and at irregular intervals for some years. This requires good liaison between primary and secondary care providers.

➤ Co-ordination and integration of services is necessary to reflect the interplay between medical, social, and functional issues.

➤ There been a lack of effective liaison for individuals with neurodisability across hospital, community and social services. Services are often fragmented, and links between specialist consultant-led facilities and primary care may be unco-ordinated. Increasingly, the management of PD is based on a multidisciplinary co-ordinated service in which the PD nurse specialist will play a pivotal role.

To plan services, commissioners will need to engage in a complicated set of activities to produce a template. This template could then be used as an exemplar for other neurological diseases. Stages include:

➤ assessment of need
➤ appraisal of the options available to meet that need
➤ review of existing or planned 'Care Pathways'
➤ evaluation of the effectiveness of interventions
➤ prioritisation of the competing needs for development or change of services.

Extrapolations from prevalence figures should make it possible to calculate the likely total population with PD. This estimate will need to be adjusted if there are any local population demographic factors differing from national norms (e.g. a disproportionately high number of elderly people). It cannot be assumed that all these people would want to use the service, even if it were made easily accessible. Within the overall need of the local population, commissioners should consider how best to spend scarce resources to enable individuals and their carers to enjoy a reasonable quality of life. Although the perception is that PD is a disease of older persons, one in seven is diagnosed before their sixtieth birthday, and one in fifty before their fortieth. Communication and cultural differences may impinge in ethnic groups, and special consideration is required in planning for those in nursing homes, where up to 10% of residents[20] may have PD.

Reviewing current services

Current provision is often very patchy, involving a number of providers and with contracts usually based upon local interests and residual facilities available as a historical legacy. It will span a wide variety of services, professional personnel, and locations. It is important to include all aspects in a comprehensive review to ascertain the current situation. The current service may include any or all of the elements set out in Table 12.5.

TABLE 12.5 Service involvement for patients with PD

There should be consultation with:

- Community and hospital nursing services through Primary Care Trusts, including general practitioners and primary healthcare teams
- Social services departments
- Community health councils
- Local Parkinson's Disease Society branch(es); user groups and other voluntary organisations, e.g. Age Concern, Carer's National Association
- Disabled Living Centres.

A wide variety of other services and organisations also have an interest in this service, and their views should be considered when planning services.

In some cases, it is difficult to obtain an overview if local services are fragmented and involve many elements and different budgets. It can be very difficult to determine how much is being spent, and what level of service is being provided. It is clear that any review of services must be multidisciplinary and must include a broader scope of primary, secondary and tertiary care. It should be noted that the key to an effective service is that services are properly co-ordinated, and that the clinicians involved have special training in the care of people with PD.

One approach that can be used in the collation of such information is the preparation of a matrix in which the services available in each health economy are plotted.

While most services are provided locally, tertiary neuroscience services are mainly provided on a regional or supra-regional basis serving a population of one million. These will include highly specialised neurology, imaging and neurosurgery (*see* Box 12.1).

It is suggested that PDNSs have a caseload of 300 patients with PD. In order to satisfy the requirements of clinical governance, the health economy should adopt a formal quality assurance system. Comprehensive evaluations of service provision will benefit greatly from the framework that an established system would provide. In recent years, a wide range of approaches to quality systems has been developed, although almost all are based on self-assessment against a specific model. Any system is only as good as the way it is used, and the culture of each service will be unique and the systems should match the culture. To retain ownership of any changes or improvements (and to be cost-effective), service users and staff should be actively involved in the implementation of any quality system. Providing a quality service should not necessarily imply higher costs as the more efficient use of resources may reduce the overall cost.

BOX 12.1 Relationships and roles: primary and secondary care

- Medical specialists, neurologists, geriatricians, rehabilitationists, psychiatrists
- Nurse specialists (PDNSs)
- Generalist and specialist nursing services, e.g. district nursing services, continence nurse specialists
- Acute hospitals for medical and rehabilitation services
- Specialist PD clinics either secondary- or primary care-based
- Day hospitals
- Physiotherapy
- Speech and language therapy
- Occupational therapy
- Dietetics
- Services for people with cognitive impairments [neuropsychiatry and Elderly Mental Infirm (EMI) services]
- Services to long-term care, respite care, residential and nursing homes
- Psychology
- Chiropody
- Voluntary sector services may provide complementary facilities
- Tertiary centre for neurological advice and neurosurgical treatment

Health outcome measures

Outcomes from PD are more diffuse and difficult to measure compared with the 'harder' indicators from, for example, coronary heart disease. Measures of well-being are individual, subjective and variable, and very much a matter a matter of perception. Naturally management of PD has focused on treating symptoms of the disease, but quality of life is also a primary concern. A Global Parkinson's Disease Survey[36] suggests that maintaining and improving quality of life is the desired outcome of any therapeutic intervention. It may therefore be more pertinent to measure the standards of service in terms of clinical governance and outcomes in terms of quality of life, rather than in terms of the strict performance indicators of disease severity which may have little bearing on the perceptions of the parkinsonian patient. A survey has shown that personal control and teaching people with PD how to improve their quality of life increases their satisfaction with the service received by up to a factor of four.[37]

Audit

An on-going or rolling audit review should be in place to satisfy clinical governance criteria. This could be undertaken using performance indicators for each for each of the four stages of PD; that is, at the diagnostic, maintenance, complex, and palliative care stages. All audits should include the views of users and carers.

Additionally, any audits should ensure that GPs and primary care staff are able to attend study days in order to review results and update their skills.

Some purchasers have found it useful to set up a multidisciplinary, inter-agency working group to review current services and plan for future needs. Such a group may meet for a short period only, or may continue to meet to monitor the contract for the PD services.

Addressing the needs of carers

Carers play a vital role in looking after people with PD, and have a right to expect that the NHS and social services will help them to fulfil this role. The National Priorities Guidance for health and social services in England issued in 1998 asked GPs, primary care team members and social services to identify carers by April 2000. Their health and ability to undertake tasks that require physical strength or stamina need particularly consideration. The carers' willingness to act as a carer may reveal emotional or mental health needs, and may vary with the progression of the disease, and their reaction to life events.

Developing a comprehensive service

A comprehensive service for people with PD should include professional and public education, comprehensive assessment and investigation facilities, a range of multi-disciplinary treatment options, and a support and management service.

Consideration needs to be given to the following.

➤ A defined method of referral by GPs, nurses, hospital staff and patients themselves.
➤ The means of access to appropriate specialist facilities and agreed time scales (as per Table 12.5).
➤ Attention to the wishes of patients and carers.
➤ A policy concerning the purchasing and supply of equipment in the community, in residential and nursing homes and in hospitals.
➤ Well-defined audit and quality assurance systems.

The structure required to achieve these aims might include a designated manager, an expert advisory panel, and a budget to provide staff with training and support services.

A neurologist or consultant with a special interest in PD may lead this service. Commissioners must consider whether there will be a single unified service to serve all areas within their remit, or whether they will purchase a separate service from each provider. Careful consideration should be given to whether the service is to be hospital- or community-based, or both. Whichever is chosen, seamless liaison across trust and community boundaries will be needed, and this can be facilitated by a PD nurse specialist.

Teamwork

A major problem in planning is that individuals can present in any healthcare setting.

No one professional group has clear overall responsibility for PD. Indeed, it spans both healthcare and social care. It is recognised that different commissioners will have different policies on involvement of providers in planning and consultation. There is potential for a conflict of interest if providers write strategies for services for which they may subsequently tender. This conflict is often outweighed by the provider's local knowledge, and desire to enhance local services.

Steering group

Trying to co-ordinate and liaise between all these different specialties presents a considerable challenge, and this should be the responsibility of a key worker designated for each individual area. It is recommended that a small steering group be appointed for the service, with representatives from commissioners, purchasers, providers and service users. This group could meet several times per year to monitor progress and review problems that arise.

Care management

Following implementation of the 1990 Community Care Act, the concept of care management for people with long-term disability has gained widespread acceptance. Care management provides an excellent forum for the inclusion of specific objectives aimed to promote independence for individuals with a long-term disability. The cost of caring can be reduced through the inclusion of a comprehensive health-promotion strategy using the care management approach. Social service departments should be encouraged to consider PD services specifically when drawing up community care plans.

Conclusions

Many of the problems experienced by patients with PD, and by their carers, can be overcome by the application of modern treatments and therapies, and by understanding the organisation and management of health, social and voluntary services. A PD team in which the PD nurse specialist has a pivotal role in areas of clinical management, liaison, and education can facilitate the co-ordination of these providers. These services need to be commissioned according to local circumstances, respecting geographical, cultural and logistical features unique to the locality. However, the principles stated in this chapter should help guide this process and allow the development of properly managed cost-effective and evidence-based services.

REFERENCES

1 Department of Health. *Supporting People with Long-term Conditions; an NHS and social care model to support local innovation and integration.* London: Department of Health; 2005.
2 Department of Health. *Creating a Patient-led NHS.* London: Department of Health; 2005.
3 Department of Health. *Your Health, Your Care, Your Say.* London: Department of Health; 2006.

4 Department of Heath. *Independence, Well-being and Choice: our vision for the future of social care for adults in England.* (Social Care Green Paper). London: Department of Health; 2005.

5 Department of Health. *National Service Framework for Older People.* London: Department of Health; 2001.

6 Department of Health. *National Service Framework for Long-term Conditions.* London: Department of Health; 2005.

7 Department of Health. *National Service Framework for Mental Health.* London: Department of Health; 1999.

8 National Collaborating Centre for Chronic Conditions. *Parkinson's Disease National Clinical Guideline for Diagnosis and Management in Primary and Secondary Care.* London: Royal College of Physicians; 2006.

9 Jones R. Self-care. *BMJ.* 2000; **320**: 596.

10 Clark NM, Gong M. Management of chronic disease by practitioners and patients: are we teaching the wrong things? *BMJ.* 2000; **320**: 572–5.

11 Greenhalgh T, Herxheimer A, Isaacs AJ, *et al.* Commercial partnerships in chronic disease management: proceeding with caution. *BMJ.* 2000; **320**: 566–8.

12 Koplas PA, Gans HB, Wisely MP, *et al.* Quality of life and Parkinson's disease. *J Gerontol Biol Sci Med Sci.* 1999; **54**: M197–202.

13 The Parkinson's Disease Task Force. *Parkinson's Aware in Primary Care.* London: Parkinson's Disease Society; 1999.

14 Hurwitz B, Bajekal M, Jarman B. Evaluating community-based Parkinson's disease nurse specialists: rationale, methodology, and representativeness of patient sample in a large randomised controlled trial project. *Adv Neurol.* 1999; **80**: 431–8.

15 Jarman B, *et al.* Effects of community-based nurses specialising in Parkinson's disease on health outcome and costs. *BMJ.* 2002, **324**: 1072.

16 Thomas S, Sweetman C. Parkinson's disease: caring for the carers. *Primary Health Care.* 2002; **12**(4): 27–9.

17 MacMahon DG, Thomas S. Practical approach to quality of life in Parkinson's disease. *J Neurol.* 1998; **245** (Suppl. 1): S19–22.

18 Goetz CG, Stebbins G. Risk factors for nursing home placement in advanced Parkinson's disease. *Neurology.* 1993; **43**: 2227–9.

19 Goetz CG, Stebbins G. Mortality and hallucinations in nursing home patients with advanced Parkinson's disease. *Neurology.* 1995; **45**: 669–71.

20 Larsen JP. Parkinson's disease as community health problem: study in Norwegian nursing homes. The Norwegian Study Group of Parkinson's Disease in the elderly. *BMJ.* 1991; **303**: 741–3.

21 de Rijk MC, Tzourio C, Breteler MM, *et al.* Prevalence of parkinsonism and Parkinson's disease in Europe: the EUROPARKINSON Collaborative Study. European Community Concerted Action on the Epidemiology of Parkinson's Disease. *J Neurol Neurosurg Psychiatry.* 1997; **62**: 10–15.

22 Mutch WJ, Dingwall-Fordyce I, Downie AW, *et al.* Parkinson's disease in a Scottish city. *BMJ.* 1986; **292**: 534–6.

23 Bennett DA, Beckett LA, Murray AM, *et al.* Prevalence of parkinsonian signs and associated mortality in a community population of older people. *N Eng J Med.* 1996; **334**: 71–6.

24 Parkinson's Disease Society UK, Royal College of Nursing, Parkinson's Disease Nurse Specialist Association. *Competencies: a framework for nurses working in Parkinson's disease.* London: PDS, RCN, PDNSA: 2006.

25 Brain R, Walton J, editors. *Brain's Diseases of the Nervous System,* 7th ed. London: Oxford University Press; 1969.

26 Thomas S, MacMahon DG. Parkinson's disease, palliative care and older people: Part 1. *Nursing Older People.* 2004; **16**(1): 22–7.

27 Thomas S, MacMahon DG. Parkinson's disease, palliative care and older people: Part 2. *Nursing Older People.* 2004; **16**(2): 22–6.

28 Hughes TA, Ross HF, Musa S, *et al.* A 10-year study of the incidence of and factors predicting dementia in Parkinson's disease. *Neurology.* 2000: **54**: 1509–602.

29 Biggins CA, Boyd JL, Harrap FM, *et al.* Prognostic features for the development of dementia in PD. *J Neurol Neurosurg Psychiatry.* 1992; **55**: 566–71.

30 Findley L, Aujla M, Bain PG, *et al.* Direct economic impact of Parkinson's disease: a research survey in the United Kingdom. *Mov Disord.* 2003; **18**(10): 1139–45.

31 Dodel RC, Berger K, Oertel WH. Health-related quality of life and healthcare utilisation in patients with Parkinson's disease: impact of motor fluctuations and dyskinesias. *Pharmacoeconomics.* 2001; **19**(10): 1013–38.

32 Haycock J. *Parkinson's Disease Society. Meeting a Need.* London: Parkinson's Disease Society; 1994.

33 MacMahon DG, Findley L, Holmes J, *et al.* The true economic impact of Parkinson's disease: a research survey in the UK. Proceedings of the Movement Disorder Society 6th International Congress of Parkinson's Disease and Movement Disorders; 2000, June; Barcelona, Spain.

34 Thomas S, MacMahon DG, Henry S. *Moving and Shaping.* London: Parkinson's Disease Society; 1999.

35 Wagner EH. Chronic disease management: what will it take to improve care for chronic illness? *Effect Clin Pract.* 1998; **1**: 2–4.

36 Findley L. Global Parkinson's Disease Survey (GPDS). Conference presentation; 1999; Vancouver, Canada.

37 Fujii C, Aoshima T, Sato S. Quality of life for patients with intractable diseases: subjective satisfaction of patients with Parkinson's disease. *Kango Kenkyu.* 1997; **30**: 11–21.

13

Parkinson's disease and the general practitioner

CATHERINE HINDLE AND JOHN HINDLE

Introduction

The general practitioner (GP) plays a unique pivotal role in the diagnosis and management of Parkinson's disease (PD). James Parkinson himself was in general practice in Shoreditch, London, following in his father's footsteps. It was the broad and eclectic interests of James Parkinson, working in the family practice, which enabled him to be aware of the cases of this syndrome.

After stroke, Parkinson's disease is the second most common cause of chronic neurological disability. The prevalence of PD in the general population is 2 per 1000.

In the elderly this increases to 2 per 100 and in nursing-home residents it may be as high as 1 in 10. Most GPs will have at least three patients under their care. PD patients develop significant co-morbidity, which can lead to greater disability and handicap unless early intervention strategies are in place.[1] Whilst specialist movement disorder services have been developed, the primary care physician or GP still plays a key role in the management of PD.

The aims of this chapter are:

> to facilitate greater understanding by GPs of their role in the management of Parkinson's disease
> to assist members of the specialist PD team in understanding the structure of primary care and the role of the GP
> to emphasise the importance to the GP of the key recommendations of national guidelines.

Although much of the discussion in this chapter relates to services in the United Kingdom (UK), the principles of development of the role of the primary care doctor and of teams linking with secondary care services should be applicable to other countries with well-developed primary care services.

The role of the primary healthcare team

In the UK the basic unit of care in the community is the general-practice-based primary healthcare team. The Royal College of General Practitioners has identified core primary healthcare team membership as consisting of general practitioners, practice nurses, community nurses, health visitors, midwives, practice managers and administrative staff. The exact composition of any primary healthcare team may depend on the particular circumstances and patients may require the services of a varying number of members of this team. The GP provides the common link with the team and usually assumes leadership. GPs have adapted their medical roles to incorporate management and business skills including the employment of some of the staff within the team. The roles of such a team relevant to conditions such as PD include the following.

> The diagnosis and management of acute and chronic conditions – in the patients' homes, when necessary.
> Prevention of disease and disability.
> Follow-up and continuing care of chronic and recurring disease.
> Rehabilitation after illness.
> Helping patients and their relatives to make appropriate use of other agencies for care and support, including hospital-based specialists.
> The co-ordination of services for those at risk, including the mentally ill, the bereaved and the elderly.
> Care during terminal illness.[2]

Features of a good team are that the members meet regularly, understand one anothers' competencies, are clear about responsibility, communicate effectively, plan together and contribute to teaching and training of each member. Time is limited in primary care and effective use of the team can compensate for time pressures on GPs.

The general practitioner's role

The GP provides the first point of contact with health services. This is at the request or demand of the patient and can be for any problem deemed medical by the patient. The GP's role is to evaluate the patient's presenting complaint to identify symptoms and signs of illness. The GP has a vital 'gatekeeper' function which helps to prevent the over-investigation of the worried but well, while ensuring that further assessment and treatment are obtained by those who require it. At present the GP has the only fully integrated medical record containing information from primary care and specialist advice in the UK although progress with the development of the NHS Care Record Service will change this.[3] GPs usually have knowledge of the patient and the family prior to the onset of the illness. They have an awareness of premorbid factors that may affect the outcome of illness and disability. They can assess the wider effects of chronic disease. GPs are able to review events in relation to a span of time rather than as individual episodes and this role continues throughout the disease. The GP is part of the wider community of which the patient is a member and may be aware of other factors that might help or hinder the patient in their disease. GPs do not normally have special expertise in the management of PD, although some have set up community PD clinics.

Parkinson's disease carries a considerable health burden, which increases with advancing stages of the disease, irrespective of age.[4] GPs are able to intervene in PD through looking holistically at the patient. When treating symptoms, practitioners need to be aware of the high level of pain, fatigue and depression associated with this condition, even in the early stages. Family relationships are affected early in the disease, indicating the importance of providing prompt referral to services such as home care, social work, therapy, counselling and PD support groups.[5] Practitioners must also be aware that caring for a spouse with PD produces considerable social, psychological and physical effects,[6] and contributes to depression in carers.[7] The GP is in an ideal position to evaluate the many effects on the sufferer and wider family. The main tool the general practitioner has at his/her disposal is the primary healthcare team.

Primary care nursing

There may appear to be a confusing variety of nursing posts within primary care teams. Community (district) nurses work outside the practice setting, often in the patients' own homes, and provide vital support for patients with advanced PD. Health visitors have a role in working with families and individuals in preventive medicine and health promotion, which is not confined only to children under the age of five years. Nurses with health visitor or district nursing qualifications are able to prescribe for their patients from a limited list of drugs and dressings. In some areas, community mental health nurses from adult teams are integrated into the primary care team but the integration of services for the elderly mentally ill is more limited. Some Primary Care Trusts and GP practices have increased the integration of team working by the direct purchasing of community nursing services and nurse specialists.

Practice nurses are employed by the GP practice. Their roles and duties vary between practices and may include immunisation, counselling, family planning advice, cervical cytology screening and the management of common chronic diseases. Some practices have enhanced this to a nurse practitioner role, which requires a higher level of education and training. This role can include a limited degree of diagnosis and management, and may set a precedent for the employment of a PD nurse specialist with responsibility for a number of practices.[8]

The document *Parkinson's Aware in Primary Care*, developed by the primary care task force of the Parkinson's Disease Society for the United Kingdom (summarised in Figure 13.1), outlines the priorities and referral requirements in the diagnostic, maintenance, complex and palliative stages of PD. This document is a useful aid to the management of patients with PD in primary care, in close liaison with specialist clinics. It envisages a key role for the PD nurse specialist.[9]

This key role is supported by the National Institute for Health and Clinical Excellence (NICE) guidelines on the diagnosis and management of PD in primary and secondary care, which state that people with PD should have regular access to the following – which may be provided by a Parkinson's disease nurse specialist:[10]

➤ clinical monitoring and medication adjustment
➤ a continuing point of contact for support, including home visits
➤ a reliable source of information about clinical and social matters of concern to people with PD and their carers.

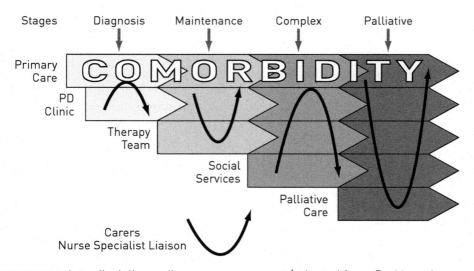

FIGURE 13.1 Interdisciplinary disease management (adapted from *Parkinson's Aware in Primary Care*).

A framework for Nurses with Special Interests has been published to encourage and guide GPs in the development of nurses with specialist roles in providing more secondary care in the community.[2]

The general practitioner consultation

The doctor–patient relationship is central to general medical practice. It is an important predictor of quality of life for patients with PD[11] and can be enhanced – but not replaced – by team working.[2] The consultation is the main process through which this relationship is established. In 2002, in the UK, more than 86% of patient contacts were face-to-face consultations in the surgery; 9% were telephone contacts, and only 5% were home visits. People aged 75–84 years accounted for many of the home visits. Patients attend the GP, on average, five times per year (women six, men four), but patients aged over 75 years attend (on average) eight times. The average duration of a surgery consultation was 13.3 minutes. Almost one-third of consultations were for respiratory conditions, while 17% were for nervous and sensory system conditions, the majority of which were due to depression and anxiety or non-specific symptoms.[12]

The frequency and intensity with which patients with PD utilise the services of the GP varies tremendously. In a survey of GPs to ascertain the frequency of consultation with PD patients, nearly half (42%) reported seeing the patients three to four times a year, with 22% seeing patients once or twice a year, and 20% only when problems arise. Few GPs saw patients more than four times per year.[13] The frequency of consultation depends upon many factors including co-morbidity, attendance at specialist clinics, severity of disease and domicile.

Perspectives on PD in practice

Although, in terms of formal neurological disease, PD is relatively common, in relation to the spectrum of neurological symptoms seen by the GP in daily practice, it is relatively rare. This was confirmed by a survey conducted through the National Hospital for Nervous Diseases in two GP surgeries over a period of one year. The incident neurological disorders were described and extrapolated to populations of 100 000 people. The relative incidence per 100 000 population of these disorders is summarised in Table 13.1.[14] The incidence of PD was estimated to be 26 cases per 100 000 per year. This same group of workers in London found, in a GP survey, that the age-adjusted prevalence of parkinsonism is 254 and of PD is 168 per 100 000 population,[15] which is similar to that found in other studies. It can be seen that the vast majority of the GP's time in relation to neurological symptomatology is taken up with non-specific illness, headaches and back syndromes.

In 2005, the Parkinson's Disease Society undertook a survey of 203 GPs, 50 geriatricians and 50 neurologists. This provided a baseline for monitoring the implementation of the NICE guidelines. Ninety-four per cent of GPs felt that they had no specialist knowledge of PD and other neurological conditions. Only half had access to a local PD nurse specialist. Just under a third do not refer people with suspected PD immediately and of those not referred, 61% are treated by the GP without referral. One in five people with PD seen by the GP are never referred to a specialist. Although nearly all patients referred to geriaticians are seen in less than 12 weeks, up to a third referred to neurologists wait more than 24 weeks.[16]

TABLE 13.1 The incidence of neurological syndromes in GP surgeries[14]

Condition	Frequency per 100 000 population
Headache	210
Back syndrome	313
Cerebrovascular disease	128
Non-specific neurological symptoms	514
Migraine	64
Parkinson's disease	26
Epilepsy	23

The early symptoms of PD may be difficult to recognise, so that the patient and GP remain unaware of the implications of the presenting complaints and the need for specialist multidisciplinary assessment. The accuracy of diagnosis by GPs has been well studied through a community register in North Wales. Parkinsonism was confirmed in 74% of cases, and clinically probable PD in 53%. The most common misdiagnoses were essential tremor, Alzheimer's disease and vascular pseudo-parkinsonism. It was concluded that diagnosing parkinsonism and PD in elderly subjects is difficult and that GPs should refer patients for specialist assessment.[17] Using this community register, the services received by patients attending a specialist PD clinic were compared with those received by patients being cared for by the GP.[18] In total, 172 patients were interviewed, of whom 102 attended a specialist clinic. Those attending the specialist clinic had significantly more contacts with therapists, social workers and, interestingly, with GPs. The utilisation of other community services was similar for both groups.[18] Attendance at specialist clinics may have stimulated an increased frequency of review by the GP or, alternatively, the patients may have had more severe disease requiring more medical input. The results suggest that there remains the need for an increased awareness within primary care of the importance of the diagnosis and multidisciplinary management of PD. The NICE guidelines emphasise that the management of PD is multidisciplinary, and patients should have access to a PD nurse specialist, physiotherapy, occupational therapy and speech and language therapy. People with PD and their carers should also be given the opportunity to discuss end-of-life issues with the appropriate healthcare professionals, including GPs.[10]

In a survey of patients with parkinsonism in a general practice in North Wales, the average number of GP attendances was seven per year which was identical to the national average for the whole population in this age group.[12] Although PD was the largest single cause of consultation, most consultations were for co-morbid problems unrelated to PD, and on average only one consultation per patient was directly related to PD. The best predictor of GP consultations was the number of co-morbid conditions, with no relationship to the severity of PD. The overall number of GP consultations was less in institutionalised patients (particularly in nursing homes), but these consultations were more likely to be home visits. Home visits were more likely with increasing age and co-morbidity.[19] The results of this survey confirm the importance of the GP in the care of patients suffering from chronic disease. Co-morbidity and institutionalisation had much more effect on the frequency of consultation than any factors related to PD. The specialist PD team and nurse specialists are only one component in the wider medical and social care of elderly PD patients managed through the primary healthcare team. Guidelines and disease management strategies used in commissioning services for patients with PD must take account of the burden of co-morbidity and the utilisation of primary care resources.

Parkinson's disease management guidelines

Most GPs will have at least three patients with PD under their care. The condition can lead to extensive disability, which affects the quality of life of the individual, family and carers, and produces a considerable economic impact. The assessment and management of PD are increasingly complex. For these reasons, the NICE guideline is designed to improve the healthcare of people with PD. The guideline reviews the diagnosis, drug and surgical treatments, the more complex non-motor features and palliative care of PD, and includes information for both primary and secondary care.[10]

Good communication is important, as are the requirements to take into account the patients' individual needs and preferences, so that they can make informed decisions about their care and treatment. The GP is likely to be the first healthcare professional to communicate the possible diagnosis of PD. It is important to be aware of recommended good practice in the communication of this diagnosis. The diagnosis is clinical and, when made by GPs, is likely to be less accurate than when made by a specialist. People with suspected PD should therefore be referred quickly and untreated to a specialist with expertise in the differential diagnosis of this condition, and patients should be seen within six weeks. The diagnosis of PD should be reviewed regularly by specialists and reconsidered if atypical features develop.[10]

Not all GPs have been happy with this guidance, particularly relating to early referral, and some have doubted whether the standards are achievable in all areas, whilst agreeing that PD can be a difficult diagnosis to make – in secondary care as well as in primary care. GPs can be faced with a lack of specialist support which may make implementation of the guidelines difficult – there may be long waiting lists for outpatient appointments and fragmentation of care.[20]

Shared care

Whilst it is widely accepted that GPs should refer all cases of possible PD and related disorders to a specialist team,[21] it is important to emphasise that the role of the GP continues through the whole of the patient's disease process, complementing the activities of the more specialised team.[22] The level of involvement of the GP in the day-to-day management of patients may vary. Some clinics will assess patients, confirm diagnosis and then refer back to the GP pending any change in the condition. Other clinics tend to review patients on a regular basis.

In recent years there has been increasing emphasis on the concept of integrated care pathways, in which one or more members of the primary healthcare team work with other specialist groups in the shared care of patients. Shared care applies when the responsibility for the healthcare of the patient is shared between individuals or teams who are part of separate organisations, or where substantial organisational boundaries exist. This sharing makes it possible to integrate patient care across organisational boundaries. Examples of shared care in general practice have included care for those with asthma and diabetes, terminal care, maternity care and health promotion. Another example is the role of GP out-of-hours co-operatives, which have expanded as a result of the new General Medical Services (GMS) contract allowing GPs to opt out of direct responsibility for out-of-hours care. With the creation of Care Trusts to provide social services and intermediate care and nurse-led Walk-in Centres, NHS Direct and GP Co-ops to provide out-of-hours services, teamwork between teams or institutions will become ever more important.[2]

The development of GPs with Special Interests (GPwSI) may make it possible to carry out more acute, elective and intermediate care in primary care, and this may include the development of specialised GP Parkinson's disease services. This could lead to greater integration of services between different practices in the same area and the blurring of the traditional practice-based team. General and specific specialist guidance for the development of GPwSI posts is available from the Royal College of General Practitioners although, as yet, there is no specific guidance on PD.[23]

Prescribing

The pharmacological management of PD is increasingly complex and choice of drugs, particularly in early disease, may affect long-term outcomes. There is no universal first choice treatment for early or late disease and choices need to take into consideration individual circumstances and co-morbidity.[10] These choices need specialist assessment. Decisions regarding the prescription of medication, or a change in the medication regime, can lead to disagreement and confusion between specialist services and general practice. In the majority of cases, medication is prescribed by the GP following specialist advice although, in some areas, drugs such as apomorphine may be part of a restricted list of medications that can only be prescribed by a specialist. It is important to remember that the responsibility for medication rests with the prescriber, so GPs must have confidence in the proposed arrangements. Many GPs prefer the clarity of hospital prescription of drugs such as apomorphine, but the practicalities of this may lead to substantial difficulties in the community. Some drugs such as clozapine can only be prescribed by a registered specialist in secondary care. Agreement and discussion with the GP prior to the commencement of new or expensive medications may clarify the issues and avert difficulties.

Whatever the local regulations, local agreement and clear guidelines for the prescription of such drugs across the boundary between specialists and primary care are needed. There must be clear arrangements for the prescription and continuation of medication, for adjustments in medication within a spectrum of doses, and for access to advice should side effects or problems occur. This is particularly important in the case of patients on apomorphine, who may develop local skin reactions and difficulty with infusion pumps, or with obtaining the medication. In many areas, easy access to advice and support for the prescription of complex medication regimes is obtained by the provision of a PD nurse specialist and PD advice lines. An appropriately trained nurse may adjust medications within stated limits, to avoid unnecessary visits or discussions with the specialist, according to guidelines agreed between primary and secondary care.

Nurse prescribing is being developed in the UK, but has been limited to items such as laxatives, disinfectants, dressings and skin preparations taken from the Nurse Prescribers' Formulary.[23] Training courses for nurse and pharmacist supplementary prescribers have been developed in order to expand this role. Community pharmacists are being integrated within the primary healthcare team (PHCT) and initiatives such as repeat dispensing, supplementary prescribing and medicines management collaboratives have enabled pharmacists to perform some traditional functions of general practitioners. The development of the electronic transfer of prescriptions programme and the building of modern primary care one-stop centres with pharmacies on site will remove some physical distinction between GP and pharmacist services.[2]

GPs should be aware of the different drug classes in order to understand the choice of treatments advised by the specialist and to aid prescribing under shared care agreements. No treatments slow the progression of the disease. There is no drug of first choice in early or late disease. The choice should take into account clinical and lifestyle characteristics, and patients' preferences after they have been informed of the short- and long-term benefits and drawbacks of different drug classes.[24] Discussion about drug treatments can be informed by the development of a joint formulary between Trusts and primary care, and through regular meetings or a prescribing forum, which could include a community pharmacist.

Patient-held record

The potential for good-quality care is enhanced when patients are in partnership with the practitioners involved in their care. Patient education is important, and patients and carers must be involved in the decision-making process. Confidence can be increased by the provision of a co-operation card, which could be held by the patient as a patient-held record. There are some commercially available cards or patient-held records, which have been adapted by many clinics. Information which should be recorded on such cards includes the names, addresses and contact numbers of the clinic, the key worker and the GP, the diagnosis and a medical alert to avoid unnecessary cessation of medication during hospitalisation. The name, dose, frequency and limit of dose adjustment of medication for PD must be included with any special instructions, particularly relating to subcutaneous apomorphine. A record of unwanted side effects or occurrence of fluctuations or dyskinesia is useful. A space for the recording of comments by the hospital or GP and the date of the next clinic appointment should be included. Such a card could be produced through utilisation of a PD register, or databases in the clinic or GPs surgery, which would make regular updating and communication with the GP possible. The development of shared records through the Connecting for Health programme and the use of single or unified assessments shared between social services and health services should improve the quality of information available on complex PD patients.[3]

Commissioning

GPs have an increasing awareness of, and involvement in, the commissioning of secondary care and community services and understand the benefits and cost of such services. Each area, servicing a population of about 100 000 people, will have around 200 patients suffering from PD, costing social and healthcare over £1 million per year.[25] The magnitude of these costs has increased interest in reducing the burden of PD. There is evidence that a PD nurse specialist can reduce the cost of social care and improve care in moderate disease.[26,27] This may provide the incentive for Primary Care Trusts to promote the appointment of PD nurse specialists.[25]

The NICE guideline identified a number of key priorities for implementation which should drive the commissioning of services for PD. These include:
➤ referral to an expert for accurate diagnosis and expert review
➤ regular access to specialist nursing care, physiotherapy, occupational therapy, and speech and language therapy
➤ discussing palliative care.[10]

The guideline covers both primary and secondary care, making its implementation particularly complex. It is useful to identify a local implementation group that includes GPs, specialists and representatives from the primary care trusts (PCTs) (Local Health Boards in Wales) to review the cost and service implications of applying the guideline using the implementation advice document and the costing template provided.

NICE considered the cost of implementing the key priorities that were judged to have significant cost implications. The average PCT with an adult population of 145 000 could expect to incur additional costs of £29 000, with estimated savings of £19 000, leading to an estimated annual net cost of £10 000. Although referrals to specialists would increase, it was thought that improving regular access to specialist nurses for day-to-day care could reduce routine follow-up and free up more time for initial specialist assessment and appropriate follow-up.[10]

'Payment by Results' for England 2006/07 (not Wales or Scotland) covers in-patient and outpatient activity commissioned from acute providers. Neurology outpatient attendance is not currently included in the 'Payment by Results' tariff, so prices would be negotiated locally. Geriatric medicine is in the mandatory tariff and prices reflect the cost of multidisciplinary assessment. Savings will arise only if the recommendations on access to nurse specialists and therapy services are fully implemented.[10]

The development of health improvement programmes and national service frameworks, including the National Framework for Long-term (Neurological) Conditions in England and the National Service Frameworks for Older People in England and Wales, drives the commissioning of services.[28,29,30,31] PD is not part of the GP Quality and Outcome Framework which includes stroke, nor part of Directly Enhanced Services which may include multiple sclerosis.

Conclusions

Neurological symptoms are commonly seen in general practice, and the GP must be aware of the symptoms and signs of PD. The GP consultation is the cornerstone of the management of PD patients through the primary healthcare team. The frequency of consultation with the GP may be affected more by the presence of co-morbidity than by factors related directly to PD. It is important that specialist services and the GP work together as key components of the interdisciplinary team in the care of patients with PD. The development of shared care protocols and the commissioning of specialist interdisciplinary services should improve the quality of care that we are able to offer PD patients in primary care. A holistic approach is essential – GPs are in a unique position to improve recognition of PD due to the frequency with which they see their patients. Many patients have multiple co-morbidities and the GP's role is critical to the diagnosis and management of the condition and co-ordination of care.[20]

REFERENCES

1 Leibson CL, Maraganore DM, Bower JH, *et al*. Co-morbid conditions associated with Parkinson's disease: a population-based study. *Mov Disord*. 2006; **21**(4): 446–55.
2 Royal College of General Practitioners. *The Primary Health Care Team*. The Royal College of General Practitioners Information Sheet. No. 21. London: Royal College of General Practitioners; October 2003.
3 The National Programme for Information Technology. NHS Care Record Service. www. connectingforhealth.nhs.uk
4 Chrischilles EA, Rubenstein LM, Voelker MD, *et al*. The health burdens of Parkinson's disease. *Mov Disord*. 1998; **13**: 406–13.
5 Whetten-Goldstein K, Sloan F, Kulas E, *et al*. The burden of Parkinson's disease on society, family and the individuals. *J Am Geriatr Soc*. 1997; **45**: 844–9.
6 O'Reilly F, Finnan F, Allwright S, *et al*. The effects of caring for a spouse with Parkinson's disease on social psychological and physical wellbeing. *J R Coll Gen Pract*. 1996; **46**: 513–9.
7 Meara J, Mitchelmore E, Hobson P. Use of the GDS-15 Geriatric Depression Scale as a screening instrument for depressive symptomatology in patients with Parkinson's disease and their carers in the community. *Age Ageing*. 1999; **28**: 35–8.
8 Royal College of General Practitioners. *Practice Nurses*. Royal College of General Practitioners Information Sheet. London: Royal College of General Practitioners; August 2004. www.rcgp.org.uk
9 Parkinson's Disease Society. *Parkinson's Aware in Primary Care: a guide for primary care teams developed by the Primary Care Task Force of the Parkinson's Disease Society United Kingdom*. London: Parkinson's Disease Society; 1999.

10 National Institute for Health and Clinical Excellence. *Parkinson's Disease: diagnosis and management in primary and secondary care.* NICE Clinical Guideline CG035; 2006. www.nice. org.uk

11 Pinder R. *The Management of Chronic Illness: patient and doctor perspectives on Parkinson's disease.* London: MacMillan; 1991.

12 Royal College of General Practitioners. *General Practitioner Workload.* Royal College of General Practitioners Information Sheet. No. 3. London: Royal College of General Practitioners; April 2004. www.rcgp.org.uk

13 Grace J. Parkinson's disease: your views. *Geriatr Med.* 1995; **June**: 28–31.

14 Cockerell OC, Goodridge DM, Brodie D, *et al.* Neurological disease in the defined population: the results of a pilot study in two general practices. *Neuro-Epidemiology.* 1996; **15**: 73–82.

15 Schrag A, Ben-Schlomo Y, Quinn NP. Cross-sectional prevalence survey of Parkinson's disease and parkinsonism in London. *BMJ.* 2000; **321**: 21–2.

16 Parkinson's Disease Society. *Treatment of People with Parkinson's Disease.* PDS research survey on file. www.pds.org.uk

17 Meara J, Bhowmick BK, Hobson P. Accuracy of diagnosis in patients with presumed Parkinson's disease. *Age Ageing.* 1999; **28**: 99–102.

18 Meara J, Hobson P. Levels of service provision for people with Parkinson's disease: a survey of community registered patients' perceptions. *J Br Assoc Service Elderly.* 1997; **64**: 3–10.

19 Hindle JV, Hindle CM, Hobson P. Co-morbidity and the frequency of general practitioner consultations in Parkinson's disease in the United Kingdom. *Mov Dis.* 2007; **22**(7): 1054–6.

20 Royal College of General Practitioners. *Royal College of General Practitioners' Statement on NICE Guidance on the Care of Patients with Parkinson's Disease.* London: Royal College of General Practitioners; June 2006. www.rcgp.org.uk

21 Bhatia K, Brooks DJ, Burn DJ, *et al.* Guidelines for the management of Parkinson's disease. *Hosp Med.* 1998; **59**: 469–79.

22 Hindle JV. Interdisciplinary care of the older PD patient. *Prog Neurol Psychiatry.* 1999; **3**: 16–21.

23 Royal College of General Practitioners. *General Practitioners with a Specialist Interest.* Royal College of General Practitioners Information Sheet. No. 11. London: Royal College of General Practitioners; January 2006. www.rcgp.org.uk

24 Department of Health. *The Report of the Advisory Group on Nurse Prescribing.* Crown Report. London: Department of Health; 1989.

25 Hindle JV. Communication is key with your Parkinson's disease patients. *Guidelines in Practice.* 2006; **9**(9).

26 Henry S. Wanted: 240 Parkinson's disease nurse specialists. *Geriatr Med.* 2000; **April**: 19–20.

27 Jarman B. The Imperial College School of Medicine Parkinson's Disease Nurse Specialist Project. Presented at 'The Science and Practice of Multidisciplinary Care in Parkinson's Disease'; 1998, June; London: The Royal College of Physicians.

28 Jarman B, Hurwitz B, Cook A. Parkinson's disease specialist nurses in primary care: a randomised controlled trial. *Mov Disord.* 2000; **15** (Suppl. 3): 860.

29 Department of Health. *National Service Framework for Long-term (Neurological) Conditions.* London: Department of Health; 2005. www.dh.gov.uk

30 Department of Health. *National Service Framework for Older People: the older person's NSF.* London: Department of Health; 2001. www.dh.gov.uk

31 Department of Health. *National Service Framework for Older People in Wales.* London: Department of Health; 2006. www.wales.nhs.uk

14

Rehabilitation and the interdisciplinary team

DOROTHY ROBERTSON, ANA ARAGON, GAY MOORE AND LIZ WHELAN

Introduction

The increasing social and financial burden of chronic disease has focused attention on the neglected area of chronic disability.[1-4] A plethora of recent government initiatives relating to chronic disease, including the National Service Framework for long-term neurological conditions,[5] gives welcome emphasis to the concept of proactive care management and 'expert' patients and carers[6] as a means of stemming the tide of hospital admissions. In the context of Parkinson's disease (PD), the NICE guidelines for PD[7] advocate multidisciplinary input and care co-ordination from a PD nurse specialist (PDNS) – yet for many patients the rhetoric remains divorced from the reality. The Policy Studies Institute surveyed the PD Society membership in 1997[8] and found little change in the proportion of members reporting ever receiving physiotherapy (27%) and occupational therapy (17%) compared with the situation in 1979.[9] The exception was speech therapy (20%, increased from 3%). It should be emphasised that questions regarding therapy input were couched in terms of 'Have you ever seen . . .?' The experience of patients with multiple sclerosis (MS), suggests that things are unlikely to have improved to any significant degree. A 2006 national audit of the MS NICE guidelines concludes that 'organizations within the NHS at all levels do not have the people, information or structures in place needed to develop and improve services for people with long-term neurologically based disability'.[10]

Within PD, developing new drugs has been viewed as the solution to improving the outlook for patients. Whilst this is important, the evidence suggests that, as in stroke,[11] attention to more mundane issues such as the organisation and delivery of care pays dividends.

Patients with PD experience a wide variety of symptoms and functional problems despite their drug therapy. Dependency is particularly high for elderly patients.[12] Under-reporting of problems is common and the evolving needs of patients and carers are often overlooked within primary care.[13] The 1997 Parkinson's Disease Society membership survey[8] gives some insight into the size of the problem. Although most patients managed the majority of their personal care unaided, 75% admitted to difficulty with at least six common activities of daily living, and 20% with sixteen such activities. The commonest reported problems, occurring in more than half the respondents were: writing; doing up buttons and zips; turning over in bed; getting in and out of a chair; opening bottles, jars and tins, and controlling the flow of saliva. These figures underestimate the situation, since patients aged over 70 years are under-represented in the sample. A community-based study in Aberdeen found a similar pattern of multiple functional problems.[14] It is clear that the traditional outpatient clinic, with its focus on pathology and drugs rather than function, has limited relevance to patients with PD who need access to a wide variety of health professionals and social services.

The past decade has seen the introduction of approaching 300 PD specialist nurses, often established with Parkinson's Disease Society support. As outlined by Noble,[15] these nurses play a key role in facilitating multidisciplinary rehabilitation, supervising medication and co-ordinating care in their locality.

Rehabilitation

Rehabilitation involves a complex and poorly understood interaction between patients, carers, health professionals and social services. The literature contains numerous definitions, as it is difficult to encapsulate the concept and philosophy in a single sentence.[16–17] A King's Fund report defines it as 'a process aiming to restore personal autonomy in those aspects of daily living considered most relevant by patients or service users, and their family and carers'.[18]

The essence is the focus on function (of the person as a whole) rather than pathology, with the aim of reducing the impact of the disease on the individual's quality of life. It follows that patients and carers must be at the centre of the process since their perception is the only truly valid outcome measure.

Good practice guidelines advocate a team approach,[19,20] but it is important to emphasise the difference between multidisciplinary input and true interdisciplinary team working.[21,22] In the former, parallel or sequential referrals occur, with each discipline evaluating the situation and providing their expertise and developing goals independently. One person – usually the doctor – makes the overall treatment decisions based on information from the various disciplines. Although superior to input from a single individual, this approach in complex situations often results in duplication of effort and conflicting advice. Problems also arise when the involvement of one discipline depends on referral from another who may not appreciate what they could contribute. In contrast, interdisciplinary working entails professionals simultaneously and co-operatively evaluating the problems and developing a joint action plan with input from the patient and carer.

Terminology and concepts in rehabilitation

The World Health Organization[23] International Classification of Functioning, Disability and Health (ICF) provides a conceptual framework which allows the overall concept of rehabilitation to be defined in terms of the targeted 'level' of component interventions. The experience of illness is categorised in relation to the underlying pathology (e.g. nigrostriatal degeneration); the resulting impairments (e.g. gait disturbance, bradykinesia, rigidity, or tremor), and their effects on activities and social participation (previously described as *disability* and *handicap*).

Whilst impairment is related to social participation, this relationship is neither linear nor predictable. Reduced facial expression in PD is insignificant in terms of 'activity', but the impact on social isolation and self-esteem can be considerable; for example when children avoid 'unfriendly' grandpa. Even health professionals are more likely to judge a person with PD as hostile, unhappy, introverted, passive and dull compared with controls matched for similar levels of disability.[24] The character of Mr Omer in Charles Dickens's novel *David Copperfield* nicely illustrates the distinction between disability and handicap. He describes his new wheelchair to David as 'an ingenious thing, ain't it? . . . and I tell you what – it's an uncommon thing to smoke a pipe in . . . I see more of the world I can assure you in this chair than I ever see out of it. You'd be surprised at the number of people who looks in of a day for a chat. You really would! There's twice as much newspaper since I've taken to this chair as there used to be.'

The WHO classification highlights the interaction with 'contextual factors' subdivided into the social and physical environment as well as the personal factors that make up the individual, such as past experience, education, lifestyle, habits, coping style, etc. – aspects which may facilitate or act as barriers to rehabilitation (*see* Table 14.1).

TABLE 14.1 Revised terminology employed by the World Health Organization in the International Classification of Functioning and Disability – ICIDH-2[23]

	Impairments at body level	Activities at person level	Participation at social level	Contextual, personal and environmental
	Body function and structure	Person's daily activities	Involvement in the situation	Features of the physical, social and attitudinal world
Positive aspects	Functional and structural integrity	Activity	Participation	Facilitators
Negative aspects	Impairment	Activity limitation	Participation restriction	Barriers

An additional facet described by Wade[25] is that of 'well-being', which equates broadly with quality of life and satisfaction with life. Some impairments such as chronic pain and anxiety will directly reduce well-being, even in the presence of minimal activity limitation and good social role function. Well-being is also affected by discrepancy between the patient's expectations and their actual situation.

The scope for inter-individual variation increases with each level. The variation at the level of 'activity' and 'participation' is immense as multiple factors relating to the physical and social environment and psychological aspects come into play. It is this variation which provides the challenge for rehabilitation staff working predominantly at the 'activity' and 'participation' end of the spectrum. Whilst the same principles underlie the approach to all patients, there are no 'off-the-peg' textbook solutions to bringing out the 'Mr Omer' in our patients.

Rehabilitation services

The National Service Framework for long-term conditions,[5] the White Paper, *Our Health, Our Care, Our Say*[4] and the recent NICE guidelines for Parkinson's disease[7] provide the basis for considering what should be in place for people with Parkinson's disease. The document *Moving and Shaping: a guide to commissioning integrated services for people with Parkinson's disease* is a helpful starting point for local discussions.[26] The following principles are particularly relevant for elderly patients with PD.

The need for regular review

Patient and carer needs evolve due to the degenerative nature of the problem and the age group primarily affected. Although some patients can be relied upon to report if they are running into problems, all too often people quietly accept the fact that, for example, it is getting more difficult to turn over in bed or that they are starting to stumble. The NICE guidelines recommend that all patients are reviewed at least 6–12 monthly and that patients with complex disease should be able to access specialist advice within two weeks.[7]

The need for a specialist team

Every patient is different! While this applies to patients in general, it is particularly the case in PD, in which the clinical picture can vary enormously both at presentation and in terms of the rate and nature of progression. In addition, many patients exhibit wide fluctuations in disability and symptoms throughout the day as part of the 'on/off' syndrome. This complicates both assessment and the delivery of care – it is much easier to plan for a fixed disability. To be effective, health professionals need to be seeing enough patients to understand the vagaries of this condition, and to develop and maintain their skills. In practice, this requires a specialist service in partnership with primary care.

Old age doesn't come alone

Since two-thirds of PD patients are over the age of 70 years, other health-related problems are to be expected. Treatment must take place in the context of their general medical background and must include regular review of all medications. Cognitive problems, depression and drug-induced psychosis are all more common in older patients[27,28] and complicate treatment.

Patient and carer needs are inter-dependent and cannot be considered in isolation. Looking after someone with PD is extremely demanding,[29,30] yet elderly patients often have elderly carers with health problems of their own. Around three-quarters of carers responding to the Parkinson's Disease Society Survey[8] mentioned at least one condition – the most common being arthritis (48%), followed by anxiety (33%) and cardiovascular disease (30%). In addition, 14% had difficulty hearing and 12% mentioned visual problems, while 27% were depressed.

A key worker is essential

The greater burden of problems in older patients can result in a bewildering array of people being involved in the care – all with their own assessment forms! It is not surprising that patients and carers can be unclear as to who is dealing with what and who to call. A key worker is essential to ensuring the right care is provided at the right time by the right person, and that the relevant people are kept informed. An example of good practice is the Northumbria Parkinson's Disease Service (contact person Dr Richard Walker, North Tyneside General Hospital, Rake Lane, North Shields, Tyne and Wear, NE29 8NH, UK). The key worker, almost invariably a Parkinson's disease nurse specialist (PDNS) has access to a 'user care guide' produced by the team such that when particular problems are encountered, the relevant section of the care guide can be provided to the patient and carer. There is also a 'professional care guide' which details standard advice and interventions, and referrals to other team members, in the event of problems such as, for example, falls. The 'user care guide' provides patient empowerment in that it will state whether referrals to other healthcare professionals are recommended in certain situations.

MULTIDISCIPLINARY ASSESSMENT FORM
Clara Cross Rehabilitation Unit, St Martin's Hospital, Bath

Patient's Name: .... DOB: .... Registration No: ....

Address/Tel: .... Date: ....

Medical assessment summary:
Diagnosis – Idiopathic PD with on/off fluctuations. Diagnosed 15 years ago. Pergolide added 2 years ago. Mini mental 28/30, no hallucinations. Has intermittent Speech Therapy review.
Husband frail with poor memory.
Main problems:
1. Erratic drug response and ? compliance problems
2. Variable mobility – tending to freeze when 'off'
3. Falls – exclude postural hypotension
4. High-risk fracture but not on osteoporosis medication
5. Back pain
6. Weight loss.

Occupational therapy assessment summary:
1. Problems with bed mobility
2. Difficulty dressing
3. Difficulty with writing
4. Problems with food preparation
5. Needs education regarding PD and coping strategies for 'off' periods
6. Needs home visit to check armchair, bed and bathing – ? rails needed by toilet
7. Safety aspects re falls
8. May need help at home – carer stress.

Physiotherapy assessment summary:
1. Flexed posture with R-sided flexion
2. Neck flexion
3. Poor righting reactions and recent falls
4. Poor gait pattern with freezing
5. Back pain
6. Problems with bed mobility.

Nursing assessment summary:
1. Difficulty hearing
2. Constipation
3. Urinary frequency and nocturia
4. Weight loss
5. Poor fluid intake
6. Difficulty eating and drinking due to neck flexion
7. Drug regime complicated – difficulty remembering drug times.

Patient/carer priorities: ....

Exercises for posture, ease back pain

Key problem areas:
1. Back pain through posture
2. Poor mobility with poor righting reactions and freezing
3. At risk further falls and high-risk hip fracture
4. Constipation
5. Assessment required to improve functional abilities at home, including bed mobility
6. Nutrition
7. Medication compliance
8. Carer stress.

Key goals:	**Dates achieved:**
1. Promote postural correction and optimise analgesia to ease back pain	....
2. Promote safe mobility and teach strategies to reduce freezing	....
3. Reduce risk of fracture	....
4. Promote healthy bowel function	....
5. Facilitate independence in functional activities	....
6. Management plan to maintain/improve nutrition	....
7. Simplify medication and determine how to improve compliance	....
8. Reduce carer concerns and stress.	....

Agreed plan:
• Physiotherapy and review of analgesia for back pain
• Exclude postural hypotension
• Exclude other medical causes of weight loss and falls, check bloods, commence calcium and vitamin D
• Monitor weight and observe feeding problems at meal times
• Advice re fluid intake and review laxatives; likely to need dietician
• Home visit and consider care package
• Education re movement strategies
• Medication review and establish plan for compliance.

To attend CCRU:

Days: Tuesday afternoons   Proposed length of attendance: 5–6 weeks

Key worker: Lesley Brooker   Review dates:

Not attend CCRU at present:
Reasons why: ....
Referral to other servics: ....

Copies to:	**GP**	**DN**	**Other**

FIGURE 14.1 Example of an integrated assessment form to facilitate interdisciplinary working. The Key Problem Areas, Key Goals and Action Plan are agreed jointly at the end of the assessment clinic. Speech Therapy and Social Work assessments are not included as unfortunately they are not part of the core team at present.

Interdisciplinary rehabilitation and team working

A central tenet of rehabilitation medicine is the importance of the 'team' as a means of delivering care in partnership with primary care. Unfortunately, applying the label 'team' will not in itself cause individuals to function as a team. Many factors can undermine team working, including managerial barriers, short-term contracts, dominance by individuals or professions (usually doctors!), tensions over professional boundaries, devotion to uni-professional notes, resistance to change and poor definition of roles and objectives.[31,32] A common problem is failure to establish (both within the team and with patients and carers) whether there is a common understanding of what is wrong; why, and what can be achieved within the limitations of the disease process.

Successful teams don't just happen – they must be developed. Sensitive leadership is required, and regular face-to-face contact is essential. Shared documentation and joint educational opportunities also promote the changes in culture and practice that team working requires.

In the context of PD, a specialist interdisciplinary team should ideally contain the following: PD specialist nurse, physiotherapist, occupational therapist, speech and language therapist, social worker, dietician and a consultant with an interest in movement disorders (usually a neurologist or geriatrician). Ready access is also needed to continence advisers, mental health services, neuropsychology, dentistry and chiropody. The actual size of the core team will vary from area to area depending on resource issues, but if gaps exist, every effort should be made to establish good channels of communication and involve more peripheral staff in education sessions and service development discussions.

TABLE 14.2 The main ingredients for an effective interdisciplinary team in Parkinson's disease

1	A shared understanding of normal basal ganglia function and what goes wrong in Parkinson's disease.
2	A common approach and language based on (1).
3	Shared patient-centred goals negotiated with patient and carer and understood by all the team.
4	Consistency of approach and reinforcement of advice by all disciplines.
5	Shared understanding and respect for team member roles.
6	Equal involvement in decision making.
7	Regular face-to-face team contact.
8	Shared PD-oriented notes.
9	Enthusiasm fired by opportunities for on-going education and staff development.
10	Administration and Information Technology support.

Blurring and overlap of roles characterise an effective team. Different combinations will provide input depending on the situation – not all patients need to see everyone.

The main ingredients for an effective interdisciplinary team in PD are listed in Table 14.2. The role(s) of the team members are outlined in the following section.

PD nurse specialist (PDNS)

The PDNS provides the link between primary and secondary care for patients, carers and the rehabilitation team. His/her roles include:

> assessment of patients' needs and problems in the home or clinic setting using a structured assessment with validated scales
> counselling and education of patients and carers and liaison with the Parkinson's Disease Society
> facilitation of access to rehabilitation and encouragement of realistic goal setting
> ongoing follow-up of care management and education issues
> serving as a point of contact for patients, carers and the primary healthcare team should new problems occur
> provision of regular follow-up to highlight new difficulties before they become established problems affecting quality of life
> advice on non-motor symptom management including urinary continence and bowel care
> advice regarding medication and supervision of drug changes
> education resource for other health professionals.

Physiotherapist

The role(s) of the physiotherapist include:

> the assessment and measurement of impairments and functional problems
> providing proactive advice to maintain/improve general fitness and avoid secondary problems
> the promotion of a home exercise regimen
> the education of patients and carers in the use of visual, auditory and cognitive cues to enhance movement
> analysis and management of balance problems to reduce the risk of falls
> the promotion of postural awareness and advice regarding walking aids.

Occupational therapist

The role(s) of the occupational therapist include:

> assessment of daily living activities (in the patient's home, when relevant)
> education of patients and carers about the nature of PD and the use of practical techniques to improve or maintain functional abilities
> advice regarding ways of reducing the impact of PD on interpersonal communication and social and recreational activities
> the promotion of safety and ergonomics in daily life
> providing advice on the selection, acquisition and use of assistance aids and

equipment to increase personal independence and/or reduce carer stress
- provision of information to facilitate access to financial and other benefits such as parking permits, attendance allowance and other support services
- liaison with Social Services.

Social worker

The role(s) of the social worker include:
- the assessment of non-medical care needs of patient and carers, including social and financial aspects
- providing advice regarding services, including voluntary organisations, nursing and home care agencies, day care and respite
- the co-ordination of service providers
- providing advice regarding eligibility for disability benefits
- providing support and advice regarding nursing-home or residential-home placement.

Speech and language therapist

The speech and language therapist is responsible for:
- analysis of communication and swallowing problems
- education of patients, carers and healthcare professionals regarding strategies to improve/maintain communication
- liaison with dieticians and advice on reducing the risk of aspiration and maintaining nutrition
- assessment for communication aids.

Dietician

The dietician has responsibilities for:
- assessment of the patient's nutritional status
- giving practical advice on the maintenance of body weight and nutrition (including calcium), and the avoidance of constipation
- liaison with speech and language therapists in the management of patients with swallowing problems.

Consultant

The consultant is responsible for:
- diagnosis of the movement disorder and assessment of the general medical context
- assessment of impairments including motor, cognitive and autonomic aspects
- reviewing medication and PD treatment modification
- providing advice to the patient, carer and team members regarding medical problems and prognosis.

Rehabilitation strategies: the theory

A shared team understanding of current concepts of basal ganglia function and what goes wrong in PD is essential when dealing with patients – not only in terms of understanding their physical and mental problems, but also to provide a rationale for rehabilitation strategies.[33–37]

Cerebral imaging studies indicate that complex movement sequences are particularly dependent on basal ganglia function, especially when they are internally driven rather than externally cued.[38–40] The basal ganglia, along with the supplementary motor area (SMA) act as an 'auto-pilot', allowing well-learned movement sequences such as walking, speech and fastening buttons to run automatically while attention is focused elsewhere. Phasic neuronal activity in the globus pallidus, within the basal ganglia, is thought to act as an internal motor cue terminating pre-movement activity in the SMA and allowing correctly timed and scaled sequences of sub-movements to occur.[41,42] The basal ganglia also contribute to cortical motor preparedness for the whole motor sequence or 'motor set'.[43,44]

In PD, degeneration of neurones in the basal ganglia impairs the ability to plan, sequence and 'run' well-learned motor skills with appropriate force generation.[45–47] This manifests clinically in problems with initiation, under-scaling of movements, motor instability as the sequence proceeds and global slowing.[34,45,48] As predicted, well-learned movement sequences such as talking and walking are particularly affected due to the defective production of internal cues. The dependence on conscious attention is most apparent when people with PD attempt to do more than one thing at a time – often at the expense of maintaining balance.[49,50]

The application of conscious attention by a person with PD enhances motor performance[51] but requires tasks to be performed one at a time. Information from positron emission tomography (PET) scanning in PD reveals selective underactivity in the SMA and dorsal prefrontal cortex, brain regions strongly linked with the basal ganglia and particularly involved in motor preparation and decision making.[52,53] In contrast, lateral premotor and parietal cortical areas are overactive, explaining why actions that are cued are generally easier in PD.[54] It appears that the use of conscious attention and visual and auditory cues facilitates a switch to non-basal ganglia-dependent nerve circuitry.[55–57]

In addition to this motor loop, the basal ganglia are involved in cognition, attention, motivation and mood via connections with frontal and limbic areas.

Depression is common in PD, and the risk of dementia increases with age.[58] However, disturbance of cognitive function is common even in the absence of dementia. Patients commonly complain about their memory and deficits in working memory are a fairly consistent finding even in early disease.[59–62] Memory problems are more marked when patients are asked to recall information without cues or context.[63] Similarly, when learning new tasks, patients are more dependent on external cues, reinforcement and correction feedback.[64,65] Information processing is slowed (bradyphrenia) and this can be misinterpreted as dementia. Mental inflexibility results from problems shifting mental set, and executive dysfunction also impairs the ability to plan, problem solve, sustain attention and allocate cognitive resources when multi-tasking.[55,66] Noradrenergic and cholinergic networks are affected early in the illness[67] and dysfunction contributes to the attention deficit problems seen in PD.[66]

The retina is dopamine rich and reduced contrast sensitivity causes subtle difficulties with depth perception and focusing.[68] More problematic for patients are the difficulties with visuospatial processing which result from frontal and temporal lobe dysfunction. Accurate perception of movement in three-dimensional space as well as the ability to selectively direct attention are crucial for daily life – and these difficulties compound the perhaps more obvious motor difficulties.[66,69]

The combined effects of these changes complicate rehabilitation and underlie many of the subtle changes in behaviour and personality described by carers such as lack of organisation and resistance to change.

In summary, these concepts form the basis for a coherent approach to rehabilitation based on awareness that conscious attention facilitates movement; dual tasks are counter-productive; 'cues' can enhance function, and breaking down sequences and information into simpler parts can be helpful. In addition, the team must understand and take account of cognitive and communication difficulties as well as the potential for both symptoms and function to vary with the time of day and environmental factors.

Interdisciplinary rehabilitation: the practice
Assessment

Depending on the patient and the stage of the illness, the initial assessment may involve one or more members of the team, and take place in a variety of settings. However, most information collected will be of relevance to the whole team at some stage and should be available in an integrated record. While this seems obvious and spares patients and carers from endlessly repeating the same information, the culture change required to achieve this should not be underestimated – but is essential for interdisciplinary working. Assessment aims to determine what the problems are, be they medical, psychological, functional or social and to establish the severity and impact on quality of life at home. The initial interview also starts the process of establishing a therapeutic relationship and informs the management plan. An example of integrated paperwork used in the Rehabilitation Unit in Bath is shown in Figure 14.1. The form summarises the individual assessments and notes patient/carer priorities on the initial visit to the unit. The key problem areas, goals and action plan are then agreed jointly by face-to-face team discussion at the end of the clinic.

Certain principles are important when interviewing patients and are relevant to all professions: allow ample time and provide a quiet environment without distractions; establish rapport and gain focused attention; gauge knowledge base and understanding, and use language accessible to the individual. It is important to explain the purpose of the interview and to establish what issues the patient and carer wish to discuss. Use short sentences and stress key words, and provide a written summary of the action plan. Avoid introducing too many new ideas in one session and, above all, allow plenty of time for responses – and listen, even if several sessions are needed to complete the assessment. Staff should also be aware and take account of factors that may confound the picture. In particular, variations which occur as part of drug timings and 'on/off' fluctuations as well as fatigue at the end of a long session. The context of the assessment is also important, since awareness of being observed increases conscious attention to the task, often enhancing performance. A spacious hospital clinic setting may similarly improve gait compared with the hesitant shuffling seen in a crowd or a confined home environment. It is a source of frustration for carers when the patient performs well during assessment despite major problems at home.

Interventions and advice

Detailed description of possible interventions by the rehabilitation team is beyond the scope of this chapter. *Parkinson's Disease: a team approach*[35] (edited by Meg Morris and Robert Iansek) draws on the wealth of practical experience within the Movement Disorders Programme in Melbourne, Australia. Other useful sources of information include the Physiotherapy, Speech and Language Therapy, Occupational Therapy and Nurse Information sections in *The Professional's Guide to Parkinson's Disease* obtainable from the Parkinson's Disease Society.[70]

The Parkinson's Aware in Primary Care initiative,[71,72] based on the clinical management algorithm of MacMahon and Thomas, outlines the issues and interventions to be considered in the diagnosis, maintenance, complex and palliative stages of the disease (*see* Chapter 12).

During the first phase, the emphasis is on confirming the diagnosis medically, education (including correction of misinformation), and helping patients and carers to accept the diagnosis and develop a positive attitude. Medication may or may not be needed yet, and functional problems will vary depending on the delay in diagnosis and any co-morbidity. Education needs at diagnosis are generally not well met in primary care or with the traditional outpatient approach,[10] and the PDNS as key worker is ideally placed to fulfil this role, with help from the Parkinson's Disease Society. In older patients, input from other disciplines is often needed even in this early stage due to functional problems.

The maintenance phase has been described as the 'honeymoon phase', implying a stable situation with improvement due to starting medication. Patients have commonly been referred back to primary care with a 'send her back if she runs into trouble' comment. However, the NICE guidelines[7] recommend that patients should remain under specialist review and the opportunities and pitfalls of this period should be emphasised. The use of the term *maintenance* is perhaps unfortunate as it implies something passive. In contrast, the clinical management algorithm describes active monitoring with defined follow-up to prevent complications and maintain health. Often patients (especially the elderly) expect to get gradually worse – after all, they have PD – and therefore don't complain. Once unhelpful changes in behaviour and family dynamics have been established in response to disability, they are very difficult to change. In contrast, establishing access and relationships with a specialist PD team allows patients and carers to acquire the understanding and skills they will need to live with this highly complex disease. The maintenance stage is about building on positive aspects in the person's circumstances and facilitating 'social participation' via timely access to medical, nursing, therapy and support resources. Expert Patient and Carer Programmes are now generally available to teach self-management skills for living with a chronic disease.[6] Points to be re-enforced by team members include general aspects of maintaining health and fitness and measures to avoid secondary problems. These include encouraging suitable exercise, good dental hygiene and nutrition, as well as the importance of a positive attitude with continuance of household activities and outside interests and hobbies. Continence problems and bowel dysfunction need active management. A variety of simple interventions such as ensuring optimum height of furniture, advice to pace and simplify the domestic routine, and the provision of grab rails or a bedside rail can help patients to maintain independence. In addition, as functional difficulties increase, the concepts underlying the more specific rehabilitation techniques outlined below should gradually be introduced, either on an individual basis or via PD-specific education modules.

Attention

Concentration is essential. The relevance of concentrating on the task in hand needs to be explained to patients and carers, and re-enforced by the team. Avoid distractions during therapy sessions and avoid chatting to patients when they are performing a task.

Avoiding simultaneous tasks

Doing two things at once should be avoided whenever possible. Again, this concept should be re-enforced by the team; for example, by advising patients to sit while dressing or making a phone call, and to 'walk, then talk'.

Cues and triggers

Patients and carers can be taught a variety of techniques to facilitate movement, such as the use of visual and auditory cues, mental rehearsal, visualisation and internal commentary. Different methods work in different situations and patients vary in their response. As there is little evidence to suggest sustained effects when cues are not used, experimentation is needed to find what is effective as well as what is acceptable and hence likely to be used in real life.[73] The optimum duration and intensity of formal physiotherapy training remains to be determined.

Visual cues

Parallel strips of tape on the floor can help to maintain stride length in areas in the home which provoke freezing or deterioration in gait (*see* Figure 14.2). Strips are placed parallel at intervals to match the individual's normal stride length (approximately 45 cm (18 inches) to 56 cm (22 inches)). Where a 90-degree turn is the problem, strips can be placed to fan around the bend. Whether the feet fall on or between the strips is not important, but such strips are only effective if the patient is able (spontaneously or with prompting) to pay attention to them. In the absence of orthopaedic or other problems, stairs rarely cause difficulties for patients with PD, since the edge of the steps seem to act as a visual cue.

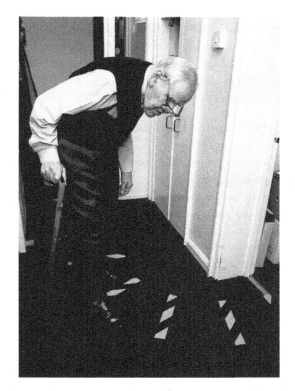

FIGURE 14.2 Visual cues for the prevention of 'freezing' and falls. Individually tailored floor markers are applied by the physiotherapist or occupational therapist in areas which provoke shuffling or freezing. A week later their effectiveness and the need for any additional markers is assessed. This patient is prone to 'freezing' with frequent falls. The visual cues significantly improved his gait, with a marked reduction in falls.

Visual environment

The environmental layout has a major impact on gait in PD,[74] and simple advice from an occupational therapist on repositioning furniture can be very effective. Central coffee tables should be moved to the side, thus allowing direct access from the armchair to the door or television. Multiple floor colours and patterns should be avoided where possible.

Auditory cues

The beneficial effects of music and rhythm on gait in PD are well known, and portable metronomes have been used to facilitate movement.[75,76] The baseline step frequency is calculated by counting the number of steps during straight-line walking over 10 metres at comfortable (preferred) speed. Setting the metronome to a cueing frequency of +10% can increase speed but a reduced frequency of −10% is more effective for improving stride length − and is advised for patients with freezing of gait.[77] Simple commands such as 'One-Two'; 'Left-Right' or 'Big Step' are also very effective. Patients poised and ready to stand may be helped by the firm command '1 . . . 2 . . . 3 . . . Stand'. Similarly, problems with swallowing may respond to reading or hearing the carer saying '1 . . . 2 . . . 3 . . . Swallow', and repeated verbal reminders to 'write big' can improve micrographia.[78]

Mental rehearsal, planning and visualisation

In patients able to master the technique and maintain concentration, attentional strategies such as visualising and then focusing on the desired step length is as effective as floor strips at improving gait.[34] Freezing can be overcome by stepping over an imaginary log or line, and negotiating a crowded supermarket will be easier if the route is first planned and visualised from the door. If patients find a particular task difficult, the illustration of sports training in which athletes visualise the precise movements involved in scoring a goal to improve their performance can be used as an analogy to encourage mental rehearsal prior to movement.

Breaking up the sequence

Long movement sequences such as getting out of bed or standing from a chair flow more easily if they are broken down into smaller parts and attention is focused on each sub-movement in turn. For example, when standing from a chair think: shuffle bottom forward, feet well back, 'nose over toes', push forwards and up to stand. Similarly, sentences should be divided into short phrases when speaking.

In practice, a mixture of techniques is used depending on the situation and the stage of the disease. For example, mental rehearsal of the individual steps for standing is combined with a running commentary out loud or internally while performing the task. Similarly, the auditory cue 'Big Step', combined with the carer placing their foot at right-angles to the patient's toes, provides an auditory and visual cue to prompt stepping when patients 'freeze'. Table 14.3 illustrates a strategy for promoting independence and safety in dressing.

As the disease moves into the 'complex' phase, more intensive input is required to manage and prevent problems. Patients are generally less able to use internal cues such as mental rehearsal and internal commentary, and are more reliant on visual, verbal and sensory cues and prompts from carers as well as on simple physical aids. Since care will involve several disciplines and probably social services, co-ordination by a key worker and communication with the primary care team is vital. Psychiatric symptoms and fluctuations in drug response often complicate management, and flexible access to medication advice is essential. In the presence of response fluctuations, it is essential for the whole team to have a clear picture of both symptoms and function during the various phases of 'off', 'on' and 'in-between'. Outpatient assessment can be misleading, as patients often manipulate their medication to be 'on' for the doctor.

A careful history is essential, and asking the patient or carer to complete an 'on/off' diary prior to clinic can be useful. A 'wearing off' questionnaire[79] and a 'non-motor symptoms of Parkinson's questionnaire'[80] can highlight issues which might otherwise be missed. A rehabilitation clinic setting is very useful in this situation as it allows the patient to be observed over a longer period of up to several hours, and problems with mobility, eating and toileting can be observed first hand.

TABLE 14.3 Strategy to promote independence and safety in dressing

1	Collect all the clothes you plan to wear, lay them in the correct order for dressing.
2	SIT DOWN on a chair or the bed close to your stack of clothes.
3	Concentrate on dressing, avoid distracting thoughts, sounds or conversations.
4	Before doing each item, imagine yourself doing it.
5	Describe each body movement while you are dressing, e.g. 'put right hand into this sleeve and pull up'.
6	Stand to pull up pants/trousers, making sure the body is well balanced.
7	Sit down to do buttons and fastenings.
	REMEMBER
	• Do only one task at a time.
	• Concentrate fully on the task.
	• Describe each movement to yourself.

Mood swings often accompany the ups and downs of motor performance, and need to be explained to carers. A vital role of the key worker is to ensure that everyone involved appreciates how the patient's physical and emotional needs vary with the 'on' and 'off' state, and adapt their care accordingly. It is particularly important to ensure that care-home staff understand about PD. In this complex phase, the team is often involved in 'brokering' compromise to try to meet the needs of both the patient and the carer. Examples are when views differ on respite or care provision or when the carer but not the patient wants continence problems to be managed with a catheter.

In the 'palliative' phase, the model emphasises relief of symptoms and distress, support for carers and maintenance of dignity. Drug side effects may require a gradual reduction in PD medication, and nursing aspects of management become increasingly important.

Clinical resources for therapists

A new multi-professional PD guide is available from the PD Society[70] – updating previous therapy and nursing information packs. The Association of Physiotherapists in Parkinson's Disease Europe (APPDE) website (http://appde.unn.ac.uk/) links to the association's newsletter as well as providing purchasing details for a video 'Common mobility problems in PD and how to address them'. The RESCUE project, a Dutch and UK collaborative research project has produced a CD-ROM 'Using cueing to improve mobility in Parkinson's Disease'. Patient information leaflets relating to cueing are also available via the website, www.rescueproject.org and an English version of the Dutch PD Physiotherapy guidelines should be available shortly via the APPDE website.

Examples of interdisciplinary working

To justify itself, an interdisciplinary approach should have more impact than the sum of its parts. The added benefit of a team approach can best be illustrated in the context of the management of falls, and also problems at night. Some of the interventions that may be needed are listed in Tables 14.4 and 14.5, and require close collaboration between the disciplines involved and re-enforcement by the whole team.

TABLE 14.4 Interdisciplinary assessment and management of falls in Parkinson's disease

- Assessment and treatment of relevant medical factors – remember osteoporosis
- Reinforce movement strategies such as the use of planning, attention and cues, and remind to do one thing at a time – e.g. 'Don't walk and talk!'
- Reinforce techniques for safe turning – don't swivel, turn 'feet first' or in a wide arc if space allows
- Examine footwear
- Balance practice in sitting, standing and walking
- Reduce clutter at home to maximise floor space
- Ensure adequate night lighting
- Consider strips on floor in areas provoking freezing
- Remove loose mats; check toilet, bed and chair heights and install grab rails at danger spots
- Assess possible need for walking aid
- Teach techniques for getting up and consider a 'life-line' to summon help
- Common-sense advice to reduce unnecessary risk taking
- Confidence building to alleviate fear of falling

Falls

Falls are a major source of anxiety, morbidity and, indeed, mortality in PD. Assessment and management lend themselves to a team approach since numerous factors may be involved (*see* Table 14.4). If 'freezing' is a problem, a careful history may determine whether this is an 'on' or 'off' phenomenon, or is unpredictable and provoked by the environmental layout. Turning is a high-risk activity in PD, because, due to faulty weight transference, the feet may cross, or 'freezing' may occur mid-turn. Other common situations provoking falls include hurrying to the toilet at night and in the dark, walking while carrying things, dressing, getting in and out of bed or a chair, walking on uneven ground, and negotiating a crowded or unfamiliar environment. Looking or reaching up without adoption of a secure stance first may result in backward falls. From the medical point of view, postural hypotension and other medical causes should be excluded, the drug therapy reviewed and osteoporosis prophylaxis[81] considered. Precipitating factors can be highlighted by the use of a 'falls diary'[82] to document the time of day, relation to medication times, where the patient was and what they were doing when they fell, as well as any associated symptoms such as dizziness. Specific patterns may emerge such as falls when 'off' or a tendency to fall when turning in the kitchen, or when carrying things, or dressing; such patterns help to target management. A randomised control trial of a home-based exercise programme targeted to PD patients who fall reduced the frequency of near falls, with a trend towards a reduction in falls. Less severely affected patients were more likely to benefit.[83]

Nocturnal problems

Problems at night are common in PD[72-74,84,85] and, if unresolved, often lead to nursing-home placement. Problems include sleep fragmentation; parasomnias, e.g. REM sleep behaviour disorder; vivid dreams/hallucinations; restlessness, and pain. Depression disrupts sleep, and poor night mobility compounds the problem of nocturia, causing incontinence. As with falls, assessment and management lend themselves to a team approach, since several interrelated factors may be involved (*see* Table 14.5).

TABLE 14.5 Interdisciplinary assessment and management of nocturnal problems in Parkinson's disease

- Medical review of medication. Consider depression and analyse why sleep is disturbed. Consider slow-release levodopa or dopamine agonist at bedtime if mobility poor or there is discomfort; reduce levodopa if hallucinations, restlessness or unpleasant dreams occur.
- Mental health input if significant psychosis/agitation or depression.
- Joint medical and nursing assessment of continence problems. Agree plan for management with patient, carer and District Nurse.
- Joint physiotherapy and occupational therapist assessment of bed mobility. Review technique and reinforce strategies including planning, attention and cues. Involve carer.
- Occupational therapist advice regarding equipment, e.g. commode, satin draw sheet, bedside rail, plus mattress elevator if arthritic or other co-morbidity demands.
- Nursing advice to avoid pressure sores.
- Assess impact on carer.
- Advice regarding Attendance Allowance, Care Agencies and Respite Care.

Conclusions

The specialist PD team functions within a wide network of people involved with the patient's care. Strong links are needed with clear channels of communication and mechanisms to serve as signposts for patients and carers, so that they can gain access to information and support as needed. Regardless of the management stage, certain principles apply; namely the need for regular review, ready access to relevant members of a specialist team, and a key worker to co-ordinate care.

REFERENCES

1 Beardshaw V. *Last on the List: community services for people with physical disabilities*. London: King's Fund Institute; 1988.

2 Davis RM, Wagner EH, Groves T. Managing chronic disease. *BMJ*. 1999; **318**: 1090–1.

3 Wagner EH. Chronic disease management: what will it take to improve care for chronic illness? *Effect Clin Pract*. 1998; **1**: 2–4.

4 Department of Health. *Our Health, Our Care, Our Say: a new direction for community services*. London: HMSO; 2006. www.dh.gov.uk/PolicyAndGuidance/OrganisationPolicy/Modernisation/OurHealthOurCareOurSay/fs/en

5 Department of Health. *National Service Framework for Long-term (Neurological) Conditions*. London: Department of Health; 2005. www.dh.gov.uk/PolicyAndGuidance/HealthAndSocialCareTopics/LongTermConditions/LongtermNeurologicalConditionsNSF/fs/en

6 Department of Health. *The Expert Patient: a new approach to chronic disease management for the 21st century*. London: HMSO; 2001. www.dh.gov.uk/assetRoot/04/01/85/78/04018578.pdf

7 National Institute for Clinical Excellence. *Parkinson's Disease: diagnosis and management in primary and secondary care*. London: NICE; 2006. www.nice.org.uk/page.aspx?o=CG035

8 Parkinson's Disease Society. *Policy Studies Institute Survey of Parkinson's Disease Society Membership*. London: Parkinson's Disease Society; 1997.

9 Oxtoby M. *Parkinson's Disease Patients and Their Social Needs*. London: Parkinson's Disease Society; 1982.

10 Royal College of Physicians of London. *NHS Services For People With Multiple Sclerosis: a national survey. An audit of commissioning, provision, and experience of services used by people with multiple sclerosis in 2005–6, against recommendations from NICE Clinical Guideline 8*. London: Royal College of Physicians of London; 2006. www.rcplondon.ac.uk

11 Collaborative systematic review of the randomised trials of organised inpatient care after stroke. Stroke trialists' collaboration. *BMJ*. 1997; **314**: 1151–9.

12 Tison F, Barberger-Gateau P, Dubroca B, *et al*. Dependency in Parkinson's disease: a population-based survey of non-demented elderly subjects. *Mov Disord*. 1997; **12**: 910–5.

13 Koplas PA, Gans HB, Wisely MP, *et al*. Quality of life and Parkinson's disease. *J Gerontol A Biol Sci Med Sci*. 1999; **54**: M197–202.

14 Mutch WJ, Strudwick A, Roy SK, *et al*. Parkinson's disease: disability, review and management. *BMJ*. 1986; **293**: 675–7.

15 Noble C. Parkinson's disease and the role of nurse specialists. *Nursing Standard*. 1998; **12**: 32–3.

16 Nocan A, Baldwin S. *Trends in Rehabilitation Policy*. London: Audit Commission; 1998.

17 Wade DT. Describing rehabilitation interventions. (Editorial). *Clin Rehabil*. 2005; **19**: 811–8.

18 Sinclair A, Dickenson E. *Effective Practice in Rehabilitation*. London: King's Fund; 1998.

19 Bhatia K, Brooks DJ, Burn DJ, *et al*. The Parkinson's Disease Consensus Working Group. Guidelines for the management of Parkinson's disease. *Hosp Med*. 1998; **59**: 469–80.

20 *Managing Parkinson's: making the difference*. University of Manchester: Health Services Management Unit; 1997.

21 Melvin JL. Interdisciplinary and multidisciplinary activities and ACRM. *Arch Phys Med Rehabil*. 1980; **61**: 379–80.

22 Davis A, Davis S, Moss N. First steps towards an interdisciplinary approach to rehabilitation. *Clin Rehabil*. 1992; **6**: 237–44.

23 World Health Organization. *International Classification of Functioning, Disability and Health (ICF)*. www3.who.int/icf/intros/ICF-Eng-Intro.pdf

24 Pentland B, Pitcairn TK, Gray JM, *et al*. The effects of reduced expression in Parkinson's disease on impression formation by health professionals. *Clin Rehabil.* 1987; 1: 307–13.

25 Wade DT. A framework for considering rehabilitation interventions. *Clin Rehabil.* 1998; 12: 363–8.

26 Thomas S, MacMahon D, Maguire J (on behalf of the PDS UK Primary Care Task Force). *Moving and Shaping: a guide to commissioning integrated services for people with Parkinson's disease.* London: The Parkinson's Disease Society UK; 2006. www.parkinsons.org.uk

27 Goetz CG, Stebbings GT. Mortality and hallucinations in nursing home patients with advanced Parkinson's disease. *Neurology.* 1995; 45: 669–71.

28 Tom T, Cummings JL. Depression in Parkinson's disease: pharmacological characteristics and treatment. *Drugs Ageing.* 1998; 12: 55–74.

29 O'Reilly F, Finnan F, Allwright S, *et al*. The effects of caring for a spouse with Parkinson's disease on social, psychological and physical well-being. *Br J Gen Pract.* 1996; 46: 507–12.

30 Carter JH. Parkinson's Disease Study Group. Living with a person who has Parkinson's disease: the spouse's perspective by stage of disease. *Mov Disord.* 1998; 3: 20–8.

31 Evers HK. Multidisciplinary teams in geriatric wards: myth or reality? *J Adv Nurs.* 1981; 6: 205–14.

32 Strasser DC, Falconer JA, Martino-Saltzmann D. The rehabilitation team: staff perceptions of the hospital environment, the multidisciplinary team environment and interprofessional relations. *Arch Phys Med Rehabil.* 1994; 75: 177–82.

33 Homberg V. Motor training in the therapy of Parkinson's disease. *Neurology.* 1993; 43 (Suppl. 6): S45–6.

34 Morris ME, Iansek R, Matyas TA, *et al*. Stride length regulation in Parkinson's disease: normalisation strategies and underlying mechanisms. *Brain.* 1996; 119: 551–68.

35 Morris M, Iansek R. *Parkinson's Disease: a team approach.* Blackburn, Australia: Buscombe Vicprint; 1997.

36 Iansek R. Interdisciplinary rehabilitation in Parkinson's disease. *Adv Neurol.* 1999; 80: 555–9.

37 Fama R, Sullivan EV. Motor sequencing in Parkinson's disease: relationship to executive function and motor rigidity. *Cortex.* 2002; 38(5): 753–67.

38 Debaere F, Wenderoth N, Sunaert S, *et al*. Internal vs external generation of movements: differential neural pathways involved in bimanual co-ordination performed in the presence or absence of augmented visual feedback. *Neuroimage.* 2003; 19(3): 764–76.

39 Seitz RJ, Roland PE. Learning of sequential finger movements in man: a combined kinematic and positron emission tomography (PET) study. *Eur J Neurosci.* 1992; 4: 154–65.

40 Brooks DJ. The role of the basal ganglia in motor control: contributions from PET. (Review). *J Neurol Sci.* 1995; 128: 1–13.

41 Brotchie P, Iansek R, Horne MK. Motor function of the monkey pallidus: 1. Neuronal discharge and parameters of movement. *Brain.* 1991; 114: 1667–83.

42 Brotchie P, Iansek R, Horne MK. Motor function of the monkey globus pallidus: 2. Cognitive aspects of movement and phasic neuronal activity. *Brain.* 1991; 114: 1685–702.

43 Robertson C, Flowers KA. Motor set in Parkinson's disease. *J Neurol Neurosurg Psychiatry.* 1991; 53: 583–92.

44 Phillips JG, Bradshaw JL, Iansek R, *et al*. Motor functions of the basal ganglia. *Psychol Res.* 1993; 55: 175–81.

45 Morris M, Iansek R, McGinley J, *et al*. Three dimensional gait biomechanics in Parkinson's disease: evidence for a centrally medicated amplitude regulation disorder. *Mov Disord.* 2005; 20(1): 40–50.

46 Berardelli A, Rothwell JC, Thompson PD, *et al*. Pathophysiology of bradykinesia in Parkinson's disease. *Brain.* 2001; 124 (Part 11): 2131–46.

47 Benecke R, Rothwell JC, Dick JPR, *et al*. Disturbance of sequential movements in patients with Parkinson's disease. *Brain.* 1987; 110: 361–79.

48 Morris ME, Iansek R, Matyas TA, *et al*. The pathogenesis of gait hypokinesia in PD. *Brain*. 1994; **117**: 1169–81.

49 Benecke R, Rothwell JC, Dick JPR, *et al*. Performance of simultaneous movements in patients with Parkinson's disease. *Brain*. 1986; **109**: 739–57.

50 Bloem BR, Grimbergen YA, van Dijk JG, *et al*. The 'posture second' strategy: a review of wrong priorities in Parkinson's disease. *J Neurol Sci*. 2006; **248**(1–2): 196–204.

51 Rochester L, Hetherington V, Jones D, *et al*. Attending to the task: interference effects of functional tasks on walking in Parkinson's disease and the roles of cognition, depression, fatigue and balance. *Arch Phys Med Rehabil*. 2004; **85**(10): 1578–85.

52 Brooks DJ. Motor disturbance and brain functional imaging in Parkinson's disease. *Eur Neurol*. 1997; **38** (Suppl. 2): 26–32.

53 Brooks DJ. Functional imaging of Parkinson's disease: is it possible to detect brain areas for specific symptoms? *J Neural Transm Suppl*. 1999; **56**: 139–53.

54 Rubenstein TC, Giladi N, Hausdorff JM. The power of cueing to circumvent dopamine deficits: a review of physical therapy treatment of gait disturbances in Parkinson's disease. *Mov Disord*. 2002; **17**: 1148–60.

55 Samuel M, Ceballos-Baumann AO, Blin J, *et al*. Evidence for lateral premotor and parietal overactivity in Parkinson's disease during sequential and bimanual movements. A PET study. *Brain*. 1997; **120**: 963–76.

56 Praamstra P, Stegeman DF, Cools AR, *et al*. Evidence for lateral premotor and parietal overactivity in Parkinson's disease during sequential and bimanual movements. A PET study. *Brain*. 1998; **121**: 769–72.

57 Cunnington R, Iansek R, Bradshaw JL. Movement related potentials in Parkinson's disease: external cues and attentional strategies. *Mov Disord*. 1999; **14**: 63–8.

58 Reid WGJ, Broe GA, Hely MA, *et al*. The neuropsychology of de novo patients with idiopathic Parkinson's disease: the effects of age of onset. *Int J Neurosci*. 1989; **48**: 205–17.

59 Foltynie T, Brayne CE, Robbins TW, *et al*. The cognitive ability of an incident cohort of Parkinson's patients in the UK. The CamPaIGN study. *Brain*. 2004; **127**: 550–60.

60 Levin BE, Katzen HL. Early cognitive changes and non-dementing behavioral abnormalities in Parkinson's Disease. *Adv Neurol*. 2005; **96**: 84–94.

61 Owen MA, Iddon JL, Hodges JR, *et al*. Spatial and non-spatial working working memory at different stages of Parkinson's disease. *Neuropsychologia*. 1997; **35**: 519–32.

62 Muslimovic D, Post B, Speelman JD, *et al*. Cognitive profile of patients with newly diagnosed Parkinson's disease. *Neurology*. 2005; **65**: 1239–45.

63 Dubois B, Pillon B. Cognitive deficits in Parkinson's disease. *J Neurol*. 1997; **224**: 2–8.

64 Vriezen ER, Moscovitch M. Memory for temporal order and associative learning in patients with Parkinson's disease. *Neuropsychologia*. 1990; **28**: 1283–93.

65 Dominey PF, Jeannerod M. Contribution of frontostriatal function to sequence learning in Parkinson's disease: evidence for dissociable systems. *Neuroreport*. 1997; **8**: iii–ix.

66 Bronnick K, Ehrt U, Emre M, *et al*. Attentional deficits affect activities of daily living in dementia associated with Parkinson's disease. *J Neurol Neurosurg Psychiatry*. 2006; **77**(10): 1136–42.

67 Braak H, Del Tredici K, Rub U, *et al*. Staging of brain pathology relative to sporadic Parkinson's Disease. *Neurobiol Aging*. 2003; **24**: 197–211.

68 Biousse V, Skibell BC, Watts RL, *et al*. Opthalmologic features of Parkinson's disease. *Neurology*. 2004; **62**(2); 177–180.

69 Davidsdottir S, Cronin-Golomb A, Lee A. Visual and spatial symptoms in Parkinson's disease. *Vision Res*. 2005; **45**(10): 1285–96.

70 *The Professsional's Guide to Parkinson's Disease*. Parkinson's Disease Society, 215 Vauxhall Bridge Rd, London, SW1V 1EJ. www.parkinsons.org.uk/PDF/PubProfessionalGuideNov07.pdf

71 The Parkinson's Disease Society. *Parkinson's Aware in Primary Care*. 3rd ed. London: The Parkinson's Disease Society; 2003. www.parkinsons.org.uk

72 MacMahon DG, Thomas S. Practical approach to quality of life in Parkinson's disease. *J Neurol.* 1998; **245** (Suppl. 1): S19–22.

73 Nieuwboer A, Kwakkel G, Rochester L, *et al.* Cueing training in the home improves gait-related mobility in Parkinson's disease: The RESCUE-trial. *J Neurol Neurosurg Psychiatry.* E-pub (accessed 22 August 2006).

74 Giladi N, McMahon D, Przedborski S, *et al.* Motor blocks in Parkinson's disease. *Neurology.* 1992; **42**: 333–9.

75 Thaut MH, McIntosh GC, Rice RR, *et al.* Rhythmic auditory stimulation in gait training for Parkinson's disease. *Mov Disord.* 1996; **11**: 193–200.

76 McIntosh GC, Brown SH, Rice RR, *et al.* Rhythmic auditory-motor facilitation of gait patients in patients with Parkinson's disease. *J Neurol Neurosurg Psychiatry.* 1997; **62**: 22–6.

77 Willems AM, Nieuwboer A, Chavret F, *et al.* The use of rhythmic auditory cues to influence gait in patients with Parkinson's disease: the differential effect for freezers and non-freezers, an explorative study. *Disabil Rehabil.* 2006; **28**(11): 721–8.

78 Oliviera RO, Gurd JM, Nixon P, *et al.* Micrographia in Parkinson's disease: the effect of providing external cues. *J Neurol Neurosurg Psychiatry.* 1997; **63**: 429–33.

79 Stacy M, Bowron A, Guttman M, *et al.* Identification of motor and nonmotor wearing-off in Parkinson's disease: comparison of a patient questionnaire versus a clinician assessment. *Mov Disord.* 2005; **20**(6): 726–33.

80 Chaudhuri KR, Martinez-Martin P, Schapira AH, *et al.* International multicenter pilot study of the first comprehensive self-completed nonmotor symptoms questionnaire for Parkinson's disease: the NMSQuest study. *Mov Disord.* 2006; **21**(7): 916–23.

81 Wood B, Walker RW. Brief report: osteoporosis in Parkinson's disease. *Mov Disord.* 2006; **20**(12): 1636–40.

82 Yekutiel MP. Patients falls records as an aid in designing and assessing therapy in Parkinson's disease. *Disabil Rehabil.* 1993; **15**: 189–93.

83 Ashburn A, Ballinger C, Fazakarley L, *et al.* A randomised controlled trial of a home-based exercise programme to reduce fall frequency among people with Parkinson's disease (PD). *J Neurol Neurosurg Psychiatry.* 2007; **78**(7): 678–84.

84 Tandberg E, Larsen JP, Karlsen K. A community-based study of sleep disorders in patients with Parkinson's disease. *Mov Disord.* 1998; **13**: 895–9.

85 Chaudhuri KR, Pal S, DiMarco A, *et al.* The Parkinson's disease sleep scale: a new instrument for assessing sleep and nocturnal disability in Parkinson's disease. *J Neurol Neurosurg Psychiatry.* 2002; **73**(6): 629–35.

15

The Parkinson's disease nurse specialist

ELIZABETH MORGAN AND MARALYN MORAN

Introduction

The first Parkinson's disease nurse specialist (PDNS) was appointed in 1989. Since then, the role has developed greatly, and it is the intention of the Parkinson's Disease Society of the United Kingdom to have one nurse in each Health Authority throughout the UK. In 2006 there were 210 nurses in post; however, if all the posts that were created were filled, this number would increase to 219.[1]

The ability of PDNSs to assess patients in a variety of settings, i.e. hospital, home and workplace, makes them important in the overall management of patients with Parkinson's disease (PD). Other authors have also commented on the vital function that PDNSs fulfil in the clinic and the ward area, in education and telephone support.[2] Indeed, the flexibility of their approach to patients and carers, and their ability to communicate effectively across the wide educational and social barriers that exist among these patients makes them popular with patients and carers alike. The PDNSs have, in conjunction with Royal College of Nursing and the Parkinson's Disease Society, looked at developing standards of care. These include standards on all aspects of case management.[3] These are valuable tools when auditing nursing practice, and assist in the knowledge and skills framework in conjunction with Agenda for Change (new contractual arrangements in the UK).

The healthcare environment is changing rapidly in response to economic factors, demographic changes and the need to provide cost-effective healthcare. These factors – when combined with the rising costs of hospital care and the need to reduce hospital waiting lists – puts extreme pressure on all community-based services. PDNSs are ideally placed to take on the challenges of these changing times, and have been clearly identified as playing a major role in the co-ordination of services and organisational aspects of patient management in both primary and secondary care teams.[4,5]

Qualifications for the post of PDNS have been identified by the Parkinson's Disease Society. PDNSs have to meet the following criteria.[6]

1. Minimum three years post-registered RGN, and currently registered to practise with the Nursing and Midwifery Council (NMC).
2. Skilled through training in the treatment and management of PD and other allied conditions.
3. Expertise will be maintained through clinical practice and education obtained in secondary and primary care. This will be facilitated through reflective practice seminars, conferences and related courses, and will be in line with the NMC.
4. Designated to have specialist clinical responsibility for the care and management of patients with PD.
5. The PDNS is central to the effective functioning of the medical and multidisciplinary team, and must aim to co-ordinate and implement the overall strategy for PD in his/her area.

A university course module at levels 2 and 3, 'Meeting the specific needs of people with Parkinson's and their carers', is now established in several universities. Employers are encouraged to support PDNS attendance at this and other relevant educational courses and meetings.

The majority of PDNSs in the UK are now qualified to first-degree level, with many working towards their MSc.

The role of the PDNS

The role of the PDNS has been described as being fundamental in co-ordination of case management, acting as a resource for information, providing access for advice, and as a catalyst for improved public awareness (*see* Table 15.1).[7]

The role is diverse and challenging and ranges from patient assessment to providing support for carers.

Direct patient and carer contact is essential at all four stages of the disease process

– diagnostic, maintenance, complex, and palliative.[8] The aim is to advise and guide towards maintaining independence for as long as possible, through minimising disabilities and maximising abilities. Advice can be offered within the primary or secondary care sector, and PDNSs can be based in either of these settings.

Once problems have been identified, a care plan is established by mutual agreement between nurse and patient, providing individual holistic care. The philosophy of a well-informed patient or carer is that they will feel empowered if they are actively involved in the management of their care.

The National Institute for Health and Clinical Excellence (NICE) has recommended that people with Parkinson's (PWP) should have regular access to the following services, which can be a part of specialist nursing:

➤ monitoring and altering medication appropriately
➤ providing a continuing point of contact for support, including home visits
➤ being a reliable source of information about clinical and social matters of concern to PWP and their carers.[9]

This recommendation is welcomed by most PDNSs; however, there are insufficient nurses in post to ensure access is equitable across the country.

TABLE 15.1 The needs of patients and the contribution of nurse specialists[7]

Need of patients and carer	Contribution of nurse specialist	Intended outcome
Counselling following diagnosis	Early identification of diagnosis	Acceptance of diagnosis
Timely/appropriate information	Provision of advice	Informed choice Empowerment Positive attitude Control
Time and attention	Continuity of care	Improved care support and quality of life
Multidisciplinary support	Co-ordination, oversight of care	Long-term planning
Regular re-assessment	Supervision, co-ordination	Symptom relief
Carer support information regarding respite care	Carer contact	Reduction in complications

Counselling

Helping to facilitate acceptance of diagnosis or addressing issues such as coping with long-term chronic illness are important features of the role. The PDNS will focus not only on the effect of the physical aspects of the disease, but also on the psychological, social and spiritual implications that this unpredictable disease may have. Chronic disease can impact on all the family members,[10] including children, and it is important for them to have a forum in which to express their views.

Studies have shown that a high proportion of patients felt that the opportunity to talk about their PD was the most important aspect of their contact with a nurse practitioner.[11] It has also been suggested that patients find discussing issues such as sexual dysfunction easier with nurse specialists.[12]

Previous surveys have looked at sexual function in patients with PD, and have shown that factors such as age, carer strain, depression and anxiety had an impact on sexual function and that such problems could be attributed not only to physical symptoms of the disease.[13] The knowledgeable and empathetic approach of the PDNS would appear to be important when dealing with such sensitive issues, since they will also know which support services – such as an erectile dysfunction clinic – are locally available.

Drug management

Parkinson's disease differs in many respects from other neurological conditions in that the disability that people experience can fluctuate unpredictably over the course of a day, or even an hour. It therefore becomes essential that professional advice on drug management is tailored to individual needs, thereby improving quality of life.

TABLE 15.2 Drug management – points to consider

- Drugs currently available do not offer a cure for Parkinson's disease.
- Drugs improve quality of life.
- Education and understanding of the effect of drugs and their side effects enables patients to manage the condition better in the long term.
- High protein diets can reduce the clinical response to levodopa.
- Any dietary changes including protein reduction should be carried out in a controlled environment.
- Small changes in dosage or frequency often bring about major improvements in the patient's condition.
- Choice of drugs should depend upon individual patient's needs and symptoms.
- A long-term treatment strategy is of paramount importance in Parkinson's disease and such a strategy should be agreed and shared by the physician, nurse and the patient.

An important aspect of the PDNS role is to advise and offer guidance/information on titration, potential side effects and dietary implications (*see* Table 15.2). A greater understanding of when and how to administer medication should result in the PD patient gaining optimum benefits from prescribed treatment. Concordance is a relatively new concept, and describes patients and prescribers agreeing, in partnership, about medicines. This collaboration can be dramatically improved once a patient has been educated about the nature of his/her disease and its treatment.[14] PDNSs are also well placed to identify adverse effects of medication and are aware of the need to complete and submit adverse incident yellow card reports to the Committee on Safety of Medicines.

Advice on medication is also extended to apomorphine – a powerful dopamine agonist that is currently available only as a subcutaneous injection. It has previously been documented that the success of an apomorphine programme depends on the continuing advice and encouragement of the PDNS.[15]

Many nurses have undertaken increased training and are now funtioning as supplementary prescribers of medication. This role has been defined by the Department of Health (DOH) as: 'A voluntary prescribing partnership between an independent prescriber and a supplementary prescriber to implement an agreed, patient-specific clinical management plan with the patient's agreement.' This new role is still evolving. The British Medical Association has been outspoken in its criticism of this new role.[16] Any indicators of potential conflict, with medical colleagues, such as lack of trust or credibility between individuals needs to be addressed by means of more effective communication and the clarification of working practices.

The results of DOH-funded research on nurse prescribing shows positive views. A two-year evaluation of extended formulary independent nurse prescribing was undertaken, and showed that nurses prescribe appropriately on a range of clinical situations. Patients cited accessibility as a major advantage when obtaining medicine from a nurse rather than a doctor.[16] (*See* Table 15.3.)

PDNSs who have not undertaken this training should consider gaining entry on the register as nurse prescribers, since this will improve their capacity to provide high-level individualised care to their patients.

TABLE 15.3 Nurse prescribing – key points in support of the role

Nurses:

- are safe and effective prescribers
- are professionally and politically well placed to undertake prescribing
- are familiar with their patients and aware of their cultural ethical and religious backgrounds
- have a knowledge of PD as a chronic disease
- provide prescribing, against a background of familiarity with patients' preferences, long term clinical history and PD related drug history
- enhance their role within the interdisciplinary team through prescribing.

Education

The role includes increasing awareness through education and training. Many PDNSs, although identifying patient care as their key role, also see education as an integral part of that role. Such education involves providing evidence-based learning to patients and their families as well as to medical staff, nurses, and other members of the multidisciplinary team. This is particularly important in situations where healthcare professionals have little experience of PD, or, equally, where there is a high turnover of staff. The information should be given in a non-threatening manner in an effort to reduce any feelings of de-skilling these members of the healthcare team.

With regard to education, the PDNS:

➢ is a catalyst to increase public awareness and reduce the incidence of misinformation

> provides ongoing education of PD to patients and carers
> is involved with other members of the team in the planning and delivery of education to patients, their families and carers, and the evaluation of such education
> is a main resource for educating medical and other healthcare professionals on up-to-date issues and effective clinical practices
> provides organisation of educational study days for health and social care professionals.

The PDNS is committed to ongoing education and to exploring new knowledge about medical advances in treatment strategies.

Audit, quality and clinical effectiveness

Quality of life is of paramount importance, and is gaining prominence with the advent of Clinical Governance. Clinical studies and clinical trials are now routinely using quality-of-life indicators.[18] It has previously been demonstrated that the PDNS can reduce the need for hospital admissions, outpatient appointments and GP consultations, as well as improve clinical outcomes and well-being for people with Parkinson's and their carers.[19] All these are important quality outcomes.

Audit is an integral part of the role and PDNSs are aware of its importance and of the need to undertake and implement audit and research findings in PD nursing issues in their area.

One of the strategies for the successful implementation of Clinical Governance is through clinical supervision. Active participation in this is a clear demonstration that individuals are exercising their responsibility under Clinical Governance. PDNSs should take every opportunity to implement clinical supervision in their working area.

The multidisciplinary team

Along with the PDNS and patient, this may consist of a neurologist or geriatrician, physiotherapist, occupational therapist, speech and language therapist, dietician and social worker. All should have a specialist interest and expertise in the field of PD. It is also important that the main carer is identified as part of the multidisciplinary team. The PDNS is the key element in co-ordinating care management, and should be responsible for liaising with the primary care team regarding co-ordination of activities.

Patients require a continuum of care, which is best provided by a multidisciplinary team approach.[20]

Contact with other healthcare professionals

Contact with other healthcare professionals may occur within either primary or secondary healthcare settings, and may involve nurses, doctors and the multidisciplinary team. Such contact often consists of giving educational support and advice as necessary. This also incorporates involvement in discharge planning, liaising with community nurses and GPs, and facilitating continuity of care.

Links with the pharmaceutical industry

The pharmaceutical industry is committed to improving patient education, and PDNSs are pro-active in creating educational packages, audio–visual aids and information sheets for both patients and carers.

The Parkinson's Disease Society has previously won awards due to the productive relationship between the pharmaceutical industry, the NHS and patient associations. These agreed that PDNSs have achieved a successful outcome, demonstrating cost savings for the NHS and providing real benefits for patients.[21]

Carer support

The impact of PD on carers should not be underestimated. It has been well documented that 'looking after a person with Parkinson's disease can be stressful and may lead to social isolation as well as physical and mental health problems'.[22] A study on carer spouses of patients with PD were shown to have worse social, psychological and physical profiles, and also showed that carers providing extensive care experienced worse health.[23] These results also have implications for targeting appropriate intervention, and identifying the needs of carers should be seen as a priority for PDNSs.

It is generally accepted that carers experience more stress as a consequence of the psychiatric manifestations of PD that occur in patients than as a result of the purely physical symptoms.[24]

Hallucinations by patients are predictive of nursing-home admission,[25] and re-assessment of the patient would be required at this stage of mental deterioration.

Sleep disturbances are also common in PD with up to 98% of patients reporting problems.[26] The added burden placed on carers who are also deprived of a good night's rest may impact on their ability to cope during the day. A formal assessment of this problem by using one of the sleep evaluation tools and providing practical as well as psychological support should be a priority. New and serious issues have emerged over the past few years regarding impulsive behaviour in some PD patients on dopaminergic drugs. These changes include hypersexuality, gambling and punding (a repetitive purposeless, prolonged behaviour).[27,28] These may have a devastating financial and personal impact on all family members. Early identification of such problems, through including questions about them in the nursing assessment, and supporting family members, may prevent such an escalation occurring.

Again, the role of the PDNS in co-ordinating care and providing increased support to carers when confronted by these serious issues should not be underestimated (*see* Table 15.4). This is of even greater importance nowadays considering the decreasing number of potential family carers.

TABLE 15.4 Action points for carers' support/counselling

- As potential carers are usually female daughters/wives, they may already have extra stress of employment, and growing families and may feel ill-equipped to take on a caring role.

- Women may be reluctant to seek out help, as society has a greater expectation on women to be carers than it does on men.

- Role reversal may be an issue, particularly when the affected partner had previously been the breadwinner in the home.

- Men may find it easier to take on the role of caring due to their previous delegation in the workplace.

- Underlying feelings of guilt when a partner is placed in care can produce strong emotional reactions.

Links with professional and voluntary organisations

The PDNS works in close contact with many agencies, including the Parkinson's Disease Society and the local PD support branches. Currently, there are approximately 250 support branches within the UK which are run by volunteers, and this creates an ideal arena for the nurse specialist to disseminate up-to-date information to patients and carers in an informal setting. There is also a national group specifically for young-onset patients, the Younger Parkinson's Network.

Conclusions

Specialisation in nursing is a dynamic and ever-changing phenomenon, and it is important for nurses to be sensitive, flexible and responsive to these changes. The PDNS is pivotal in providing a service in healthcare, bridging a gap where the previous provision was lacking.

The move towards an advanced nursing practitioner level is currently being debated in the UK.[29] Studies on nurse attitudes to the expansion of their clinical role have found that extending the nurses' role could be beneficial as it improves continuity of care. However, inappropriate proliferation of these roles may be a result of doctors unloading what they consider to be 'mundane' tasks. There has been long-standing concern that extended roles lead to nurses being used to cut costs in the work force.[30] PDNSs may find it more acceptable to continue to demonstrate their autonomy and develop within the parameters and boundaries of nursing practice through gradual expansion of their role.

Providing effective healthcare, improving quality, evaluation and research, leading and developing practice, innovation, self-development and cross-boundary working are all essential for the implementation of higher-level nursing practice.[31] Future purchasers of healthcare – from Health Authorities through to Primary Care Trusts (Local Health Boards in Wales) – will be looking for cost-effectiveness and PDNSs must continue to demonstrate clinical effectiveness and functioning at the highest level of clinical practice in order to ensure continued funding.

It is clear that the PDNS has an extremely important role in the holistic management of the PD patient and his/her family. This role has evolved steadily over the past decade, and the logical progression from registered practitioner to senior practitioner and finally consultant practitioner is inevitable, presenting new and exciting challenges for the PDNS who has chosen to work in the rapidly expanding field of Parkinson's disease.

REFERENCES

1 Carter L. Manager of Nurse Development, Parkinson's Disease Society, London. Personal correspondence, 2006.
2 Macmahon D. A paradigm for geriatric medicine. *Care of the Elderly.* 1994; **April**: 51–8.
3 Royal College of Nursing. *The Developing Role of the Parkinson's Disease Nurse Specialist.* London: Royal College of Nursing; 1998.
4 Marsden D. *Managing Parkinson's: making the difference.* Manchester: Health Services Management, University of Manchester; 1997.
5 Bhatia D, Brooks DJ, Burn DJ, *et al.* Guidelines for the management of Parkinson's disease. *Hosp Med.* 1998; **59**: 467–79.
6 Parkinson's Disease Society. *The Development of the Parkinson's Disease Nurse Specialist.* London: Parkinson's Disease Society; 1998.
7 Noble C. Parkinson's disease and the role of nurse specialists. *Nurs Stand.* 1998; **12**(22).
8 Macmahon D, Thomas S. Practical approach to quality of life in Parkinson's disease: the nurse's role. *J Neurol.* 1998; **45**: 19–22.
9 National Institute for Health and Clinical Excellence. *Parkinson' Disease Diagnosis and Management in Primary and Secondary Care.* NICE Clinical Guideline CG035; 2006. www.nice.org.uk
10 Peace G. Living under the shadow of illness. *Nurs Times,* 1996; **92**: 46–8.
11 Whitehouse C. A new source of support. The nurse practitioner role in Parkinson's disease and dystonia. *Professional Nurse.* 1994; **April**: 448–51.
12 Calne S. Nursing care of patients with idiopathic Parkinson's. *Nurs Times.* 1994; **90**: 38–9.
13 Brown RG, Jahanshahi M, Quinn N, *et al.* Sexual function in patients with Parkinson's disease and their partners. *J Neurol Neurosurg Psychiatry.* 1990; **53**(6): 480–6.
14 Nyatanga B. Psychosocial theories of patient non-compliance. *Prof Nurse.* 1997; **12**: 331.
15 Colzi A, Turner K, Lees AJ. Continuous subcutaneous waking day apomorphine in the long-term treatment of levodopa-induced interdose dyskinesias in Parkinson's disease. *J Neurol Neurosurg Psychiatry.* 1998; **64**: 573–6.
16 British Medical Association. *BMA calls for urgent meeting with Patricia Hewitt on plans to extend prescribing powers.* Press release, 10 November 2005. www.bma.org.uk (accessed 15 November 2005).
17 Latter S, Maben J, Myall M, *et al. An Evaluation of Extended Formulary Independent Nurse Prescribing.* Southampton: Department of Health, University of Southampton; 2005.
18 Findley L. Global Parkinson's Disease Survey. Quality of life. Presented at the 13th International Congress on Parkinson's Disease; 1999, July; Vancouver, Canada.
19 Parkinson's Disease Nurse Specialist website: www.pdnsa.org.ukrole/keypoints.asp
20 Quinn N. Drug treatment of Parkinson's disease. *BMJ.* 1995; **310**: 575–9.
21 Parkinson's Disease Society. *PDS wins award for development of PDNSs.* News release, July 1999. London: Parkinson's Disease Society; 1999.
22 Maguire R. Parkinson's disease. *Prof Nurse.* 1997; **13**: 33–7.
23 O'Reilly F, Finnan F, Allwright S, *et al.* The effect of caring for a spouse with Parkinson's disease on social, psychological and physical well being. *Br J Gen Pract.* 1996; **46**: 507–12.

24 Miller E. Caring for someone with Parkinson's disease: factors that contribute to distress. *Int J Geriatr Psychiatry*. 1996; **11**: 263–8.
25 Goetz CG, Stebbins GT. Risk factors for nursing home placements in advanced Parkinson's disease. *Neurology*. 1993; **43**: 2227–9.
26 Comella C. Sleep disturbance in Parkinson's disease. *Curr Neurol Neurosci*. 2003; **Rep 3**: 173–80.
27 Seedat S, Kesler S, Niehaus DJH, *et al*. Pathological gambling emergence secondary to treatment of PD with dopaminergic agents. *Depress Anxiety*. 2000; **11**(4): 185–6.
28 Evans AH, Katzenschlager R, Paviour D, *et al*. Punding in Parkinson's disease: its relation to the dopamine dysregulation syndrome. *Mov Disord*. 2004; **19**(4): 397–405.
29 Magennis C, Slevin E, Cunningham J. Nurses' attitudes to the extension and expansion of their clinical roles. *Nurs Stand*. 1999; **13**: 46–53.
30 Higgins M. Developing and supporting expansion of the nurse's role. *Nurs Stand*. 1997; **11**: 41–4.
31 Skyte S. Rigorous but not elitist. *Nurs Stand*. 1999; **13**: 21–3.

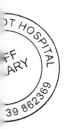

16

Drug therapy

JEREMY PLAYFER

Introduction

Drug therapy is central to the management of patients with Parkinson's disease (PD). The primary aim of therapy is to relieve symptoms and improve function. As part of chronic disease management, it is important to avoid longer-term complications of therapy, particularly motor fluctuations and psychiatric side effects. Ideally, the treatment should modify the progression of the disease by providing neuroprotection. The current edition of the *British National Formulary* lists eighteen drugs recommended specifically for PD.[1] These have two general modes of action: (1) drugs which enhance dopaminergic transmission, either singly or in combination, and (2) drugs which affect non-dopaminergic transmitter systems, notably anti-muscarinic drugs which reduce central cholinergic activity and drugs which modify glutamate transmission.

TABLE 16.1 Options for initial pharmacotherapy in early PD

Initial therapy for early PD	First-choice option	Symptom control	Risk of side effects	
			Motor complications	Other adverse events
Levodopa	✓	+++	↑	↑
Dopamine agonists	✓	++	↓	↑
MAO-B inhibitors	✓	+	↓	↑
Anticholinergics	✗	Lack of evidence	Lack of evidence	Lack of evidence
Beta-blockers	✗	Lack of evidence	Lack of evidence	Lack of evidence
Amantadine	✗	Lack of evidence	Lack of evidence	Lack of evidence

Key

+++ = Good degree of symptom control

++ = Moderate degree of symptom control

+ = Limited degree of symptom control

↑ = Evidence of increased motor complications/other adverse events

↓ = Evidence of reduced motor complications/other adverse events

The evidence base for therapies in PD is incomplete. Most major therapeutic trials are sponsored by the pharmaceutical industry and are designed for proof of purpose. The populations studied do not reflect the population that requires therapeutic treatment. In particular, the average age of patients in therapeutic trials is lower than that of the average patient suffering from the disease, and the exclusion criteria, such as cognitive impairment, will lead to a lower propensity to psychiatric side effects within groups studied.[2] There have been a number of attempts to collate and apply current literature to provide algorithms and guidelines to assist physicians in making appropriate clinical decisions.[3,4,5] The most recent guidelines, at the time of writing, are those of the National Institute of Health and Clinical Excellence (NICE), which provide a comprehensive review of the management of PD.[6] They are noticeably patient centred and take into consideration frailty and old age in their recommendations. Pharmacological intervention is divided into early disease intervention, defined as for people who have developed some functional disability and require symptomatic treatment, and later disease intervention, which refers to people on levodopa who have developed motor complications. The recommendations are based on a comprehensive review of available information and recognise that it is not possible to identify one drug of first choice to initiate treatment in PD. The choice of initial drug therapy has to take into account a variety of clinical factors and the emphasis should be on informing the patient of the short- and long-term benefits and risks of particular drug classes. It is recognised that a combination of drugs is often required in later disease. As levodopa is almost always required at this stage, guidelines provide advice on adjunct pharmacotherapy at this stage in the disease. The NICE guidelines provide useful tables summarising the relative merits of the different drug treatments in both early (*see* Table 16.1) and later disease (*see* Table 16.2).[6]

PD is a chronic progressive condition with a clear age-related distribution. General considerations for prescribing to the elderly apply for PD. Patients are more likely to have other illnesses and therefore have to take other prescribed medicines, leading to problems of polypharmacy associated with increased adverse reactions.

Most patients' anti-Parkinson regimes are complex – and therapy compliance is reduced by complex drug regimes.[7] Most people with PD do not adhere to their prescribed regime, and in particular the timing of anti-Parkinson's drugs is variable for nearly all patients. The timing of medication may be disturbed by hospitalisation and there can be serious consequences from abrupt withdrawal of anti-Parkinson medication, which may not be recognised easily in an older patient.

TABLE 16.2 Options for adjuvant pharmacotherapy in later PD

Adjuvant therapy for later PD	First-choice option	Symptom control	Risk of side effects	
			Motor complications	Other adverse events
Dopamine agonists	✓	++	↓	↑
COMT inhibitors	✓	++	↓	↑
MAO-B inhibitors	✓	++	↓	↑
Amantadine	✗	NS	↓	↑
Apomorphine	✗	+	↓	↑

Key
+++ = Good degree of symptom control
++ = Moderate degree of symptom control
+ = Limited degree of symptom control
↑ = Evidence of increased motor complications/other adverse events
↓ = Evidence of reduced motor complications/other adverse events
NS = Non-significant result

Age increases the sensitivity and susceptibility to adverse drug reactions. Ageing of the nervous system also makes the patient more vulnerable to neurotoxicity and this is evident in the high prevalence of drug-induced parkinsonism.[8,9,10] Drugs such as prochlorperazine (commonly prescribed for dizziness), given outside their licence indication of short-term use, have a high probability of producing extra-pyramidal side effects, including parkinsonism. Patients who are already parkinsonian will find that such drugs antagonise the effects of anti-parkinsonian drugs.

The pharmacokinetics of many drugs used in PD are complex. Pharmacokinetics can be changed by intercurrent illness, especially sudden changes in renal function. An unexpected variation in response to drugs may be due to pharmacokinetic factors, such as timing of levodopa dose relative to meals, or the taking of drugs affecting gastric motility.[11] There is evidence that the pharmacodynamics of anti-Parkinson drugs may be modified by age. This explains in part the increased susceptibility of older people to psychiatric side effects, and a lessening propensity to develop motor fluctuations.[12]

Dopaminergic drugs in PD

Levodopa

The rationale for levodopa in the treatment of PD centres around the notion that the symptoms of the disease result from a deficiency of the neurotransmitter dopamine in the striatum; this occurs as a result of progressive degeneration of the pigment-containing cells of the pars compacta of the substantia nigra. Levodopa is a precursor of dopamine and, when made available, is avidly taken up by depleted dopaminergic neurones where it undergoes decarboxylation in the presynaptic terminal to dopamine, which is then incorporated into the presynaptic vesicle. This helps to replace the endogenous neurotransmitters lost because of progressive pathology in the pars compacta.[13]

PD was the first neurodegenerative disease to be treated by neurotransmitter replacement. To date, no other drug has been shown to be more effective than levodopa at relieving the symptoms of Parkinson's disease. Levodopa is used almost universally in combination with a decarboxylase inhibitor, either carbidopa or benserazide. These compounds prevent the conversion of levodopa to dopamine outside the central nervous system and thus reduce the nausea and vomiting and the postural hypotension that are associated with levodopa monotherapy. They also increase the availability of levodopa in the brain. The introduction of decarboxylase inhibitors during the early 1970s was a major step forward in controlling the early complications of levodopa.

Efficacy

The effectiveness of levodopa was shown in clinical studies during the late 1960s and early 1970s.[14,15] Only one randomised controlled trial, the ELLDOPA study, has compared levodopa with a placebo.[16] This was a recent large multicentre study randomising 361 patients into four treatment groups: three at different doses of levodopa – 150, 300, 600 mg daily combined with a decarboxylase inhibitor – and a fourth group being a placebo group. All patients enrolled had not been previously given anti-Parkinson medication. The trial lasted forty weeks, followed by a two-week washout period at the end of the trial. Clinical assessment was using Unified Parkinson's Disease Rating Scale (UPDRS) and imaging of dopamine transporters. The results of this study were complex and have been the subject of much debate. The study showed that there was a dose response curve in symptomatic relief in PD. Following a two-week washout period, the patients who had received levodopa did not deteriorate to the level of those who had received placebo. This result could be interpreted as showing a protective effect of levodopa, or at least a lack of a deleterious effect on clinical disease progression. In contrast with this, the percentage decrease in dopamine transporter uptake and, by inference, the loss of presynaptic dopaminergic terminals appeared to be greater in the levodopa group than in the placebo group. This could be interpreted as showing a deleterious effect of levodopa on the presynaptic nerve terminal.

Possible explanations of these conflicting results include: the washout phase being too short to show the full extent of deterioration off levodopa; the possibility that dopamine transporter imaging is not reflective of disease severity. Side effects, particularly dyskinesias, were commoner at higher doses. Generally the drug was well tolerated. At the dose of 300 mg of levodopa a day, the rate of dyskinesias was lower than in previous studies of levodopa. Overall the results are reassuring and confirm that the use of low doses of levodopa gives good clinical benefit with no evidence of acceleration of disease progression and low rates of dyskinesia.[16]

In the early stages of Parkinson's disease, virtually all patients will show an initial clinical improvement on levodopa, and failure to do so raises a question mark about the diagnosis. The drug has greatest benefit in akinesia and rigidity, although there is some effect on tremor, but this is often disappointing. Heightened response in initial therapy is due to suprasensitivity from long-term denervation. At the early stages of the disease, there is preserved capacity for the presynaptic nerve terminals to store dopamine. The clinical benefit, therefore, of each levodopa dose lasts for several hours – significantly longer than would be expected from the very short half-life that plasma levodopa levels demonstrate.

As the disease progresses, the population of functional nigrostriatal neurones is reduced and with it the capacity to store dopamine. Some of the initial suprasensitivity to dopamine is also lost. The theoretical disadvantages of levodopa, which are not evident initially, become more evident. Levodopa has poor bioavailability. In particular, its gastric absorption is irregular and can be affected by competition with other large neutral amino acids. The plasma half-life is shorter than would be desirable. Consequently, the first detrimental symptom to emerge is usually end-of-dose deterioration of response, or the 'wearing-off' phenomenon. Patients with a good response to drugs can usually pinpoint precisely when the drug begins to work and also when it wears off. Over time, the kinetics of levodopa change, with a reduced nerve terminal storage capacity for dopamine together with compensatory changes in modulation of synaptic and post-synaptic mechanisms involving regulation of dopamine receptors. These changes lead to an increasingly unpredictable response to levodopa.[17] Once 'wearing off' occurs, the patient usually notices the symptoms becoming worse over time, eventually progressing to experience more unpredictable phenomena such as motor fluctuations, dyskinesias and 'on/off' syndrome. In addition to motor fluctuations, non-motor fluctuations such as mood change, anxiety, fatigue, pain, sensory problems, and autonomic symptoms including sweating and cognitive impairment are described.[18]

Motor side effects

Dyskinesias most commonly begin to appear at between three and five years after commencement of treatment with levodopa. For the elderly population, dyskinesias appear to be less common than for younger patients.[18] The most common form of dyskinesia is peak–dose dyskinesia, when plasma levels of levodopa are high. Biphasic dyskinesia occurs secondary to a rapid change of plasma level as patients switch between 'on' and 'off'. To complicate matters, dystonic phenomena often occur when plasma levels are low, and are particularly likely to occur in the early morning when patients may complain of painful curling dystonic movements of the feet. Once fluctuations in clinical response including dyskinesias and dystonia emerge on levodopa, the main focus is to try to reduce these unpleasant side effects.

There is little evidence of benefit of strategies such as fragmenting treatment into smaller, more frequent doses or the use of controlled-release preparations of levodopa.[6] Adjunctive therapies with dopamine agonists, MAOB inhibitors, COMT inhibitors and eventually apomorphine need to be considered.

How one can sustain the benefit of levodopa while reducing the long-term complications has been much debated in the management of PD over the past ten years or more. PD is as much a psychiatric condition as a motor condition with a range of phenomena being described, from mild cognitive impairment and mood disorders, to acute confusional states, hallucinosis and frank psychotic states. Drug treatment can exacerbate mental features, particularly the tendency to acute confusional states or hallucinosis and can precipitate frank psychotic disorders. These symptoms are more likely to arise with the escalation of treatment doses in order to control problems such as freezing and prolonged 'off' periods.[19]

Dopamine is a neuromodulatory transmitter, and in most circumstances its release in the striatum is continuous (tonic) rather than pulsatile (phasic). Experiments using intravenous administration of levodopa or duodenal infusions to maintain constant levels of the drug in the plasma (Continuous Dopaminergic Stimulation) have been shown to abolish fluctuations. This has led to efforts to modify the formulation of the drug, resulting in the development of controlled-release preparations.

There has been a long-running debate as to whether levodopa itself may be toxic to dopaminergic neurones. This thought has encouraged the use of much lower doses of levodopa than were usual 10–15 years ago. There is a theoretical risk that levodopa may increase oxidative stress and thereby accelerate nigral cell death. One advantage of using a lower dosage has been a reduction in the emergence of motor fluctuations. Indeed, a consensus seems to be developing that the total daily dose of levodopa should be limited to 600 mg or less.[6]

Formulations

There are two sustained-release formulations of levodopa: one is based on Madopar™ (levodopa and benserazide) and uses an osmotic principle; the other is based on Sinemet™ (levodopa and carbodopa) and uses an eroding matrix.[20,21] The matrix system appears to give more consistent stable plasma levels over a wide range of dosage.[22]

The 'CR first' study group undertook a five-year multicentre study comparing immediate-release and controlled-release Sinemet™ in PD.[23] This study was unusual in finding a very low prevalence of motor complications, which made it difficult to distinguish statistically between the two preparations. A sub-analysis of the study results showed benefits of the controlled-release preparation in quality of life and reduced adverse reactions, and also an improvement in nocturnal symptoms.[24] Open studies have consistently shown an increase in 'on' time on controlled-release preparations. Thus it was surprising that this was not confirmed in the controlled trial. Controlled-release forms of levodopa are more expensive and reduce the bioavailability and peak-dose plasma levels. The pharmacokinetic profile shows a slower rise to a peak level which persists for longer. Patients accustomed to an immediate effect from conventional-release levodopa often miss the 'kick-start' that this produces and their treatment may need supplementation by conventional doses.

The NICE guidelines, which quote three other studies on the effectiveness of modified-release levodopa, concluded that there is no value in using existing preparations in early disease. They confirm that these preparations may be useful for nocturnal problems later in the disease.[6]

The interaction with levodopa and dietary protein has been the subject of a number of studies.[26] Administering levodopa on an empty stomach at least 30 minutes before a meal reduces drug competition with dietary protein absorption from the gut and competition with transfer across the blood–brain barrier. Although there are claims that this improves the response to levodopa, it can also result in an increase in dyskinesias. Protein restriction is not to be recommended in elderly patients, since symptoms of progression of the disease often include weight loss and dietary problems.

Swallowing disorders are common in PD and in response to these, formulations of levodopa dispersible in liquid have been developed; notably a dispersible version of Madopar™, which is available in the UK. This formulation has a very quick onset of action and maybe useful in supplementing other forms of levodopa. However, there is no indication from studies that 'on' time is increased by the use of such preparations. The swallowing of fluid formulations can be just as difficult for PD patients as swallowing solid forms of levodopa.

COMT inhibitors

Enzymes control the metabolism of levodopa and dopamine (*see* Figure 16.1), with levodopa being converted to dopamine by the enzyme dopa decarboxylase. Dopamine itself is metabolised by methylation, transamination or oxidation.

Once peripheral decarboxylation is inhibited by using a peripheral decarboxylase inhibitor in Madopar™ or Sinemet™, COMT (catechol-O-methyl transferase) accounts for most of the extra cerebral metabolism of levodopa, resulting in increased levels of metabolite, 3-O-methyldopa. This metabolite competes with levodopa for absorption and transport across the blood–brain barrier into the central nervous system where it may compete with dopamine binding at the dopamine receptors. The effect of inhibiting the enzyme is to produce sustained and stable plasma levels of levodopa and reduce the production of 3-O-methyldopa.[25] Two COMT inhibitors – tolcapone and entacapone – are licensed for use in the UK.

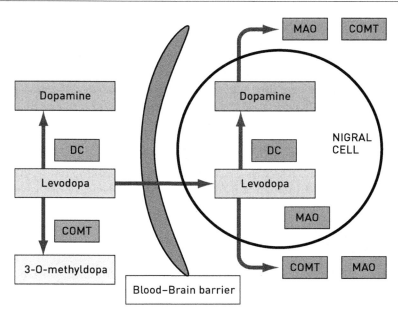

FIGURE 16.1 Levodopa enzyme actions.

Tolcapone was the first COMT inhibitor to enter clinical practice in England and Wales but its European product licence was withdrawn in November 1998 after three cases of fatal hepatic toxicity. However, after further clinical experience in other markets and a forced switch from entacapone to tolcapone study, it has recently been re-introduced in Europe.[27] The licence was reinstated in 2005 with specific restrictions. It is currently licensed for people who have failed on entacapone at a dose of 100 mg three times a day. There is mandatory liver-function test monitoring at two-week intervals for the first year of treatment. Its use should be avoided in the presence of dyskinesia.

Animal studies have confirmed that entacapone increases both plasma and brain levels of levodopa, when combined with levodopa decarboxylase inhibitor, while reducing 3-O-methyldopa levels.[25]

Phase I and II clinical studies have shown that the pharmacokinetics of entacapone and levodopa are similar. This led to the co-administration of entacapone with levodopa preparations (Stalevo™). Neither age nor renal function changed the pharmacokinetic profile. Patients with severe hepatic impairment showed enhanced drug levels but no evidence of exacerbation of already existing liver disease. Animal studies with entacapone showed no evidence of hepatotoxicity,[28] in contrast to tolcapone. Clinical studies using 200 mg doses of entacapone, combined with standard doses of levodopa/decarboxylase inhibitors, have shown that the plasma level of levodopa is sustained without changes to the peak concentration (C^{max}).[29]

The time concentration curve is flattened such that less dose-to-dose variation occurs. In theory, avoidance of the rapid cycling of plasma levels should reduce motor complication by simulating continuous dopaminergic stimulation. Randomised placebo-controlled trials have been undertaken with entacapone as adjunct therapy in patients with complicated late-stage PD: the 'Nomicomt' study in Scandinavia and the 'See Saw' study of North America.[29,30] These studies have provided consistent results with an average increase in 20% 'on' time in patients treated with entacapone, and with good tolerability. Beneficial effects on motor function and activities of daily living were demonstrable. The use of a COMT inhibitor allowed a reduction in levodopa dosage of, on average, 100 mg per day.

Entacapone is well tolerated with only two highlighted side effects. Firstly, an increase in dyskinesias, which is a reflection of increased dopaminergic activity; secondly, an increased incidence in diarrhoea. This is usually not severe and is tolerated by most patients and easily controlled by codeine. Where it is persistent, however, the drug needs to be stopped.

Entacapone has the unusual property of chelating iron and, therefore, is contra-indicated in patients taking oral iron preparations. Patients should be warned that their urine may be an unnaturally bright yellow and that this effect is harmless.

Entacapone is licensed for adjunctive treatment combined with levodopa for the indication of end-of-dose wearing off. It can be given in fixed combination with levo-dopa, available as Stalevo™, where 200 mg of entacapone can be combined with 50, 100, 150 mg of levodopa with, respectively, 12.5 mg, 25 mg and 35 mg of carbidopa. Entacapone can be prescribed safely with other anti-parkinsonian drugs. It needs to be used with caution with apomorphine.[31] There are potential interactions with methyl-dopa, antidepressants, dopamine and dobutamine, adrenaline and noradrenaline – in all cases enhancing the effects of these drugs.

The evidence base for the use of COMT inhibitors in motor fluctuations has been subjected to a Cochrane Review and also evaluated by NICE.[28,6] The Cochrane Report drew attention to fourteen trials, including the LARGO trial.[32] Although there were methological difficulties in some of the trials, particularly lack of randomisation and allocations concealment methods, they do conclude that COMT inhibitors have a use in reducing motor complications in people with later PD. NICE advises that the triple preparation Stalevo™ may improve concordance and should be the method of choice of using entacapone.

The placebo-controlled COMT-inhibitor trials document the efficacy of these agents in reducing 'off' time and levodopa dose, whilst improving 'on' time, motor impairments and disability. This is at the expense of increased dopaminergic adverse events such as nausea, vomiting and dyskinesia.

MAO-B inhibitors (monoamine oxidase type B inhibitors)

MAO-B inhibitors can be used both in early disease and as adjunct to levodopa in later disease. By inhibiting monoamine oxidase type B, this class of drug reduces the breakdown of dopamine, prolonging its activity centrally (*see* Figure 16.1). By reducing dopamine metabolism to potentially toxic products and by also reducing free-radical generation, there is a rationale for this class of drug to be neuroprotective. The drugs may also have anti-apoptotic effects, thus reducing cell loss. The DATATOP study demonstrated that starting therapy with selegiline could delay the need to introduce levodopa.[33] Although this was originally interpreted as neuroprotection, the mild symptomatic benefit of the drug had not been taken into account, so weakening the claim.

Selegiline was used widely as initial therapy for PD until the 1995 report of the UK Parkinson's Disease Research Group (PDRG) study on the effect of mortality data in levodopa and levodopa combined with selegiline.[34] This study indicated an increased complication and mortality rate on selegiline. The NICE guidelines recognise two meta-analyses and a randomised-controlled trial which address this issue.[35,36]

The Cochrane Review predominantly on selegiline refuted the UK PDRG study, showing no excess mortality between MAOB-inhibitor-treated individuals and PD with controls. The conclusion from the analysis demonstrated a symptomatic effect in early disease with MAOB inhibitors. It showed no change in mortality. Delayed onset of motor fluctuations with MAOB's was comparable with the effect of starting on dopamine agonists and it was felt that this was likely to be a levodopa sparing effect, rather than a distinct pharmacological action.

The novel delayed start design randomised controlled trial of rasagaline against placebo, then delayed rasagaline therapy,[37] showed that the benefit of early use was not caught up by those patients on the delayed start. Whether this is evidence of neuro-protection is open to question and will require further data to support the claim.

Rasagaline has been shown to be well tolerated in older patients.[37] It has the advantage that, unlike selegeline, its metabolic pathway does not generate L-methyl amphetamine. The TEMPO trial demonstrated the drug's efficacy in early mono-therapy use with an effect equivalent to selegiline.[38]

The LARGO study compared rasagaline against entacapone with levodopa.[37] It demonstrated that rasagaline was well tolerated in a single daily dose with its effects on 'wearing off' similar to those of entacapone. The age distribution within the LARGO and the TEMPO trials suffered from the defect of most trials, in that the trials did not include sufficient numbers of older people.

The use of selegiline and rasagaline as adjunct therapy is established in the NICE guideline recommendations. These guidelines point out that the size and quality of the trials of adjunct selegiline were poor and that the two large rasagaline trials provided more convincing evidence for the efficacy and safety of MAOB inhibitors in later PD.[6] However, all studies were of short duration, so that we cannot be secure in longer-term benefits. The size and quality of the adjuvant selegiline trials were poor, so it is impossible to reach firm conclusions about selegiline's efficacy and safety in later PD. The more recent study with the buccal formulation of selegiline and two large oral rasagaline trials provide more convincing evidence for the efficacy and safety of MAOB inhibitors in later PD. However, all studies were of short duration, so no comments on the long-term benefits and drawbacks of these agents can be made.

The oral fast-melt preparation Zelopar™, a formulation of selegiline avoiding first fast metabolism in the liver and given in a dose of 1.25 mg, is supported by a single ran-domised placebo-controlled trial demonstrating its efficacy in reducing 'off' time.[39]

Anti-muscarinic drugs

Muscarinic receptor blockade was first used by Charcot in the nineteenth century in the form of belladonna. Dopamine deficiency results in the failure to inhibit the excitatory effect of acetylcholine. Excess cholinergic stimulation is thought to contribute to the generation of tremor, and anti-muscarinic drugs have been shown to have significant anti-tremor effects.[40] These drugs have less effect in the core disabling signs of rigidity and bradykinesia. Anti-muscarinic drugs have been shown to have significant adverse effects on cognitive function. Although these effects are more evident in older patients, they are not limited solely to the elderly and one study showed that 70% of patients prospectively placed on anticholinergic drugs develop worsening cognitive function.[41]

Drugs which have incidental anti-muscarinic effects (e.g. oxybutinin used to control hyper-reflexia of the bladder) have also been shown to worsen cognitive and psychiatric functions in PD patients.[42] It has been shown that this class of drug can impair memory even in young, healthy volunteers.[43] This drug class also carry a high risk of side effects including dry mouth, difficulty in swallowing and constipation due to autonomic blockade. Anti-cholinergic drugs should not be recommended in the older patient.

It is a common misconception that these drugs are effective in preventing Parkinson's signs and tardive dyskinesias in patients on neuroleptic drugs, whereas in fact they may worsen both of these conditions.[44] Procyclidine and benzatropine, when given parenterally, have been shown to be effective as an emergency treatment for acute drug-induced dystonic reactions, and this is probably now their main indication for use.[45]

The NICE review concluded that there was insufficient data from the three randomised controlled trials available on the efficacy and safety of use of anticholinergics in PD. Use should be limited to younger patients, in early PD, with severe tremor.[6]

Amantadine

Amantadine is an unusual drug. Its anti-parkinsonian effect was discovered by chance when it was being used as an anti-viral agent.[46] Pharmacologically amantadine resembles anticholinergic drugs. It also appears to have effects modulating dopamine re-uptake and the releasing of dopamine stores. More recently amantadine has been shown to have anti-NMDA receptor activity, blocking the action of glutamate within the basal ganglia circuitry.[47] There are reports that it may be beneficial in reducing levodopa-induced dyskinesias.[48] The recommended dose for amantadine is 100 mg daily, increased after one week to 100 mg twice daily to a maximum of 400 mg. The drug must be used in caution with the elderly and a daily dose over 200 mg has a significant risk of psychiatric side effects. Amantadine is best used as adjunct therapy. It can give a short-term boost to anti-Parkinson treatments on special occasions for the patient. There are many cautions and potential interactions with this drug. In particular, it should be avoided in patients with hepatic or renal impairment. It may cause significant fluid retention. Gastro-intestinal disturbances, insomnia and anxiety, vasculitis (livedo reticularis) and visual disturbance are side effects which frequently curtail the use of amantadine. In longer-term use it is difficult to withdraw and side effects such as weight loss, cognitive impairment and hallucinations become more evident.

The Cochrane Systematic Review included six studies and a total sample size of 215 people with PD.[49] The major study included 100 patients, dated from the 1970s, and had significant methodological limitations.[50] The NICE guidelines advise that amantadine can be used in early PD but is not a drug of first choice.[6] The weakness of the evidence base and the high adverse drug reaction mitigate against widespread use of this drug in older people for initial treatment.

The NICE guidelines also advise that amantadine can be used to reduce dyskinesia in later disease.[6] Although dyskinesia is less common in older patients, if it is problematic then amantadine may be helpful, providing it is tolerated. Clinical experience suggests that even a small dose of 100 mg may suppress dyskinesia enough to help the patient's daily life.

Dopamine agonists

Dopamine agonists have been available to treat Parkinson's disease for more than 20 years. These drugs have the theoretical advantage that they act directly on postsynaptic receptors and, unlike levodopa, are not dependent on the degenerating presynaptic nigrostriatal neurones. Like many other neurotransmitters, dopamine fulfils more than one function in the brain. This heterogeneity of action and tissue distribution is reflected by the different classes and sub-types of dopamine receptor (D1–D5). The dopamine receptors are classified into two major classes: D1-like receptors (D1 and D5), and D2 microceptors (D2, D3 and D4). The caudate nucleus and putamen contain a high density of D1 and D2 receptors, which are concerned with motor function – the D1 receptor being involved in the direct motor loop and the D2 receptor in the indirect motor loops. The main dopamine pathways concerned with movement are in the neostriatum.

D3 receptors are localised in the limbic systems and have effects on behaviour, mood and emotion. D3, D4 and D5 receptors are also expressed in other areas of the brain but their function is less clearly understood than that of D1 and D2 receptors.[51] The ideal dopamine agonist would target simply motor function. Unfortunately, most dopamine agonists available have non-motor side effects, particularly effects on cognitive function and a tendency to produce hallucinosis. Nevertheless the potential for selective dopamine receptor activation is an important consideration in choosing drugs to treat Parkinson's disease.[52]

Because dopamine agonists reduce turnover endogenous dopamine, they theoretically have a mechanism for promoting neuroprotection by reducing oxidative stress generated by the metabolism of dopamine. There is strong research effort to demonstrate that dopamine agonists are neuroprotective and these studies include cell culture and animal models. NICE found eight clinical studies addressing the neuroprotective effects of dopamine agonists versus levodopa therapy in PD.[6] Most interesting of these studies were the REAL-PET study of ropinirole and the CALM-PD involving pramipexole. These studies measure the decline of radioactive tracer uptake in the striatum using dopamine transporters binding radioactive ligands.[53,54] Both studies demonstrated that there was an apparent reduction in the rate of tracer loss, indicating preservation of pre-synaptic cells with dopamine transporters. There has been a major debate about the significance of this work. It is unclear whether dopamine agonists delay motor complications by a fundamental neuroprotective effect or because of longer half-lives and a purely pharmacokinetic effect.

The exact indication of using dopamine agonists in older patients remains hotly debated and controversial. Recent trial work has concentrated on dopamine agonists as initial therapy, against their traditional use as adjunct therapy. Initial use of dopamine agonists reduces motor complications in later PD.[55] However, dopamine agonists give less symptomatic benefit than levodopa. There is a significant increase in psychiatric side effects, particularly hallucinations on dopamine agonists. Excess somnolence and oedema occur more frequently with dopamine agonists.[56]

The strength of evidence that dopamine agonists compared with levodopa in initial treatment of Parkinson's disease reduce motor complications is now established beyond doubt. Out of the eight trials supporting this, two are of major importance in determining clinical practice. These are the OO56 study comparing initial treatment with ropinirole against L-Dopa and the CALM-PD study comparing pramipexole against L-Dopa.[57,58] Although the studies were well designed and conducted, they are difficult to translate into clinical practice in geriatric medicine.

The average age of patients in both studies was 62 years, i.e. below the average age of presentation of the disease. With two-thirds of patients receiving treatment for PD being over the age of 70, the study samples do not reflect the therapeutic community. Both these studies excluded any patients with cognitive impairment, and the finding that the subjects had three times the rate of hallucinations and significantly increased somnolence is worrying if these drugs are to be adopted for first-line use in older patients. The propensity of older patients to develop motor complications is less, while their propensity to develop psychiatric side effects is greater.[2] Given that the symptomatic benefit is less on dopamine agonists, the evidential warrant for using these drugs for initial use in the frailer older patient is significantly deficient.[2] Selection of patients for initial therapy with dopamine agonists requires an intuitive judgement as to the robustness of the patient and their susceptibility to either motor or psychiatric side effects. An important determinant is their expectation of life and presence of co-morbidity. Patients with cognitive impairment, significant cardiovascular morbidity or hallmarks of physical frailty are probably best treated with levodopa.

Robust elderly have expectations of life of seven or more years. The benefits of initial use of dopamine agonists and the evidence should be discussed with each patient to ensure the right decision of the best initial therapy for each individual. Both the OO56 and CALM-PD studies allowed supplementation with levodopa and it has to be recognised that the vast majority of patients will need levodopa therapy in addition to the dopamine agonists in the first few years of treatment.

The case for using ergot-derived dopamine agonists – bromocriptine, pergolide and cabergoline – has been weakened by the complications of valvulopathy and pleura-pulmonary and peritoneal fibrosis.[59,60] These drugs now require a protocol for follow-up, including monitoring of ESR, chest X-ray, lung functions and echocardiogram. Although pergolide has been shown to be a strongly effective dopamine agonist, its use is now declining rapidly. Cabergoline, which has the advantage of once-daily dosage and the ability to achieve continuous dopaminergic stimulation with good compliance, also needs to be used with great caution and only as a second line to non-ergot agonists. Liseride has never had widespread use because of its increased rate of psychiatric side effects. Its use parentally is no longer required because of alternatives such as apomorphine or rotigotine patch.

Non-ergot agonists

Two oral dopamine agonists remain widely used in older patients: pramipexole and ropinirole.

Pramipexole is a highly selective D2 and D3 receptor agonist. It has a half-life of twelve hours.[61] It has been studied in major double-blind controlled multicentre trials, which support its use in both advanced and early disease.[58,62,63] Pramipexole is effective in symptomatic control of motor problems in Parkinson's disease with a reduction – as compared with levodopa – of motor fluctuation and dyskinesias. Pramipexole appears to have particular benefit in both mood and tremor.[64–67] In the treatment of depression, pramipexole has efficacy comparable with fluoxetine; this is potentially useful in treatment of elderly patients in whom depression is common.[68] Specific efficacy against tremor has a weaker evidential base. Pramipexole has been implicated in causing day-time somnolence and was cited in the Frucht study as a cause of sudden sleepiness whilst driving.[69] Patients taking this drug are advised not to drive if they experience sudden-onset sleepiness.

Pramipexole is an effective adjunct therapy to producing significant reductions in 'off' time and reduction in the dose of levodopa. Given in a dose divided into three sub-doses, it achieves close to continuous dopaminergic stimulation.[70]

Renal function should be checked prior to commencement of pramipexole, with reduction of the dose in the case of renal impairment. In older frail people there is a risk of producing hypotension so the drug requires slow titration: initially a dose of 125 micrograms three times a day. The dose is doubled at weekly intervals until effective control of motor symptoms is achieved or until the dose is limited by toleration or emergence of side effects. Three-step titration to a dose of 1.5 mg is often sufficient to establish therapeutic effect. Titration up to the maximum recommended dose of 4.5 mg gives flexibility as the disease progresses. All the doses given above are in the salt form of pramipexole; confusion can occur as the doses and strengths are sometimes expressed as the base form – with 88 micrograms of base equivalent to 125 micrograms of salt. This complication of prescribing should not deter use of this highly effective agonist. The nausea may need to be controlled in initial stages by giving domperidone for the first two weeks of treatment.

Ropinirole has a D2-specificity with particular high affinity with D3 receptor.[61] There is strong evidential support for both its initial use and its treatment of long-term complications of Parkinson's disease where its efficacy in increasing 'on' time and in reducing dyskinesias and motor fluctuations is similar to that of pramipexole.[70] Long-term follow-up with ten-year studies on ropinirole[71] confirm it is an effective treatment with low motor complications. Excessive somnolence and ankle oedema can be a problem with ropinirole use, and patients must be warned about driving if they suffer excess sleepiness.[72,73] Ropinirole has the advantage of ease of use with starter and follow-on packs, which allow titration up to 3 mg (starter pack) and 9 mg (follow on pack) respectively. Many patients require higher doses to get effective relief of symptoms, so the drug may be used up to a maximum of 24 mg. A 24-hour prolonged-release form of ropinirole (Ropinirole XL) has recently undergone trials and will be licensed in Europe.[74]

The use of both the non-ergot agonists has been associated with disorders of impulse control, particularly pathological gambling. These problems are rare and are more likely to occur in younger patients.[75]

Apomorphine

Apomorphine is a unique drug for use in late-stage PD. It is the most effective dopamine agonist and has clinical efficacy almost equivalent to levodopa. It is given by the subcutaneous route by intermittent injection using a Penject injection. The intermittent injection rescues the patient from the 'off' state within 5–15 minutes of administration, and the effects last for about one hour. In more advanced cases, where more than eight 'rescue' injections are needed each day, apomorphine can be given by continuous subcutaneous infusion using an ambulatory syringe driver. The dosage of apomorphine needs to be titrated for individual patients. The dose range is very wide, from a few milligrams per day by intermittent injection up to 150 mg a day by continuous infusion (the current licence recommends up to 100 mg). Continuous infusion over a period of months, together with reduction of other dopaminergic drugs, may significantly reduce dyskinesias.[76] Most patients ultimately progress from intermittent injections to continuous infusion of apomorphine.

Apomorphine is selective for D1, D2 and D3 receptors and has no opiate or addictive properties.[77] It cannot be used orally because of extensive hepatic first pass metabolism.

Formulations using other routes of administration have been piloted (e.g. rectal, sublingual or inhaled) but none is currently available commercially.

In order to establish apomorphine therapy, an apomorphine challenge test is necessary to ascertain whether the patient responds to the drug and to determine the individual threshold dose. In addition, careful monitoring for side effects such as postural hypotension or neuro-psychiatric symptoms must be undertaken. Before a patient is exposed to apomorphine it is necessary to prescribe domperidone 30 mg orally every eight hours for at least three days. Domperidone blocks the very strong emetic effects that previously limited the use of apomorphine. The patient is initially induced into an 'off' state by withdrawing oral medication overnight. In order to avoid hypotensive episodes, it is best to perform the tests with the patient recumbent. An initial dose of 1.5 mg of apomorphine is given subcutaneously, after which the patient's motor responses are observed for up to 30 minutes.

If there is no response, a subsequent dose of 3 mg is given 40 minutes later, followed by 1.5 mg incremental steps until a response is seen. If no response is seen by the time 7.5 mg is administered, the patient is classified as a non-responder and is unlikely to benefit from apomorphine.

The hourly infusion rate of continuous infusion can be established by using the threshold dose from an apomorphine challenge test, or by transferring the intermittent dose to an hourly rate. In frail patients in whom there are concerns about performing a challenge test, a low-dose infusion of 1 mg/h can be started after pre-treatment with domperidone, but without withdrawal of any other oral therapy. This infusion rate can be gradually increased hourly or even daily, depending upon the patient, until a response or unacceptable side effects are seen. During any assessment of apomorphine treatment, it is useful to assess patients using a motor scale such as UPDRS, or alternatively to video patients. The sites of injection must be rotated in order to minimise local skin reactions and formation of subcutaneous nodules. Nodule formation can be reduced by scrupulous technique, and ultrasound of local nodules can help reduce their size. The needle site for infusions should ideally be changed daily, but some patients prefer to change on alternate days.

Apomorphine treatment is quite demanding, and the support of a PD nurse specialist is valuable in instructing the patient or carers in intermittent subcutaneous injection or infusion pump techniques. The side effects of apomorphine include dyskinesias, confusion, hallucinations, postural hypotension and sleepiness.[78] Eosinophilia associated with myalgia, and haemolytic anaemia (usually in conjunction with levodopa treatment) has also been described. It is recommended that a haemological blood count be performed every six months in patients receiving apomorphine.[79]

Apomorphine is useful in pre- and post-operative situations such as gastric surgery, where oral medication may be discontinued. It can also be used in the case of other withdrawal symptoms from dopaminergic therapy, such as the rare malignant neuroleptic syndrome. Apomorphine now has a very firm place in the treatment of advanced PD and is certainly suitable for the older patient, provided that sufficient supervision and support can be given with the PDNS as key worker.[76]

Rotigotine

The range of treatments available to PD patients has increased with the introduction of the dopamine agonist rotigotine which is delivered by a transdermal patch. The rotigotine transdermal patch was initially licensed in the UK for monotherapy in early disease but then acquired a licence for adjunctive therapy in 2007. Rotigotine is a non-ergot dopamine agonist, which has a broad spectrum of dopamine receptor activity. Pharmacokinetic studies are particularly impressive as this drug closely approaches continuous dopaminergic stimulation.

The drug has been trialled on more than 1000 patients in early-stage PD and demonstrated significant improvements in patients' UPDRS motor scores, regardless of age, gender and disease duration.[80] The patches have a similar range of side effects to those of other dopamine agonists.

Rotigotine is applied once daily. It requires titration through 2 mg, 4 mg, 6 mg, and – if needed – 8 mg patches, in monotherapy, and can be increased up to 16 mg in adjunctive therapy. When applied, the patch must be held on the skin for 30 seconds to improve adherence. The patches must be rotated through different skin sites over a 14-day cycle and are difficult to use in very hirsute subjects.

It remains to be seen whether this mode of delivery proves popular with patients. Its use may be very valuable in patients with dysphagia or who are unable to tolerate oral administration for other reasons. Rotigotine was not licensed in the UK and no research studies were reviewed at the time when the searches were done for the NICE guidelines. Therefore, although a promising treatment, the place of this new therapy in the treatment of older people with PD has yet to be established.

Duodopa™

In advanced, complicated Parkinson's disease where patients cannot tolerate apomorphine and surgery is contra-indicated, a new alternative has been developed to achieve continuous dopaminergic stimulation and relieve the more severe manifestations of motor fluctuations. Duodopa™ (L-Dopa and Carbidopa) returns to basics, using levodopa combined with a decarboxylase inhibitor as the basis for therapy, formulated as a gel, which is delivered directly into the jejunum. A percutaneous endoscopic gastrostomy (PEG) is performed, and a specially designed pigtail jejunal extension is fitted and connected to a portable pump system. This method, pioneered by Aquilonius and Nyholm, allows flexible regulation of the delivery of levodopa and is the closest approach yet to continuous dopaminergic stimulation. The Nyholm series (the DIREQT study) shows extremely good results with very few side effects.[81] There is a demonstrable improvement in the quality of life and function of patients whose severe motor fluctuations could not previously be controlled. Duodopa™ is classified as an orphan drug – i.e. one which will only be used in very rare cases and thus for individual use is very expensive. It is estimated it will cost about £30 000 a year to support somebody on Duodopa™. One would hope that the cost would come down to more realistic levels the more patients use this therapy.

The cost is driven by two factors: (1) the gel is not stable at room temperature and therefore has to be replaced on a daily basis, and (2) there also needs to be support for nursing and pump technology, which are provided as part of the cost of the treatment.[81]

Future developments of anti-parkinsonian medication

The potential worldwide market for anti-Parkinson's drugs is growing with an ageing population. There is a significant number of compounds under development for the treatment of PD. Increasing understanding of the pathophysiology of PD has led to new pharmacological targets.[82] It is always very difficult to predict which areas of research will be fruitful and bring new products to the market place. At the most fundamental level, we should eventually be able to exploit our knowledge of the pathophysiology with drugs that alter the progression of the disease. Neuroprotection has been the target for Parkinson's drug treatment for some time but claims made in this regard with present therapy are far from established. Among the currently researched drug classes with possible neuroprotective mechanisms are: (1) mitochondrial protectors (coenzymeQ10, creatine); (2) anti-apoptotic agents (CEP-1347); (3) anti-inflammatory agents; (4) monoamine oxidase inhibitors (rasagiline, safinamide); (5) protein aggregation inhibitors, and (6) neurotropic agents.[83]

Beyond neuroprotection, neuro-rescue with the regeneration of dying neurones is a possibility, particularly with the use of nerve growth factors such as glial cell line-derived neurotrophic factor (GDNF).[84] More radical neuro-restoration will depend on techniques of cell biology, including gene therapy and surgical cell implantation of stem cells or nerve growth factors. These fall outside the remit of this chapter.

Current symptomatic treatments have major limitations. Although motor function can be improved, it does not return to normal. The increasingly recognised non-motor symptoms do not have established or effective treatments. Loss of efficacy and long-term motor complications plague the management of this chronic disease. Future pharmaceutical approaches include three categories: firstly, the refinement of dopaminergic medication; secondly, drugs designed to effect modulatory neurotransmitters outside the dopamine system, including targeting of non-motor symptoms and dyskinesias, and, thirdly, disease-modifying drugs which are both neuroprotective and symptom relieving.

It is increasingly apparent that the key to reducing motor complications is continuous dopaminergic stimulation.[85] The major advantage of dopamine agonists is their longer half-life and it is likely that this pharmacokinetic parameter is more important than any putative neuroprotection. The short half-life of levodopa and its erratic absorption leads to pulsatile stimulation of the dopaminergic receptors in the striatum, and in long-term use this causes compensatory dysregulation in the glutaminergic striatal medium spiny neurones. If this can be avoided from an early stage in management, the late motor complications are likely to be reduced. This is now established beyond reasonable doubt in animal studies.[55] There is a variety of new systems of delivering continuous dopaminergic stimulus either based on levodopa or on dopamine agonists in development. Particularly exciting are the slower-release forms of dopamine agonists such as ropinirole.[75] The STRIDE study using Stalevo™ will decide whether L-Dopa plus COMT-inhibition as initial therapy can achieve reduction in motor complications. Several smart dopamine agonists which have actions on other neurotransmitters are in development and offer promise of ameliorating non-motor complications. I suspect that most of the new drug developments in the next ten years will be drugs which modify non-dopaminergic pathways. Current active research areas include glutaminergic, serotonergic, adrenergic and adenosine A2A receptor modulation. Agents such as adenosine A2A receptor antagonists are already at a late stage of development. A2A receptors modulate the release of GABA.[86] These drugs have downstream effects on both cholinergic and dopaminergic systems. The animal models show promise that this class of drug is useful in reducing motor complications. Istradefylline is a novel adenosine A2A receptor antagonist that has reached phase 3 clinical trials.[87]

Anti-glutamate antagonists and NMDA receptor antagonists have efficacy in controlling dyskinetic movements. Drugs such as such riluzole and remacemide have so far produced disappointing results in clinical trials.[88,89] Idazoxan and alpha-adrenergic antagonists have been studied for their anti-dyskinetic activity and are now under clinical trials.[90] Drugs that may modify free-radical generations, such as spin trap agents or antioxidants, continue to be widely researched in animal models. Drugs targeting opioid and cannabinoid receptors are at an early stage of development.[91]

In addition to Duodopa™, with jejunal delivery, other novel methods of delivery to give continuous stimulation are in development.[92] Further transdermal patches to deliver dopamine agonists are likely, while specialised sublingual preparations including methyl and ethyl esters of levodopa and newer systems of controlled release are all being developed.

Management of the frail elderly PD patient

Making the best use of available evidence on drug therapy and applying it to the individual patient is more difficult when there are confounding factors such as frailty, cognitive impairment, and co-morbidity. These factors are the rule rather than the exception in managing the older patient. The individual clinician has to interpret and apply available evidence within a management plan, which includes non-pharmacological interventions. Clinical evidence derived from commercial sources is difficult to apply to patients treated in normal practice, since confounding factors are excluded from trials. The age distribution of patients treated in practice is much wider than the age distribution of subjects within proof-of-purpose trials. Older patients should not be denied innovations of treatment but there needs to be caution where lack of evidence can increase risk.[2]

The use of dopamine agonists in older patients very clearly illustrates these points. It would seem appropriate to give agonists to robust elderly patients without confounding factors, who would thus benefit from the reduction in long-term motor complications, whereas it would be inappropriate to give these drugs to patients who were at a high risk of psychiatric or cardiovascular morbidity. Such decisions rest with the individual clinician. The essential decisions in management of Parkinson's disease are:
- Is the diagnosis idiopathic PD which will respond to anti-parkinsonian medication?
- When should we start treatment?
- Which drug should be prescribed for initial use?
- How should drug effect be maintained?

Is the diagnosis idiopathic PD which will respond to anti-Parkinsonian medication?

Many patients are treated with anti-parkinsonian drugs unnecessarily, particularly patients with arteriosclerotic, pseudo-PD or essential tremor. Modern aids to diagnosis such as DAT scans are helpful in reducing error. Careful use of strict clinical criteria and avoidance of patients with drug-induced parkinsonism will undoubtedly reduce the mistakes in this area.

When should we start treatment?

Whether treatment should be started immediately on diagnosis or delayed until the disease is causing symptoms which require alleviation remains an open question. Decisions have to be taken on an individual basis and it depends very much on the lifestyle and preference of the patient as guided by the physician. The primary effect of drug treatment is to provide symptomatic relief and improve function.

Delaying the introduction of treatment is a frequently exercised option to delay the complications of levodopa. There is increasing evidence that delaying the introduction of levodopa does not necessarily delay levodopa complications. The original study by Markham and Diamond[94] has been supported by the more recent ELLDOPA trial.[14] It is often wise to give the patient a period of time to come to terms with the diagnosis and have a chance to discuss fully the implications of drug treatment. Such a delay of two or three months may empower the patient by giving a sense of ownership of the treatment.

Which drug should be prescribed for initial use?[6]

The NICE guidelines tackle this difficult problem with some degree of wisdom: 'it was evident from reviewing the evidence base that there is no single drug of choice in the initial pharmacotherapy of early PD. Further trials are required to compare initial treatment of PD with levodopa, dopamine agonists and MAO-B inhibitors, preferably using quality-of-life and healthy economic outcome measures. The UK PD MED trial will attempt to address these comparisons. The choice of initial therapy should be based on the clinical and lifestyle characteristics and patient preference when the patient has been informed of the short- and long-term benefits and drawbacks of drug classes.'

There is, however, a rule of thumb which – although crude – is practical, namely that the frailer the patient is, the more likely one is to initiate with levodopa rather than a dopamine agonist. In starting a patient on a dopamine agonist as initial therapy, it has to be recognised that most patients will require levodopa within the first two years. Combined preparations of levodopa and decarboxylase inhibitor are effective for symptom relief, easy to titrate, well tolerated and inexpensive. Dopamine agonists have the promise of reducing long-term motor complications but have slightly less efficacy and tolerability than levodopa and can require more complicated titration to achieve a therapeutic dose. They may, however, modify the disease process.[93] They are significantly more expensive than levodopa. Given life expectancy and a reduced propensity to develop motor complications, with low doses of levodopa, most patients over 75 can avoid the long-term levodopa syndrome. Where there is any degree of frailty, co-morbidity or psychiatric complications, there is a strong argument for initiating treatment with levodopa.

How should drug effect be maintained?[6]

Both levodopa and dopamine agonists have limitations in long-term use and require adjunct therapy. Both COMT inhibitors and MAO-B inhibitors are now well established at supporting levodopa treatment in the longer term. The tolerability of both entacapone and rasagaline in older patients has been demonstrated with a low rate of psychiatric side effects. Dopamine agonists, however, are very effective in supplementing levodopa for motor problems. Maintenance therapy, as far as drugs are concerned, usually involves combinations of medication and the objectives of treatment shift from purely symptomatic relief of symptoms to avoiding complications of medication. Once again the recommendations of NICE fairly reflect current practice. 'It is not possible to identify a universal first choice of adjunct drug therapy with late PD. The choice of adjuvant drug first prescribed should take into account clinical and lifestyle characteristics and patient preference after the patient has been informed of the short- and long-term benefits and drawbacks of drug classes.' NICE also warns against sudden withdrawal and the need to replace dopaminergic therapy when patients are admitted with emergencies into hospital, often using parenteral treatment such as apomorphine to cover surgery. Dopamine dysregulation syndrome, an uncommon disorder in which dopaminergic medication misuse (particularly that of dopamine agonists), is associated with abnormal behaviours including hyper-sexuality, pathological gambling and stereotypic motor acts, and it needs to be recognised. While this syndrome was originally felt to be much more frequent in younger patients, it is now being described in older patients.

The real challenge of later disease in older patients is dealing with the problems caused by the increasing prevalence of dementia, depression, hallucinations, autonomic problems such as difficulty with bladder function and swallowing, speech difficulties, constipation and orthostatic hypertension. In most of these areas evidence is lacking, although treatment of the psychiatric complications is dealt with in Chapter 6. One rare example of effectiveness evidence, specifically for Parkinson's disease, is the treatment of constipation where a double-blind control study of movicol has substantiated its use to prevent chronic constipation in PD patients.[95]

Care must be taken in avoiding drugs which may exacerbate the Parkinson's disease. The most common of these are metoclopramide, prochlorperazine and cinnarizine. Anti-psychotic drugs worsen or cause Parkinson's symptoms (even atypicals in high doses).

It needs to be recognised that Parkinson's disease is a progressive disease and at the very late stage in the disease when it is complicated by dementia and severe swallowing disorders, retreat from drug therapy may be necessary with recognition that one is managing the case palliatively.

Conclusions

Parkinson's disease remains a complex disorder, and we are fortunate to have effective drug therapy to relieve symptoms. Skill and judgement in the individual case is essential to maximise the benefit of drug therapy within a rehabilitation plan.

Balancing the benefits to symptoms with a reduction of risks of side effects is changed by the age and frailty of the patient. Although two-thirds of patients are over 70 years of age, most of the evidence on drug treatment pertains to a younger group. The choice of initial treatment is biased towards levodopa in the older patient, but most patients require a complex regime, eventually with adjunctive therapy. Expensive supportive treatment such as apomorphine and Duodopa™ should not be denied to the elderly on the ground of age alone.

REFERENCES

1 British Medical Association, Royal Pharmaceutical Society. *British National Formulary*, No. 52. London: British Medical Association and Royal Pharmaceutical Society; 2006.

2 Playfer JR. Ageing and Parkinson's disease. *Pract Neurol*. 2007; 7(1): 4–5.

3 Bhatia K, Brooks DJ, Burn DJ, *et al*. Updated guidelines for the management of Parkinson's disease. *Hosp Med*. 2001; **62**: 456–70.

4 Olwanow CW, Watts RL, Koller WC. An algorithm (decision tree) for the management of Parkinson's disease (2001): treatment guidelines. *Neurology*. 2001; **56** (Suppl. 5): SI–S888.

5 Primary Care Task Force. *Parkinson's Aware in Primary Care: a guide for primary care teams developed by the Primary Care Task Force for PDS (UK)*. London: Parkinson's Disease Society; 1999.

6 National Institute for Health and Clinical Excellence (NICE). *Parkinson's Disease Diagnosis and Management in Primary and Secondary Care*. London: NICE; 2006. www.nice.org.uk/CG035

7 Grosset KA, Bone I, Grosset DG. Suboptimal medication adherence in Parkinson's disease. *Mov Disord*. 2005: **20**: 1502–7.

8 Mena MA, de Yebenes JG. Drug induced parkinsonism. *Expert Opin Drug Saf*. 2006; 5(6): 759–71.

9 Hirose G. Drug-induced Parkinson's: a preview. *J Neurol*. 2005; **253** (Suppl. 3): iii 22 to iii 24.

10 Stephen PJ, Williamson J. Drug-induced parkinsonism in the elderly. *Lancet*. 1984; **ii**: 1082–3.

11 Simon N, Gantcheva R, Bruguerolle S, *et al*. The effects of a normal protein diet on levodopa kinetics in advanced Parkinson's disease. *Parkinsonism Relat Disord*. 2004; 10(3): 137–42.

12 Katzenschlager R, Lees AJ. Treatment of Parkinson's disease: levodopa as the first choice. *J Neurol*. 2002; **249** (Suppl 2): 19–24.

13 Cotzias GC, Woert MHV, Schiffer LM. Aromatic amino acids and modification of Parkinson's disease. *N Eng J Med*. 1967; **276**: 374–9.

14 Cotzias GC, Papavasillou PS, Steck A, *et al*. Parkinsonism and levodopa. *Clin Pharmacol Ther*. 1971; 12(2): 319–22.

15 Cotzias GC. Levodopa in the treatment of Parkinsonism. *JAMA*. 1971; **218**(13): 1903–8.

16 Fahn S, Oakes D, Shoulson I, Parkinson's Disease Study Group. Levodopa and the progression of Parkinson's disease. *N Eng J Med*. 2004; **351**(24): 2498–508.

17 Chase TN, Mouradian MM, Engber TM. Motor response complications and the function of the striatal efferent systems. *Neurology*. 1993; **43** (Suppl. 9): 523–7.

18 Schrag A, Quinn N. Dyskinesias and motor fluctuations in Parkinson's disease: a community-based study. *Brain*. 2000; **11**: 2297–305.

19 Papapetropoulos S. Drug-induced psychosis in Parkinson's disease: phenomenology and correlations among psychosis rating instruments. *Clin Neuropharmacol*. 2005; **28**(5): 215–9.

20 Crevoisier C, Hoevels B, Zurcher G, *et al*. Biovailability of L-dopa after Madopar HBS administration in healthy volunteers. *Eur Neurol*. 1987; **27** (Suppl. 1): 36–46.

21 Juncos JL, Fabbrini G, Mouradian MN, *et al*. Controlled-release levodopa treatment of motor fluctuations in Parkinson's disease. *J Neurol Neurosurg Psychiatry*. 1987; **50**(2): 194–8.

22 Pahwa R, Busenbark K, Huber SJ, et al. Clinical experience with controlled-release carbidopa/levodopa in Parkinson's disease. *Neurology*. 1993; **43**(12): 677–81.

23 Block G, Liss C, Reines S, et al. CR First Study Group. Comparison of immediate-release and controlled-release carbidopa/levodopa in Parkinson's disease. *Eur Neurol*. 1997; **37**: 23–7.

24 Grandas F, Marinez-Martin P, Linazasoror G, on behalf of the STAR Multicentre Study Group. Quality of life in patients with Parkinson's disease who transfer from standard levodopa to Sinemet CR: The STAR Study. *J Neurol*. 1998; **245** (Suppl. I): S31–3.

25 Bonifatis V, Meco G. New, selective catechol-O-methyltransferase inhibitors as therapeutic agents in Parkinson's disease. *Pharmacol Ther*. 1999; **81**(1): 1–36. (Ref ID: 19766).

26 Frankel JP, Kempster PA, Bovingdom M. The effects of oral protein on the absorption of intra-duodenal levodopa and performance. *J Neurol Neurosurg Psychiatry*. 1989; **52**: 1063–7.

27 Entacapone to Tolcapone Switch Study Investigators. Entacapone to tolcapone switch: multicenter double-blind, randomized, active-controlled trail in advanced Parkinson's disease. *Mov Disord*. 2007; **22**(1): 14–9.

28 Dean KHO, Spieker S, Clarke CE. Catechol-O-methyltransferase inhibitors for levodopa-induced complications in Parkinson's disease (Cochrane Review). *The Cochrane Database of Systematic Reviews*. 2004; **4**: CD004554. (Ref ID: 19624).

29 Rinne UK, Larsen JP, Siden A, et al. Entacapone enhances the response to levodopa in parkinsonian patients with motor fluctuations. *Neurology*. 1998; **51**: 1309–14.

30 Parkinson Study Group. Entacapone improves motor fluctuations in levodopa-treated Parkinson's disease patients. *Ann Neurol*. 1997; **42**: 747–55.

31 Zijmans JC, Debily B, Rascol O, et al. Safety of entacapone and apomorphine coadministered in levo-treated Parkinson's disease patients: pharmacokinetic and pharmacodynamic results of a multicenter, double-blind, placebo-controlled, cross-over study. *Mov Disord*. 2004; **19**(9): 1006–11.

32 Rascol O, Brooks DJ, Melamed E, et al. Rasagiline as an adjunct to levodopa in Parkinson's disease patients with motor fluctuations (LARGO study): a randomised, double-blind, parallel-group trial. *Lancet*. 2005; **365**: 947–954. (Ref ID: 19840).

33 Parkinson Study Group. Effect of deprenyl on the progression of disability in early Parkinson's disease. *N Eng J Med*. 1989; **321**: 1364–71.

34 Lees AJ, on behalf of the Parkinson's Disease Research Group of the United Kingdom. Comparison of therapeutic effects and mortality data of levodopa and levodopa combined with selegiline in patients with early, mild Parkinson's disease. *BMJ*. 1995; **311**: 1602–7.

35 Ives NJ, Stowe RL, Marro J, et al. Monoamine oxidase type B inhibitors in early Parkinson's disease: meta analysis of 17 randomised trials involving 3525 patients. *BMJ*. 2004; **329**(7466): 593–596. (Ref ID: 2739).

36 Macleod AD, Counsell CE, Ives N, et al. Monoamine oxidase B inhibitors for early Parkinson's disease. *The Cochrane Database of Systematic Reviews*. 2005; **3**: CD004898. (Ref ID: 20026).

37 Parkinson Study Group. A controlled randomised delayed-start study of rasagiline in early Parkinson's disease. *Arch Neurol*. 2004; **61**(4): 561–6. (Ref ID: 2764).

38 Parkinson Study Group. A randomised placebo-controlled trial of rasagiline in levodopa-treated patients with Parkinson disease and motor fluctuations: the PRESTO study. *Arch Neurol*. 2005; **62**(2): 241–8. (Ref ID: 19833).

39 Waters CH, Sethi KD, Hauser RA, et al. Zydis selegiline reduces 'off' time in Parkinson's disease patients with motor fluctuations: A 3-month randomized, placebo-controlled study. *Mov Disord*. 2004; **19**(4): 426–32. (Ref ID: 428).

40 Duvoisin RC. Cholinergic-anticholinergic antagonism in Parkinsonism. *Ann Neurol*. 1967; **17**: 124–6.

41 Katzenschlager R, Sampaio C, Costa J, et al. Anticholinergics for symptomatic management of Parkinson's disease (Cochrane Review). *The Cochrane Database of Systematic Reviews*. 2002; **3**: CD003735. (Ref ID: 92).

42 Donnellan CA, Fook L, McDonald P, *et al*. Oxybutin and cognitive deficits in Parkinson's disease. *BMJ*. 1997; **315**: 1363–4.

43 Dubois B, Dange F, Pilln B. Cholinergic dependent cognitive deficits in Parkinson's disease. *Ann Neurol*. 1987; **22**: 26–30.

44 Parkes JD, Bedard P, Marsden CD. Chorea and torsion in Parkinson's disease. *Lancet*. 1976; **2**(7977): 155.

45 Quinn N. Drug treatment in Parkinson's disease. *Drugs*. 1994; **28**: 236–62.

46 Schwab RS, England AC, Young RR. Amantadine in the treatment of Parkinson's disease. *JAMA*. 1969; **208**(7): 1168–70.

47 Bibbiana F, Oh JD, Kielaite A, *et al*. Combined blockade of AMPA and NMDA glutamate receptors reduces levodopa-induced motor complications in animal models of PD. *Exp Neurol*. 2005; **196**(2): 422–6.

48 Verhagen Metman L, Del Dotto P, van den Munekhof P, *et al*. Amantadine as treatment for dyskinesias and motor fluctuations in Parkinson's disease. *Neurology*. 1998; **50**: 1323–6.

49 Crosby N, Deane KHO, Clarke CE. Amantadine in Parkinson's disease (Cochrane Review). *The Cochrane Database of Systematic Reviews*. 2003; **1**: CD003468. (Ref ID: 51).

50 Schwab RS, Poskanzer DC, England AC, *et al*. Amantadine in Parkinson's disease. Review of more than two years' experience. *JAMA*. 1972; **222**(7): 792–5.

51 Strange PD. Dopamine receptors in the basal ganglion: relevance to Parkinson's disease. *Mov Disord*. 1992; **8**: 263–70.

52 Playfer JR. A short history of Dopamine agonists. *Geriatric Med*. 2007; **7**(4): 59–65.

53 Whone AL, Watts RL, Stoessl AJ, *et al*. Slower progression of Parkinson's disease with ropinirole versus levodopa: the REAL-PET study. *Ann Neurol*. 2003; **54**(1): 93–101. (Ref ID: 808).

54 Marek K. Dopamine transporter brain imaging to assess the effects of pramipexole vs levodopa on Parkinson disease progression. *J Am Med Assoc*. 2002; **287**(13): 1653–61. (Ref ID: 809).

55 Olanow CW. Present and future directions in the management of motor complications in patients with advanced PD. *Neurology*. 2003; **61** (6 Suppl. 3): 524–33.

56 Olanow CW. The scientific basis for the current treatment of Parkinson's disease. *Ann Rev Med*. 2004; **55**: 41–60.

57 Rascol O, Brooks DJ, Korczyn AD, *et al*. A five-year study of the incidence of dyskinesias in patients with early Parkinson's disease who were treated with ropinirole or levodopa. *N Eng J Med*. 2000; **342**(20): 1484–91. (Ref ID: 2540).

58 Parkinson Study Group. Pramipexole vs levodopa as initial treatment for Parkinson's disease: a randomised controlled trial. *JAMA*. 2000; **284**(15): 1931–8.

59 Horvath J, Fross RD, *et al*. Severe multi-valvular heart disease: a new complication of the ergot derivative dopamine agonists. *Mov Disord*. 2004; **19**(6): 656–62.

60 Baseman DG, O'Suilleabhain PE, Reimold SC, *et al*. Pergolide use in Parkinson disease is associated with cardiac valve regurgitation. *Neurology*. 2004; **63**(2): 301–4.

61 Kvernmo T, Hartler S, Burger E. A review of the receptor-binding and pharmacokinetic properties of dopamine agonists. *Clin Ther*. 2006; **28**(8): 1065–78.

62 Clarke CE, Speller JM, Clarke JA. Pramipexole for levodopa-induced complications in Parkinson's disease (Cochrane Review). *The Cochrane Database of Systematic Reviews*. 2000; **2**: CD002261. (Ref ID: 58).

63 Moller JC, Oertel WH, Koster J, *et al*. Long-term efficacy and safety of pramipexole in advanced Parkinson's disease: results from a European multicenter trial. *Mov Disord*. 2005; **20**(5): 602–10.

64 Barone P, Scarzella L, Marconi R, *et al*. Depression/PD Italian Study Group. Pramipexole versus sertraline in the treatment of depression in Parkinson's disease: a national multicenter parallel-group randomized study. *J Neurol*. 2006; **253**(5): 601–7.

65 Rektorova I, Rektor I, Bares M, *et al*. Pramipexole and pergolide in the treatment of depression in Parkinson's disease: a national multicentre prospective randomised study. *Eur J Neurol*. 2003; **10**(4): 399–406.

66 Pogarell O, Gasser T, van Hilten JJ, *et al*. Pramipexole in patients with Parkinson's disease and marked drug resistant tremor: a randomised double-blind placebo-controlled multicentre study. *J Neurol Neurosurg Psychiatry*. 2002; **72**(6): 713–20.

67 Navan P, Findley LJ, Undy MB, *et al*. A randomly assigned double cross-over study examining the relative anti-parkinsonian tremor effects of pramipexole and pergolide. *Eur J Neurol*. 2005; **12**(1): 1–8.

68 Corrigan MH, Denahan AQ, Wright CE, *et al*. Comparison of pramipexole, fluoxetine, and placebo in patients with major depression. *Depress Anxiety*. 2000; **11**(2): 58–65.

69 Frucht S, Rogers JD, Green PE, *et al*. Falling asleep at the wheel: motor vehicle mishaps in persons taking pramipexole and ropinirole. *Neurology*. 1999; **52**: 1908–10.

70 Clarke CE, Deane KHO. Ropinirole for levodopa-induced complications in Parkinson's disease (Cochrane Review). *The Cochrane Database of Systematic Reviews*. 2001; **1**: CD001516. (Ref ID: 60).

71 Korczyn A, De Deyn P, Rascol O, *et al*. Incidence of dyskensia in a 10-year follow-up of patients with early Parkinson's disease (PD) initially receiving ropinirole compared with L-dopa. *Neurology*. 2005: **64** (Suppl.): 396.

72 Stacy M. Sleep disorders in Parkinson's disease: epidemiology and management. *Drugs Aging*. 2002; **19**(10): 733–9.

73 Etminian M, Samil A, Takkouche B, *et al*. Increased somnolence with the new dopamine agonists in patients with Parkinson's disease: a meta-analysis of randomised controlled trials. *Drug Saf*. 2001; **24**(11): 863–8.

74 Pahwa R, Stacy MA, Factor SA, *et al*. Ropinirole 24-hour prolonged release: randomized, controlled study in advanced Parkinson disease. *Neurology*. 2007; **68**(14): 1108–15.

75 Voon V, Thomsen T, Mivaski JM, *et al*. Factors associated with dopaminergic drug-related pathological gambling in Parkinson's disease. *Arch Neurol*. 2007; **64**(2): 212–6.

76 Katzenschlager R, Hughes A, Evans A, *et al*. Continuous subcutaneous apomorphine therapy improves dyskinesias in Parkinson's disease: a prospective study using single-dose challenges. *Mov Disord*. 2005; **20**(2): 151–7. (Ref ID: 19993).

77 Lees AJ, Richardson CL, Turner K. *Treatment of Parkinson's Disease with Apomorphine: shared care guidelines*. 3rd ed. London: University College London Hospitals NHS Trust; 1999.

78 Deleu D, Hanssens Y, Northway MG. Sub-cutaneous apomorphine: an evidence-based review of its use in Parkinson's disease. *Drugs Aging*. 2004: **21**(11): 687–709.

79 Youdim MBH, Gassen M, Gross A, *et al*. Iron chelating, antioxidant and cytoprotective properties of the dopamine receptor agonist apomorphine. *J Neural Transmission-suppl*. 2000; **58**: 83–96.

80 Guldenpfennig WM, Poole KH, Sommerville KW, *et al*. Safety tolerability and efficacy of continuous transdermal dopaminergic stimulation with rotigotine patch in early stage idiopathic Parkinson disease. *Clin Neuropharm*. 2005; **28**: 106–10.

81 Nilsson D, Nyholm D, Aquilonius SM. Duodenal levodopa infusion in Parkinson's disease: long-term experience. *Acta Neurol Scand*. 2001; **104**: 343–8.

82 Wu SS, Frucht SJ. Treatment of Parkinson's disease: what is on the horizon? *CNS Drugs*. 2005; **19**(9): 723–43.

83 Bonuccelli U, Del Dotto P. New pharmacological horizons in the treatment of Parkinson's disease. *Neurology*. 2006; **67** (Suppl. 2): S30–8.

84 Olanow CW. The scientific basis for the current treatment of Parkinson's disease. *Ann Rev Med*. 2004; **55**: 41–60.

85 Nyholm D. Pharmacological optimisation in the treatment of Parkinson's disease: an update. *Clin Pharmacokinet*. 2006; **45**(2).

86 Chen JF. The adenosine A(2A) receptor as an attractive target for Parkinson's disease treatment. *Drug News Perspect*. 2003; **16**(9): 597–604.

87 Jenner P. Istradefylline, a novel adenosine A2A receptor antagonist, for the treatment of Parkinson's disease. *Expert Opin Drugs*. 2005; **14**(6): 729–38.

88 Jankovic J, Hunter C. A double-blind placebo-controlled and longitudinal study of riluzole in early Parkinson's disease. *Parkinsonism Relat Disord.* 2002; 8(4): 271–6.

89 Shoulson I, Parkinson Study Group. A randomised controlled trial of remacemide for motor fluctuations in Parkinson's disease. *Neurology.* 2001; 56(40): 455–62.

90 Rascol O, Arnulf J, Peyro-Saint PH, *et al.* Idazoxan, an alpha-2 antagonist and L-Dopa-induced dyskinesias in patients with Parkinson's disease. *Mov Disord.* 2001; 16(4): 708–13.

91 Fox S, Henry B, Hill M, *et al.* Stimulation of cannabinoid receptors reduces levo-induced dyskinesia in the MPTP-lesioned nonhuman primate model of Parkinson's disease. *Mov Disord.* 2002; 17(6): 1180–7.

92 Johnston TH, Fox SH, Brotchie JM. Advances in the delivery of treatments for Parkinson's disease. *Expert Opin Drug Deliv.* 2005; 2(6): 1059–73.

93 Schapira A. Disease modification in Parkinson's disease. *Lancet Neurol.* 2004; 3: 362–8. (Ref ID: 19537).

94 Diamond SG, Markham CH, Techiokas LJ. A double-blind comparison of levodopa, Madopar and Sinemet in Parkinson's disease. *Ann Neurol.* 1978; 3: 263–7.

95 Eichorn TC, Oertel WH. Macrogol 3350/electrolytes improves constipation in Parkinson's disease and multi system atrophy. *Mov Disord.* 2001; 16: 1176–7.

17

Neurosurgery

THELEKAT VARMA AND ANDREAS KOUYIALIS

Historical aspects

The past decade has seen a phenomenal expansion in the use of surgery to treat movement disorders. However, this field of neurosurgery is not new but has a long history during which there has been a gradual evolution towards the new techniques and methodology that are available today.

Early procedures involved open surgical techniques and while many of these offered varying degrees of benefit, they often had a high morbidity, especially with regard to the neurological deficits that they induced. The surgical procedures ranged from cortical excision[1] to section of spinal nerve roots.[2] Open surgery of the subcortical structures included transventricular resection of the caudate nucleus,[3] pedunculotomy[4] and open pallidotomy.[5] Spiegel and Wycis (1947) are widely credited with the introduction of stereotactic surgery into neurosurgery.[6] In the absence of satisfactory pharmacological treatment, the 1950s and 1960s saw the widespread introduction of stereotactic surgery in the treatment of Parkinson's disease (PD). Both thalamotomy and pallidotomy procedures were carried out in large numbers and while some patients undoubtedly benefited from surgery, a combination of poor patient selection and limited technology resulted in a high morbidity. The introduction of levodopa during the early 1960s saw a dramatic downturn in the use of stereotactic surgery for PD.

The renewed interest for surgical therapy of PD has been a result of several developments:

➤ recognition that long-term L-Dopa therapy declines in effectiveness and often leads to debilitating drug-induced dyskinesias and motor fluctuations

➤ greater understanding of basal ganglia circuits and their malfunction in PD, providing a better scientific rationale for previously utilised procedures and new targets

➤ use of advanced imaging techniques to visualise intracranial structures and the introduction of computer technology into stereotactic surgery has simplified the procedures and treatment planning[7,8]

➤ The introduction of implanted deep-brain stimulators for the treatment of movement disorders in the 1990s[9–13] now provides an attractive alternative to the irreversible ablative techniques that were previously used.

Targets for surgery in PD

Thalamus

Hassler is credited with having carried out the first thalamotomy in 1954[14] and since then the ventrolateral (VL) nucleus of the thalamus has been one of the most commonly used target sites in stereotactic surgery. Cells firing at the tremor frequency (tremor cells) can be recorded by microelectrodes in the ventralis intermedius (Vim) part of the ventrolateral nucleus in parkinsonian patients, and lesions or stimulators placed at this site give excellent control of tremor.[15,16] The anterior (VOA) part of the ventrolateral nucleus receives inputs from the basal ganglia and lesions here reduce rigidity and bradykinesia though the effects are rarely as dramatic as the abolition of tremor by lesions placed in Vim.

Globus pallidus

The serendipitous observation by Cooper in 1953 that ligation of an accidentally damaged anterior choroidal artery resulted in a dramatic improvement in parkinsonian symptoms focused attention on the pallidum as a target for surgery.[17] Leksell, in Sweden, identified the ventral and posterior part of globus pallidus interna (GPi) as the optimum site in the pallidum and this procedure was popularised by Laitinen and co-workers.[18]

In experimental and human PD there is increased activity in the GPi due to the reduced inhibitory drive from the corpus striatum and increased excitatory drive from the subthalamic nucleus (STN). Following pallidotomy, the interruption of activity in the motor region of GPi decreases the inhibitory influence on the motor thalamus.[12]

The most consistent and predictable effect of pallidotomy is the alleviation of levodopa-induced dyskinesias – this has been reported to be as high as 77% and sustained for at least four years on the side opposite to surgery; and as high as 43% on the ipsilateral side, sustained for at least two years.[19,20] There is also increased 'on'-state time and the reduction in dyskinesia allows an increase in levodopa intake.[21-26] While improvement in tremor[22,23,26,27] has been reported in various studies, this is in the author's experience not as good as with thalamic surgery. Most studies have also shown 'off'-state improvements in contralateral bradykinesia, with a 30% reduction in the Unified Parkinson's Disease Rating Scale motor scores (UPDRS-III) and disability scores.[22,23] Improvements in akinesia, axial symptoms and gait are, however, less predictable.[28]

Bilateral pallidotomy, even though attempted in the past, has been abandoned nowadays due to the uncertainty of benefits and the high incidence of major cognitive and speech defects.[29]

To treat patients with bilateral disease, bilateral GPi deep-brain stimulation (GPi-DBS) was introduced in 1993. This procedure has been shown to result in a 39% improvement in the 'off' medication UPDRS-III at four years after surgery, with improvement in all major PD symptoms (85% improvement in tremor; 38% in rigidity; 30% in hypokinesia, and 28% in gait[30]), without the high incidence of complications associated with bilateral pallidotomy.

Subthalamic nucleus

Experimental studies using the MPTP (1-methyl-4-phenyl-1, 1, 2, 3, 6-tetrahydropyridine) primate model showed increased cellular activity in the STN and that lesioning of the STN would reverse the cardinal symptoms of the disease.[31-33] However, surgeons were reluctant to lesion the STN in the human parkinsonian patient because of the risk of inducing intractable hemiballismus.[34,35] The Grenoble group was the first to report the results of bilateral electrical stimulation of the STN and the dramatic improvement in parkinsonian symptoms and signs.[36-38] Subsequently several groups have reported similar results and this remains one of the most significant advances in surgery for PD.

STN stimulation five years post-surgery has been shown to increase 'on' time; improve UPDRS motor scores while 'off' medication by 54%; activities of daily living by 49%; tremor by 75%; rigidity by 71%, and akinesia by 49%. Painful 'off'-period dystonia, sleep quality, postural stability and gait were also improved and most patients were independent, while prior to surgery most were fully dependent on a caregiver.[39]

There is still some ongoing debate on whether STN or GPi is the best target for the treatment of PD symptoms. Both targets have been proven effective against the motor symptoms of the disease. GPi has superiority over the STN in treating levodopa-induced dyskinesias directly, while it is also associated with a lower incidence of neuropsychological and cognitive impairment and mood disturbances.[30]

STN, on the other hand, has an indirect effect on drug-induced dyskinesias because it allows reduction in levodopa intake after the procedure and has a better effect on akinesia.[40] Improvement in the cardinal symptoms of PD also favours STN over GPi and these effects seem to be more long lasting. Finally, STN stimulation requires less energy consumption than GPi and along with medication reduction makes this target more cost effective.

In the absence of definite data concerning the superiority of one target over the other, target selection should be based on the patient's most disabling symptoms, response to medication and treatment goals.

Indications and patient selection

While it is obvious to clinicians that current surgical techniques are not a cure for PD, patient and carer expectations are often unrealistic and careful counselling is required. Most patients would have already undergone a wide range of pharmacological treatments before being considered for surgery and would have been either resistant to or intolerant of medication. Careful discussion between the physicians and surgeon is needed in this matter.

The diagnosis of Parkinson's disease should be established conclusively as the results of surgery for Parkinson's-like or Parkinson's plus syndromes are generally poor. A minimum of 40% improvement in the UPDRS-III from the 'off' state in response to levodopa treatment is considered a good clinical indicator of the patient's response to surgery.[41]

Tremor, which is often resistant to drug therapy, responds consistently well to surgery[9,10,42,43] aimed at the Vim nucleus of the thalamus. However, as STN stimulation improves not only tremor but also other motor symptoms of PD, it is now the preferred treatment option in the majority of patients but in older patients with stable tremor-dominant PD, thalamic stimulation can be a treatment option.[44]

Surgery offers no benefit in cognitive and psychological symptoms of the disease and the onset of dementia or the presence of active untreated depression is a contra-indication to surgery.[36–38]

There is uncertainty as to the exact stage at which surgery should be considered, but it provides little benefit to patients in the end stages of the disease. The proven safety and efficacy of this procedure has led several authorities to suggest earlier operations, before severe impairment of the quality of life occurs.[45] Advanced age by itself is not a contraindication to surgery but some studies have shown a poorer response to surgery in older patients and a higher risk of cognitive impairment after the age of 70 years.[41,46]

Surgery involves a prolonged operation under local anaesthesia and frail patients with intercurrent illnesses may have difficulty in tolerating the procedure. The presence of cognitive dysfunction makes intra-operative assessment difficult and can increase morbidity. The presence of significant cardiovascular or respiratory disease is a relative contraindication to surgery.

The need for a team approach in patient selection and management cannot be over-emphasised. Most departments undertaking such surgery will have a multi-disciplinary team that includes neurosurgeons, neurologists, neurophysiologists, neuropsychologists, neuroanaesthetists, nurse specialists and therapists to assess and manage patients before, during and after surgery.

Surgical techniques

Surgical techniques vary, but surgery is generally performed in three stages:
1. radiological localisation
2. physiological localisation
3. ablation or implantation of deep-brain stimulators.

Radiological localisation

This initially involves the fixation of a stereotactic localiser to the skull under local anaesthesia so that imaging can be performed under stereotactic conditions. In the past, ventriculography was the radiological technique used to identify reference points in the brain, but in most centres this has been replaced by CT or MRI. A short anaesthetic is sometimes administered to avoid patient movement during imaging. The position of the target site is calculated using measurements obtained from stereotactic atlases of the human brain, with reference to identifiable structures in the brain such as the anterior and posterior commissures. With good-quality MRI it is now possible to visualise directly the pallidal and subthalamic targets, though the thalamic nuclei remain invisible and have to be located indirectly.

Sophisticated computer software programmes are now available that facilitate the use of multiple image data sets and digitised atlases which help in the calculation of target co-ordinates.

Physiological localisation

When radiological studies have been completed, the patient is returned to the operating theatre and the radiological localiser is replaced with the stereotactic frame. Under local anaesthesia, a small opening is made in the skull and the stereotactic arc system is used to guide recording or stimulating electrodes to the chosen target.

Despite modern imaging methods, the final localisation of the target site has to be achieved using neurophysiological methods. These may include microelectrode recordings, somatosensory-evoked potentials, impedance measurement and electrical stimulation. Extensive neurophysiological localisation can be prolonged and opponents consider them unnecessarily time-consuming with added risk, while proponents view them as essential for accurate localisation.[16,47-49]

The final position of the target is decided on the physiological recordings and the patient's response to electrical stimulation of the target site. Unexpected or unwanted responses to stimulation will also warn the surgeon of erroneous positioning of the electrode.

Ablation or implantation of deep-brain stimulators

There are currently two treatment options available once the target site has been identified – ablation or chronic deep-brain stimulation.

Ablation of the appropriate area by creating a thermal lesion has for a long time been the standard method of treatment. A radiofrequency current is applied which heats the tip of the lesioning electrode and creates an irreversible thermal lesion in the tissue.

In the past there has been considerable discussion as to the choice between ablation and stimulation but currently DBS is the mainstay of surgery for PD. The disadvantages of cost, hardware problems and prolonged care are amply compensated for by the lower morbidity, reversibility and greater effectiveness of DBS.

Chronic deep-brain stimulation (DBS)

High-frequency stimulation of the target site has always been used as a method of identifying the targets during stereotactic surgery for movement disorders. Stimulation of the Vim nucleus at frequencies above 100 Hz was noted to arrest contralateral tremor and this effect was reversed as soon as stimulation was discontinued. Chronically implanted deep-brain stimulators had been used extensively in the treatment of chronic pain.[50,51] Following publication of the first studies of the use of this technology in the treatment of movement disorders[9–11] there has been a massive resurgence in stereotactic surgery. This has been coincident with technical improvements in the electrodes and pulse generators used for DBS.

The initial target localisation is similar to that used for ablative surgery, but once the target has been identified the tracking electrode is replaced by an implantable quadripolar DBS electrode that is firmly anchored to the skull. The system is internalised by connecting the electrode to a battery-powered pulse generator similar to a cardiac pacemaker placed subcutaneously in the infraclavicular fossa. The stimulator can be programmed, and stimulation parameters altered using an external programmer. The patient has some control of the system using a hand-held programmer that can be used to alter some of the stimulation parameters and to turn the device on or off.

Even though the efficacy of DBS is indisputable, the exact mechanism of action is still unclear. The following three different explanations have been proposed.
➤ Block of local neuronal activity by conduction block, thus producing effects similar to destructive lesioning.
➤ Preferential activation of inhibitory axon terminals.
➤ Excitation of projection neurons and increase in their firing rate, driving them at regular frequencies that override the rhythmic firing patterns associated with tremor, or the irregular firing patterns associated with PD.

Cost-benefit analysis of DBS

DBS surgery requires implantation of expensive hardware and this inevitably raises questions concerning treatment costs. Studies of cost-benefit analysis comparing STN DBS with medication treatment[52] have shown that costs for PD treatment may rise up to 32% following the first year after surgery, because of the implanted hardware, in-patient hospitalisation costs and the increased need for patient follow-up in order to adjust stimulation parameters. Reduction in the overall treatment costs become obvious from the second year post-surgery and may decrease by between 43% and 54% annually, due mainly to reduction in required medication, while the patient will also enjoy the benefits from surgery.

Other surgical procedures

At present, nigral and adrenal tissue transplants, gene therapy and the use of selective neurotrophic or neurotoxic agents remain experimental and are not in routine clinical use. However, these approaches hold hope in perhaps finding a surgical cure for PD. Furthermore, as our understanding of the pathophysiology of PD increases, new targets will become available and may provide better results in alleviating the symptoms of the disease.

Risks and morbidity of neurosurgery for PD

The mortality rate of stereotactic surgery is low (<1%), and is usually the result of unexpected intracranial haemorrhage. Unexpected neurological deficits occur with varying frequency, depending on the site of the lesion, and are often due to inaccurate localisation of the target. Short periods of confusion sometimes occur, especially when the procedure has been prolonged. There is also a small risk of post-operative epilepsy. Transient or permanent hemiparesis can be seen after thalamotomy or pallidotomy if the lesion encroaches on the internal capsule. The risks of cognitive dysfunction, speech deficits and dysphagia are higher after bilateral procedures (up to 18%).[53]

With DBS, side effects of stimulation can occur in up to 30% of patients and include paraesthesia, dysarthria and ataxia. These are, however, often transient and can be reversed by altering the stimulation parameters.[11]

Specific risks associated with STN DBS include behavioural changes and persistent changes in cognitive, emotional, mental and psychic functioning attributed to current spread to surrounding structures.[45] Depression and apathy, also known as 'loss of psychic self-activation', has been described and is attributed to the reduction in levodopa. Other side effects include hypomania, emotional lability, eyelid apraxia, weight gain and diminished verbal fluency.[41]

Hardware-related complications include skin erosion, infection, electrode migration or fracture and battery depletion. The incidence of wound infection is low but if it does occur, it may be necessary to remove the implanted hardware.

With increasing expertise and improving technology, the risks of modern stereotactic surgery for PD are low, and surgery can offer considerable benefit in what is a severely disabling disease.

REFERENCES

1 Bucy PC. Cortical extirpation in the treatment of involuntary movements. *Am J Surg.* 1948; **75**: 257–63.

2 Foerster OH. Resection of the posterior spinal nerve roots in the treatment of gastric crises and spastic paralysis. *Proc R Soc Med.* 1911; **3**: 226–54.

3 Meyers HR. Surgical procedure for postencephalitic tremor. *Arch Neurol Psych.* 1940; **44**: 455–9.

4 Cooper IS. Surgical treatment of parkinsonism. *Ann Rev Med.* 1965; **16**: 309–30.

5 Guiridi J, Lozano A. A brief history of pallidotomy. *Neurosurgery.* 1997; **41**: 1169–80.

6 Spiegel EA, Wycis HT, Marks M. Stereotactic apparatus for operations on the human brain.

Science. 1947; **106**: 349–50.

7 Hardy TL, Smith JR, Brynildson LRD, *et al.* Magnetic resonance imaging and anatomic atlas mapping for thalamotomy. *Stereotact Funct Neurosurg.* 1992; **58**: 30–2.

8 Kall BA, Goerss SJ, Kelly PJ. A new multimodality correlative imaging technique for VOP/VIM (VL) thalamotomy procedures. *Stereotact Funct Neurosurg.* 1992; **58**: 45–51.

9 Benabid AL, Pollack P, Gervason C, *et al.* Long-term suppression of tremor by chronic stimulation of the ventral intermediate thalamic nucleus. *Lancet.* 1991; **337**: 403–6.

10 Blond S, Siegfried J. Thalamic stimulation for tremor and other movement disorders. *Acta Neurochir Suppl.* 1991; **52**: 109–11.

11 Limousin P, Speelman JD, Gielen F, *et al.* Multicentre European study of thalamic stimulation in parkinsonian and essential tremor. *J Neurol Neurosurg Psychiatry.* 1999; **66**: 289–96.

12 Starr PA, Vitek JL, Bakay RA. Ablative surgery and deep-brain stimulation for Parkinson's disease. *Neurosurgery.* 1998; **43**: 989–1015.

13 Blond S, Caparros-Lefebvre D, Parker F, *et al.* Control of tremor and involuntary movements by chronic stimulation of the ventral intermediate thalamic nucleus. *J Neurosurg.* 1992; **77**: 62–8.

14 Hassler R, Riechert T. Indikationen und Lokalisations-methode der gezielten Hirnoperationenen. *Nervenarzt.* 1954; **25**: 441–7.

15 Lenz FA, Tasker RR, Kwan HC, *et al.* Selection of the optimal lesion site for the relief of Parkinsonian tremor on the basis of spectral analysis of neuronal firing patterns. *Appl Neurophysiol.* 1987; **50**: 338–43.

16 Fukamachi A, Ohye C, Narabayashi J. Delineation of the thalamic nuclei with a microelectrode in stereotactic surgery for parkinsonism and cerebral palsy. *J Neurosurg.* 1973; **39**: 214–25.

17 Cooper IS. Ligation of the anterior choroidal artery for involuntary movements in Parkinsonism. *Psychiatr Q.* 1953; **27**: 317–9.

18 Laitinen LV, Bergenheim AT, Hariz MI. Leksells posteroventral pallidotomy in the treatment of Parkinson's disease. *J Neurosurg.* 1992; **76**: 53–61.

19 Krack P, Poepping M, Weinert D, *et al.* Thalamic, pallidal, or subthalamic surgery for Parkinson's disease? *J Neurol.* 2000; **247** (Suppl. 2): 122–34.

20 Baron MS, Vitek JL, Bakay RA, *et al.* Treatment of advanced Parkinson's disease by unilateral posterior GPi pallidotomy: 4-year results of a pilot study. *Mov Disord.* 2000; **15**(2): 230–7.

21 Iacono RP, Shima F, Lonser RR, *et al.* The results, indications and physiology of posteroventral pallidotomy for patients with Parkinson's disease. *Neurosurgery.* 1995; **36**: 1118–26.

22 Dogali M, Fazzini E, Kolodny E, *et al.* Stereotactic ventral pallidotomy for Parkinson's disease. *Neurology.* 1995; **45**: 753–61.

23 Lozano AM, Lang AE, Galvez-Jimenez N, *et al.* Effects of GPi pallidotomy on motor function in Parkinson's disease. *Lancet.* 1995; **346**: 1383–7.

24 Sutton JP, Couldwell W, Lew MF, *et al.* Venteroposterior medial pallidotomy in patients with advanced Parkinson's disease. *Neurosurgery.* 1995; **36**: 1112–7.

25 Scott R, Gregory R, Hines N, *et al.* Neuropsychological, neurological and functional outcome following pallidotomy for Parkinson's disease: a consecutive series of eight simultaneous bilateral and twelve unilateral procedures. *Brain.* 1998; **121**: 659–75.

26 Lang AE, Lozano A, Montgomery E, *et al.* Posteromedial pallidotomy in advanced Parkinson's disease. *N Eng J Med.* 1997; **337**: 1036–42.

27 Baron MS, Vitek JL, Bakay RA, *et al.* Treatment of advanced Parkinson's disease by posterior GPi pallidotomy: 1-year results of a pilot study. *Ann Neurol.* 1996; **40**: 355–66.

28 Starr PA, Vitek JL, Bakay RAE. Pallidotomy: clinical results. In: Germano IM, editor. *Neurosurgical Treatment of Movement Disorders.* Lebanon, New Hampshire: The American Association of Neurological Surgeons; 1998.

29 De Bie RM, Schuurman PR, Esselink RA, *et al.* Bilateral pallidotomy in Parkinson's disease: a retrospective study. *Mov Disord.* 2002; **17**(3): 533–8.

30 Rodriguez-Oroz MC, Obeso JA, Lang AE, *et al.* Bilateral deep-brain stimulation in Parkinson's disease: a multicentre study with 4 years follow-up. *Brain.* 2005; **128** (Part 10): 2240–9.

31 Aziz TZ, Peggs D, Sambrook MA, *et al.* Lesions of the subthalamic nucleus for the alleviation of 1-methyl-4-phenyl-1, 2, 3, 6-tetrahydropyridine (MPTP) induced parkinsonism in the primate. *Mov Disord.* 1991; **6**: 288–92.

32 Benazzouz A, Gross C, Féger J, *et al.* Reversal of rigidity and improvement of motor performance by subthalamic high-frequency stimulation in MPTP-treated monkeys. *Eur J Neurosci.* 1993; **5**: 382–9.

33 Bergman H, Wichmann T, DeLong MR. Reversal of experimental parkinsonism by lesions of the subthalamic nucleus. *Science.* 1990; **249**: 1436–8.

34 Andy OJ, Jurko MF, Sias FR. Subthalamotomy in the treatment of Parkinsonian tremor. *J Neurosurg.* 1983; **46**: 107–11.

35 Obeso J, Alvarez L, Macias RJ, *et al.* Lesion of the subthalamic nucleus (STN) in Parkinson's disease (abstract). *Neurology.* 1997; **48** (Suppl.): A138.

36 Limousin P, Pollak P, Benazzouz A, *et al.* Effect on parkinsonian signs and symptoms of bilateral subthalamic nucleus stimulation. *Lancet.* 1995; **345**: 91–5.

37 Moringlane JR, Ceballos-Baumann AO, Alesch F. Long-term effect of electrostimulation of the subthalamic nucleus in bradykinetic-rigid Parkinson's disease. *Minimal Invasive Surg.* 1998; **41**: 133–6.

38 Pollak P, Benabid AL, Limousin P, *et al.* Subthalamic nucleus stimulation alleviates akinesia and rigidity in parkinsonian patients. *Adv Neurol.* 1996; **69**: 591–4.

39 Krack P, Batir A, Van Blercom N, *et al.* Five-year follow-up of bilateral stimulation of the subthalamic nucleus in advanced Parkinson's disease. *N Eng J Med.* 2003; **349**(20): 1925–34.

40 Welter ML, Houeto JL, Tezenas du Montcel S, *et al.* Clinical predictive factors of subthalamic stimulation in Parkinson's disease. *Brain.* 2002; **125** (Part 3): 575–83.

41 Schupbach WM, Chastan N, Welter ML, *et al.* Stimulation of the subthalamic nucleus in Parkinson's disease: a 5 year follow up. *J Neurol Neurosurg Psychiatry.* 2005; **76**(12): 1640–4.

42 Matsumoto K, Shichijo F, Fukami T. Long-term follow up review of cases of Parkinson's disease after unilateral or bilateral thalamotomy. *J Neurosurg.* 1984; **60**: 1033–44.

43 Kelly PJ, Gillingham FJ. The long-term results of stereotaxic surgery and L-Dopa therapy in patients with Parkinson's disease. *J Neurosurg.* 1980; **53**: 332–7.

44 Okun MS, Vitek JL. Lesion therapy for Parkinson's disease and other movement disorders: update and controversies. *Mov Disord.* 2004; **19**(4): 375–89.

45 Benabid AL, Chabardes S, Seigneuret E. Deep-brain stimulation in Parkinson's disease: long-term efficacy and safety – What happened this year? *Curr Opin Neurol.* 2005; **18**(6): 623–30.

46 Saint-Cyr JA, Trepanier LL, Kumar R, *et al.* Neuropsychological consequences of chronic bilateral stimulation of the subthalamic nucleus in Parkinson's disease. *Brain.* 2000; **123**: 2091–108.

47 Taren J, Guiot G, Derome P, *et al.* Hazards of stereotactic thalamectomy: added safety factor in corroborating X-ray target localization with neurophysiological methods. *J Neurosurg.* 1968; **29**: 173–82.

48 Favre J, Taha JM, Nguyen TT, *et al.* Pallidotomy: a survey of current practice in North America. *Neurosurgery.* 1996; **39**: 883–92.

49 Hosobuchi Y. Subcortical electrical stimulation for control of intractable pain in humans: a report of 122 cases (1970–1984). *J Neurosurg.* 1986; **64**: 543–53.

50 Gol A. Relief of pain by electrical stimulation of the septal area. *J Neurol Sci.* 1967; **5**: 115–20.

51 Bejjani B, Damier P, Arnulf I, *et al.* Pallidal stimulation for Parkinson's disease: two targets? *Neurology.* 1997; **49**: 1564–9.

52 Meissner W, Schreiter D, Volkmann J, *et al.* Deep-brain stimulation in late stage Parkinson's disease: a retrospective cost analysis in Germany. *J Neurol.* 2005; **252**(2): 218–23.

53 Osenbach RK, Burchiel KJ. Thalamotomy: indications, techniques and results. In: Germano IM, editor. *Neurosurgical Treatment of Movement Disorders.* Lebanon, NH: The American Association of Neurological Surgeons; 1998.

18

Complementary and alternative medicine

RICHARD BROWN

Introduction

Existing medical and surgical treatments for Parkinson's disease are only partially effective in relieving the motor and non-motor symptoms, leaving all patients with the prospect of increasing disability and dependency. Little wonder that many look for extra help from outside the realms of conventional medicine. Today it is not hard to find information about complementary and alternative approaches to health. From supermarket shelves to glossy magazines, we find material promoting the health potential of vitamins, dietary supplements and herbal preparations. Notice boards in public libraries advertise the services of aromatherapists and reflexologists. The internet is awash with discussion groups and websites devoted to alternative and complementary health practices. Patients discuss amongst themselves the latest news, views and personal endorsements of a particular therapy. Patients are therefore far from under-informed, even if that information is often partial and of poor quality.

It is against this background that patients will often ask advice of their GP or physician, wanting to know whether or not they should be taking Vitamin E, trying acupuncture, learning the Alexander technique or practising yoga. What should we say to patients in these circumstances? The purpose of this chapter is to consider what we know of the use of complementary approaches to health in those with Parkinson's disease and the little evidence that is currently available.

The use of complementary and alternative medicine (CAM) by patients with Parkinson's disease

In 1997 the Parkinson's Disease Society (PDS) UK[1] carried out a survey of its membership of around 25 000, and received over 2000 replies. The low response rate and the potential bias mean that the results should be interpreted with caution. However, the results are consistent with subsequent smaller-scale surveys that point both to a high level of interest in, and use of, CAM therapies, with similar choices and preferences being made.[2-4]

In the PDS survey the respondents' mean age was 61.5 years (±10.4), with an approximate duration of illness of 7.7 years (±6.1). As such they are fairly typical of the patients seen in a specialist movement disorders clinic, although younger than those seen within a geriatric service. The majority (51.4%) had little or only mild restriction in normal activity. Of the remainder, most (30.9%) had moderate disability, while only 17.9% had severe disability or were totally dependent.

Just over one-third (34.9%) were currently trying or had previously tried at least one CAM therapy for problems related to their Parkinson's disease. The majority of these were under the age of 65, suggesting a bias for the younger patients in the use of complementary approaches to health, perhaps because of differences in attitude or for reasons of finance. The latter may be particularly relevant, as 43% of those trying a complementary therapy had paid £100 or more in the preceding year, with almost 10% paying over £500 (based on 1997 prices).

Table 18.1 shows the list of therapies covered in the survey, together with the proportion of the sample that had experience of them. Most of the mainstream therapies are represented in the 'top 10', probably reflecting their availability. One trend that emerged was the change in choice of therapy as patients became more disabled. While yoga, relaxation therapy and meditation topped the list of the least disabled patients, aromatherapy and herbal medicine were likely to be chosen by the most disabled. There was no clear trend for therapy preference with increasing age.

Table 18.2 shows the subjective responses for the ten most widely used therapies, each tried by at least 90 patients. Yoga was the most positively endorsed, with two-thirds feeling that they had obtained 'considerable' or 'extreme' benefit. As interesting as the degree of benefit was the nature of the benefit that respondents reported. Across all therapies, the main ones reported related to psychological relaxation, stress relief, improved sense of 'well-being' and 'energy'. In terms of symptomatic relief, rigidity, stiffness and pain relief were the most commonly reported areas in which people found benefit.

TABLE 18.1 PDS UK Survey of CAM use
Rank order of the most commonly tried therapies

Therapy	% of total sample (N=2273)	% of those with experience of CAM (N=793)
Reflexology	9.3	27.0
Aromatherapy	9.2	26.7
Shiatsu/Massage	8.8	25.5
Relaxation/Meditation	8.5	24.7
Acupuncture/Acupressure	7.6	21.8
Yoga	6.7	19.4
Herbal medicine	6.5	18.9
Osteopathy/Chiropractic	6.5	18.9
Healing	6.3	18.3
Homeopathy	5.6	16.2
Alexander technique	3.2	9.3
Conductive education	2.8	8.1
Dietary therapy	2.7	7.8
Hypnotherapy	2.0	5.8
Tai Chi	1.7	4.9
Cranial osteopathy	1.3	3.8
Biofeedback	0.5	1.5
Feldenkrais	0.1	0.3
Others (total)	1.0	2.9

The 'evidence'

This and similar published surveys, while of interest, fail to provide the information appropriate for evidence-based management of Parkinson's disease. In common with CAM approaches in other health conditions, the evidence base from formal clinical trials of CAM in PD is sparse. The majority of the most popular therapies used by patients have either had no formal evaluation or only single, often methodologically weak, trials. The evidence, such as it is, must be interpreted with caution.

Traditional non-Western medical systems have their own long-standing approaches to the treatment of PD. The Indian system or Ayurveda (*see* reference 5) treats *Kampavata* (the clinical entity closest to Parkinson's disease) with the seeds of *Mucuna pruriens*. This concentrated natural source of levodopa has been shown to produce clinical benefit in a small-scale randomised controlled trial (RCT).[6] Another natural source of levodopa is the broad bean *Vicia faba* which can have antiparkinsonian effects and raise blood dopa levels.[7] However, while there may be a clinical effect of such products, neither has been tested formally against conventional synthetic levodopa to show that they are superior in efficacy or produce fewer side effects. Genghe[8] carried out an open trial of traditional Chinese medicine on 50 patients. He reported 'marked subjective improvement' in 30% after three months of herbal treatment and acupuncture, while 22% showed no benefit. However, while encouraging, such results do not yet reach acceptable standards of evidence. Acupuncture and other non–herbal traditional treatments have been the subject of two small open-label trials in PD.[9,10] While showing no positive effect on motor symptoms, some benefits were reported in sleep, mood and quality of life. Intriguingly, a recent study using DAT scan has shown a statistically significant effect of acupuncture on striatal DAT activity over a six-week period.[11] Furthermore, recent animal research is pointing towards possible neuroprotective effect of acupuncture, offering encouragement to further clinical studies.[12,13]

TABLE 18.2 PDS UK Survey of CAM use
Subjective benefit of 10 most commonly used therapies, with rank order of satisfaction in square brackets. Remaining % is accounted for by complaints of negative or adverse outcomes

Therapy	Considerable or extreme benefit	Slight or no benefit
Reflexology	36.6% [8]	62.6%
Aromatherapy	41.4% [4]	57.9%
Shiatsu/Massage	51.9% [2]	48.1%
Relaxation/Meditation	41.1% [5]	58.9%
Acupuncture/Acupressure	28.9% [9]	67.8%
Yoga	66.5% [1]	33.5%
Herbal medicine	36.7% [7]	62.0%
Osteopathy/Chiropractic	39.8% [6]	55.9%
Healing	42.8% [3]	57.2%
Homeopathy	28.5% [10]	68.5%

The potential value to health of compounds occurring naturally in our diet is a growing area of scientific enquiry, with opportunities offered by enhanced supplementation of such compounds for those with disease or as neuroprotection. The value of the antioxidant vitamin α-tocopherol was evaluated in the DATATOP study as a possible neuroprotective agent, one of the few large-scale trials of its type to date. Despite the size of the study, no significant effect of α-tocopherol was found,[14] although population studies offer some support for a neuroprotective action of dietary Vitamin E.[15] More promising preliminary short-term trial evidence comes from a small trial of the supplement Co-Enzyme Q10 which showed a slowing in rate of decline in early PD compared with placebo.[16] Such evidence, however, remains insufficient to recommend routine use by patients.

There is an abundance of more physical therapies and approaches available, from within both traditional systems (e.g. Yoga, Tai Chi, Qigong) and those based on more Western approaches (e.g. Dance Movement Therapy, Music Therapy), offering opportunities for improvement in areas such as mobility, posture, breathing and aerobic capacity, and promoting relaxation. Few, however, have been evaluated empirically and their superiority (or even equivalence) to more conventional physiotherapy or speech and language therapy is unproven. Nevertheless, participation in such activities is generally seen as positive, if only for the non-specific effects of exercise and social interaction on general health and well-being.

Some of those approaches have been the subject of trials (mostly small and unreplicated). A study comparing aerobic fitness training and Qigong exercises provided support for aerobic exercise in improving measures of respiratory and cardiovascular function, although neither form of exercise had any impact on motor function, mood or quality of life.[17] Another trial of Qigong exercise was similarly negative.[18] Of the more formal physical therapies, Alexander technique has been shown to have some benefits in a small-scale RCT,[19] while Dance Movement Therapy has been shown to be superior to simple exercise in improving in movement initiation, at least within session.[20] A trial of active Music Therapy reported superior effects on bradykinesia and mood than a non-music based physical therapy control.[21] Finally, massage or massage therapy, is a popular CAM approach used by people with PD, particularly those with more advanced disease. Small open-label studies offers some support for its use[22,23] possibly for the management of tremor.[24,25]

What advice can we give to patients?

While sometimes encouraging, such results do little to satisfy the need for answers by both patients and their clinicians. Virtually none of the evidence available is adequate to advise patients either to try a therapy or to avoid it. Patients are left to make choices on the basis of hearsay and hope. What practical advice *can* we give to patients at this stage? The following points are all important when discussing CAM approaches with our patients.

➤ Any CAM method tried should definitely be seen as a complement and not as an alternative to conventional approaches. Most carry cautions that should be discussed with the patient.

➤ In the absence of empirical evidence, the patient should seek information from others that have tried a particular approach.

➤ The patient should look at the therapies available and choose one that seems to have at least face value in the managing the target problem, and that fits their personal likes and ideas about health.

➤ They should consider the costs, both before starting, and in evaluating the value of any benefits.

➤ When choosing a practitioner, the patient should examine their qualifications and their expertise.

➤ Ideally, they should choose a therapist that is familiar with Parkinson's disease.

> The patient should have a clear idea about what benefits they hope for or expect – whether specific symptom relief or general improved health and well-being.
> The therapist should be able to say what benefits may be expected and how long they will take to appear (if the therapy is to be judged worthwhile).
> The patient should personally evaluate a therapy after trying it for a reasonable amount of time before deciding whether or not to continue.
> In such evaluation they should consider any differences between feeling good during a treatment, and any more lasting benefit.

Clearly, many patients see a role for CAM approaches in the overall management of their Parkinson's. For some, it is more of a lifestyle choice to enhance more general health and well-being. For others it may be motivated by a hope for a cure or major symptom relief. The clinician has a role in serving as an objective and impartial adviser to help patients make rational choices when considering CAM approaches. It is no more helpful for a clinician to unreservedly endorse a therapy in the absence of evidence, as it is for them to advise strongly against it. While waiting for empirical evidence, we can help our patients best by discussing their options and providing them with what guidance we can. The PDS produce an excellent booklet to help patients and health professional,[26] also available directly from its website (www.parkinsons. org.uk).

REFERENCES

1 Brown RG, Members of the Complementary Therapy Working Group. *The use of complementary therapy in Parkinson's disease: report on a survey of members of the Parkinson's Disease Society (UK)*. 1997. (Ref type: Unpublished work).

2 Tan LC, Lau PN, Jamora RD, et al. Use of complementary therapies in patients with Parkinson's disease in Singapore. *Mov Disord*. 2006; **21**(1): 86–9.

3 Ferry P, Johnson M, Wallis P. Use of complementary therapies and non-prescribed medication in patients with Parkinson's disease. *Postgrad Med J*. 2002; **78**(924): 612–4.

4 Rajendran PR, Thompson RE, Reich SG. The use of alternative therapies by patients with Parkinson's disease. *Neurology*. 2001; **57**(5): 790–4.

5 Manyam BV, Sanchez-Ramos J. Traditional and complementary therapies in Parkinson's disease. In: Stern G, editor. *Parkinson's Disease*. London: Raven; 1999, pp. 565–74.

6 Katzenschlager R, Evans A, Manson A, et al. *Mucuna pruriens* in Parkinson's disease: a double blind clinical and pharmacological study. *J Neurol Neurosurg Psychiatry*. 2004; **75**(12): 1672–7.

7 Rabey JM, Vered Y, Shabtai H, et al. Improvement of parkinsonian features correlate with high plasma levodopa values after broad bean (*Vicia faba*) consumption. *J Neurol Neurosurg Psychiatry*. 1992; **55**(8): 725–7.

8 Genghe L. Clinical analysis of Parkinson's disease treated by integration of traditional Chinese and Western medicine. *J Tradit Chin Med*. 1995; **15**: 163–9.

9 Shulman LM, Wen X, Weiner WJ, et al. Acupuncture therapy for the symptoms of Parkinson's disease. *Mov Disord*. 2002; **17**(4): 799–802.

10 Eng ML, Lyons KE, Greene MS, et al. Open-label trial regarding the use of acupuncture and yin tui na in Parkinson's disease outpatients: a pilot study on efficacy, tolerability, and quality of life. *J Altern Complement Med*. 2006; **12**(4): 395–9.

11 Jiang XM, Huang Y, Li DJ, *et al.* Effect of electro-scalp acupuncture on cerebral dopamine transporter in the striatum area of the patient of Parkinson's disease by means of single photon emission computer tomography. *Zhongguo Zhen Jiu.* 2006; **26**(6): 427–30.

12 Wang YC, Ma J, Wang H. Effects of Shuanggu Yitong needling method on proliferation and differentiation of nerve stem cells in the Parkinson's disease model rat. *Zhongguo Zhen Jiu.* 2006; **26**(4): 277–82.

13 Park HJ, Lim S, Joo WS, *et al.* Acupuncture prevents 6-hydroxydopamine-induced neuronal death in the nigrostriatal dopaminergic system in the rat Parkinson's disease model. *Exp Neurol.* 2003; **180**(1): 93–8.

14 Shoulson I. DATATOP: a decade of neuroprotective inquiry. Parkinson Study Group. Deprenyl and tocopherol antioxidative therapy of parkinsonism. *Ann Neurol.* 1998; **44** (3 Suppl. 1): S160–S166.

15 De Rijk MC, Breteler MM, den Breeijen JH, *et al.* Dietary antioxidants and Parkinson disease: the Rotterdam Study. *Arch Neurol.* 1997; **54**(6): 762–5.

16 Shults CW, Oakes D, Kieburtz K, *et al.* Effects of coenzyme Q10 in early Parkinson disease: evidence of slowing of the functional decline. *Arch Neurol.* 2002; **59**(10): 1541–50.

17 Burini D, Farabollini B, Iacucci S, *et al.* A randomised controlled cross-over trial of aerobic training versus Qigong in advanced Parkinson's disease. *Eura Medicophys.* 2006; **42**(3): 231–8.

18 Schmitz-Hubsch T, Pyfer D, Kielwein K, *et al.* Qigong exercise for the symptoms of Parkinson's disease: a randomized, controlled pilot study. *Mov Disord.* 2006; **21**(4): 543–8.

19 Stallibrass C, Sissons P, Chalmers C. Randomized controlled trial of the Alexander technique for idiopathic Parkinson's disease. *Clin Rehabil.* 2002; **16**(7): 695–708.

20 Westbrook BK, McKibben H. Dance/movement therapy with groups of outpatients with Parkinson's disease. *Am J Dance Therapy.* 1989; **11**: 27–38.

21 Pacchetti C, Mancini F, Aglieri R, *et al.* Active music therapy in Parkinson's disease: an integrative method for motor and emotional rehabilitation. *Psychosom Med.* 2000; **62**(3): 386–93.

22 Paterson C, Allen JA, Browning M, *et al.* A pilot study of therapeutic massage for people with Parkinson's disease: the added value of user involvement. *Complement Ther Clin Pract.* 2005; **11**(3): 161–71.

23 Hernandez-Reif M, Field T, Largie S, *et al.* Parkinson's disease symptoms are differentially affected by massage vs progressive muscle relaxation: a pilot study. *J Bodywork Movement Therapies.* 2002; **6**: 177–82.

24 Steefel L. Massage therapy as an adjunct healing modality in Parkinson's disease. *Alternative and Complementary Therapy.* 1996; **2**: 377–82.

25 Miesler DW. Massage and Parkinson's disease. *Massage Therapy.* 1996; **35**(377): 382.

26 Parkinson's Disease Society. *Complementary Therapies for Parkinson's Disease.* London: Parkinson's Disease Society of the United Kingdom; 2005.

19

Caring for the carers

ROSANNA COUSINS, ANN DAVIES, JEREMY PLAYFER AND
CHRISTOPHER TURNBULL

Introduction

Most research on Parkinson's disease (PD) has focused on the person with the diagnosis. In recent years, however, there has been a move towards recognising that PD, as a chronic and progressive illness, has a major impact upon the spouse and other family members who assume the responsibility for giving care to the person with the diagnosis. As PD is both a movement disorder and a neuropsychological disorder, carers of people with PD are faced with a variety of challenges from physical and psychological symptoms of the illness. Addressing the needs of the PD patient in the community places demands on carers that warrant them being described as 'the hidden patients'[1] for 'caregiving is potentially a fertile ground for persistent stress'.[2] The accumulation of evidence that family carers are an 'at risk' population has resulted in a National Strategy for Carers,[3] which aims to support carers in terms of information and practical assistance. Interventions to improve quality of life for people with PD must therefore include in their focus the welfare of the caregiver, and outline the current UK government commitment to 'caring about carers'.

Background

Developments in medicine and technology in the last century have led to a dramatic change in lifespan. Coupled with increases in the number of older adults are increases in the number of older adults with functional disabilities, chronic impairments and progressive diseases such as PD where age is a proven risk factor. To remain in the community, the frail elderly need support in activities of daily living, which, for the large part, is provided by the family. They provide nursing care, task-related assistance and also moral support. However, there is a cost. Study after study indicates that unpaid, unanticipated care of the elderly is a stressful life event.

The focus of much caregiving research has been to provide predictors of distress, depression, burden and, more lately, well being.[4–12] These studies have clearly shown that there are caregiving-specific predictors of carer distress, as well as non-specific predictors such as an emotional personality. As caregiver distress is a multidimensional concept, interventions should be targeted to a carer's particular needs.[13] This is especially true in PD, which, as a progressive illness, impacts upon carers differentially according to stage. For example, following from diagnosis, distress may follow from uncertainty and fears for the future due to lack of knowledge of PD. In contrast, in advanced PD, the volume of help required may distress carers and impact on their social life. For the 'new' carer then, an effective intervention would be good information, and opportunity to have their questions answered. In the case of the 'advanced' carer, their needs are more likely to revolve around practical help, and perhaps respite care. It is critical that carers are afforded effective formal interventions to support their informal care in order to reduce the need for institutionalisation.[14–18] It was reported as early as 1972 that when institutionalisation does occur, it is usually because of a breakdown in caregivers' health.[19]

Who is a carer?

The formal Department of Health definition is that 'a carer is anyone who gives regular and substantial unpaid care to a partner, relative or friend'. An individual may provide care for a range of personal reasons, from family ties to the lack of adequate alternative care. Some carers are happy to take on full-time caregiving; others report that they have little choice. Family obligations and love are the driving force of informal care of people with PD.[20-21] Nevertheless, acting in love does not negate the reality that complying with the demands of PD will have consequences on their own lives. While this remains the case, there is a necessity to address carer distress alongside the needs of the person with PD. PD provides a critical family illness situation in which both the patient and their carer have legitimate requirements for quality of life, and the needs of both individuals need to be finely balanced for mutual benefit. That is, carer well-being has as much an effect on patient well-being as the other way round.

Model of the illness situation

The notion that PD is a family illness can be illustrated by an adaptation of Young's model of illness in later life (*see* Figure 19.1 below). Young[22] argues that the consequences of illness in the family should be conceptualised as a mutual encounter, since both the patient's response and the carer's response to the illness situation, in turn, affect the situation. The patient-caregiver interaction model shows the way in which quality of life in PD is dictated by the complex dynamic interplay of patient and caregiver responses to the illness situation.

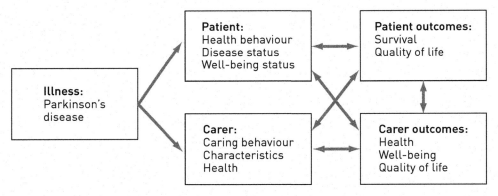

FIGURE 19.1 The patient–caregiver model.

The illness

PD is characterised by an insidious onset. Prognosis is variable, as progression and symptomatology are variable. A diagnosis of PD constitutes a fundamental threat to quality of life and emotional well-being for the patient. The need for care increases alongside physical deterioration in particular, and also in the presence of intellectual deterioration.

Patient behaviour

Besides being a motor disorder, Parkinson's disease is associated with a variety of subtle cognitive impairments and an increased risk of dementia.[23-25] About a third of PD patients will experience hallucinations in the advanced stages.[20] Depression is a serious and frequent problem for Parkinson's patients,[26–28] as are communication issues,[29] and there are changes in personality.[20–21] About half of carers perceived personality change and hence changes in behaviour in the people with PD (PPD). There are common themes in the changes reported: apathy, withdrawal and deterioration in communication; also a reduction in confidence, and an increase in worrying and agitation. Patients note such changes themselves.[29–30]

Carer behaviour and outcomes

Carers of PPD are generally family members. There is substantial evidence that indicates that if a spouse is alive and well, they will assume the responsibility for the welfare of an incapacitated elder. Where there is no spouse, close relatives are preferred to distant ones; any relative is preferred to no relative, and female relatives are preferred to male relatives.[31]

A decline in health is the starting point of the complex interactions between patient and carer, as in any illness situation. The carer addresses both physical and psychological needs, taking on a job with ever-increasing hours as demand grows alongside progression of illness. The use of dopaminergic medication brings some initial relief, but then sooner or later the 'honeymoon' is over and the medication may even bring additional problems to deal with. Patient depression is a potent predictor of carer depression;[32] the decrease in communication from the patient – conversation and interactions more generally – is a notable challenge for many carers.[20]

There are specific aspects of caregiving that are important to carer outcomes.[20,33]

1. The time demands of PD caregiving – high time demands equate to negative consequences on carers' social life; they are also associated with burden, depression, and poor psychological health.
2. High physical demands from the limitations of PD are strongly associated with all aspects of carer distress.
3. Demands resulting from psychological change in a PPD (personality change, the presence of depression, declining mental status, experience of hallucinations) are associated with an impact on the dyadic relationship, emotional burden and lowered life satisfaction in carers.

Carers bring their own characteristics into the caring situation. As indicated in the model, carer characteristics have an affect on outcomes,[34] as well as on their response to the demands of the PPD. Carers' emotionality and coping style are major predictors of caregiver outcomes.[20,33] Coping style, however, is amenable to change. There is also evidence that relationship strain predicts caregiver depression and negative health outcomes.[35] Carers are not well informed about PD, particularly the psychological aspects of the disease. Objective tests of physical demand and psychological demand indicate that those carers who look after more advanced PPD are those who know more, suggesting that they are learning 'on the job'. A judicious explanation of likely prognosis based on current symptoms should be available, perhaps through PD nurse specialists.

Patient outcomes

Patient survival and quality of life are determined by the interaction of their own disease status and behaviour, carer characteristics and behaviour and carer outcomes.[22,35] Where the carer has taken on the responsibility for medication delivery, however, a minority of carers were prepared to withhold medication for a short periods, to keep the PPD immobile, thus enabling them to complete other tasks (e.g. basic housework).

This particular example demonstrates how outcomes for patients are bound up with ethical issues that arise in caring. If one considers that there are three broad goals of caring activity:
1. to carry on living as before
2. to achieve well-being for the care-receiver
3. to achieve well-being for the carer (self),

then dilemmas can arise when actions are perceived to serve one goal, but not another. Therefore carers are called on to prioritise and make choices that are not mutually beneficial.

For example:
➤ 'It is easier for me to do things, than to let PPD struggle'
➤ 'I sometimes feel "on edge"' when I let PPD do things himself/herself
➤ 'Sometimes I have to override PPD's wishes to get things done'
➤ 'I am afraid to leave PPD alone while I go out'
➤ 'I dress PPD and choose his/her clothes every day'
➤ 'The constant demands of caring for PPD limits the needs of someone else.'

Each of these examples demonstrates ethical conflicts that constantly arise in caring. A problem arises when welfare outcomes for the PPD and their carer differ. A perceptive carer reported, 'Sometimes I do want to do things for Colin, just to help him because he might be struggling a bit. But then I think, "No, it helps him if he can do it himself".' We found that there were frequent situations where slowness caused great frustration and irritation. The dilemma centres on when to help, and when to stand back.

Because in PD caring is typically a family affair that is not overseen by others, there is the potential for conflicts in determining personal autonomy: the freedom to determine one's own actions. In family caregiving, intrusion upon autonomy can go unchecked and unseen. Care can slip into control, not from malevolence, but in the guise of good intentions. The carer takes over and this can ultimately induce a dependency situation. Alternatively, the situation can arise where the carer is totally at the PPD's beck and call – 'From the moment he opens his eyes in the morning to the time he shuts them at night, I am on call. He will not do anything for himself, and he will not be left.' The position is that carers constantly have to make judgements about the value of the consequences of their actions. Carer's judgements will adjust as information and experience is accumulated, but ultimately their actions result from the application of their own code of ethics. The handling of ethical dilemmas and issues surrounding personal autonomy is a neglected area in caring.

What public support is available for carers?

The 2001 Census showed that 5.2 million people provide informal care in England and Wales, and about a fifth, just over 1 million carers, provide over 50 hours of care per week. An acknowledgement that caregiving is a public health issue has prompted a move towards developing better carer support services. Interest in the plight of carers, and their recent rise in status to a group that requires public recognition and support, has not emerged without a challenge. Criticism has come from the disability movement for what it views as a disproportionate emphasis on the needs of carers at the expense of those for whom they care.[36–37] The assertion is that the goal of public policy should be to enable disabled people to live independently and therefore do away with the need for caring relationships. The thrust of the argument is that to focus on the carer's needs distracts attention from the (by implication) greater needs of the disabled person. However, the social base of the disability movement is among younger people with physical disability, and therefore reflects its ideals and aspirations.[38] It was feared that the energy of this movement might serve to direct attention away from the needs of carers of the elderly and especially of those who care for people with neuropsychological illness who are not in the position to strike for independence. Pertinent to this discussion, the progressive nature of Parkinson's disease means that people with PD have to expect to get to a stage where they can only remain at home with the support of a 'full-time' carer.

However, in the past ten years there has been a greater acknowledgement by the government of the contribution of carers to society, including enabling people with chronic illnesses and disabilities to stay in their own homes, and to remain independent. This has been manifested in the following three important pieces of legislation.

1. The Carers (Recognition and Services) Act 1995 was a major step forward, giving carers new rights and a clear legal status for the first time. Briefly, under the 1995 Act, PD (and other) carers are entitled to request an assessment of their ability to give care. Specifically, carers should have their needs taken into account when Social Services departments – who have the responsibility for arranging support services – plan the support offered to PPD. Before the 1995 Act was passed, Social Services were focused entirely on the person with PD, without any consideration of context.
2. The Carers and Disabled Children Act 2000 made four changes to the 1995 Act:
   a. Eligible carers (those providing a substantial amount of care on a regular basis) have the right to be assessed *independent* of the community care assessment of the person with PD
   b. Local authorities were empowered to make direct payments to carers for the services that meet their own assessed needs
   c. Social Services departments were able to run short-term voucher schemes to offer flexibility in the choice and timing of carers' breaks

d. Local authorities were given power to charge carers for the services they receive.

3. The Carers (Equal Opportunities) Act 2004, which commenced April 2005, gave carers more choice and better opportunities to lead a more fulfilling life by giving more information about their assessment rights. Critically, there is a recommendation that local authorities develop an information strategy to ensure that carers are being told of their rights and that the large numbers of unknown or 'hidden' carers are reached. In addition, the 2004 Act determines that assessments should consider the carer's wishes in relation to participating in leisure, education, or training activities and whether they want to work. It also provides for co-operation between different public authorities in relation to the planning and provision of services that may help support the carer in their caregiving role.

4. In addition to, and associated with, the above, in 1999, a cross-government National Carers Strategy *Caring about Carers*[3] was published. The strategy was developed in consultation with carers and organisations that represent them. It is essentially a substantial policy package whose main objective is to enable carers to continue caring through legislation and financial support for services. The document provides illustrations of best practice in the public support of carers. Further information of current initatives by local authorities can be seen on the Department of Health's carers website (www.direct.gov.uk/en/Caring for Someone/DG-071391).

Conclusion

Carers are important to the management of Parkinson's disease: a breakdown in caregiving leading to institutionalisation is as likely to be the result of a breakdown in the caregiver's health, as to be caused by the PPD being too ill to be cared for. We have presented a model to illustrate that PD in the community is a family illness. Patient symptoms and behaviour have an effect on the carer, and the characteristics and behaviour of both patient and carer predict carer distress levels. Patient outcomes are influenced, naturally by the illness itself, but also by the care they receive. Therefore it is imperative that carers are recognised as being part of the illness process, and do not remain hidden patients. There is increasing recognition of the importance of the caring for carers as a society, and the fact that many of them need high-quality, reliable and responsive support from statutory or voluntary services[3] to continue their role and maintain their own health and well-being. To date, however, there are no standardised instruments to put into effect these emerging aims. The answer does not all lie at the door of increased resources for public services, however, but also in a thorough understanding of the illness situation at the family level.

REFERENCES

1 Fengler AP, Goodrich N. Wives of elderly disabled men: the hidden patients. *Gerontologist.* 1979; **19**: 175–83.

2 Pearlin LI, Mullan JT, Semple SJ, *et al.* Caregiving and the stress process: an overview of concepts and their measures. *Gerontologist.* 1990; **30**: 583–94.

3 Department of Health. *Caring about Carers: a national strategy for carers.* London: Department of Health; 1999.

4 Aarsland D, Cummings JL, Larsen JP. Neuropsychiatric differences between Parkinson's disease with dementia and Alzheimer's disease. *Int J Geriatric Psychiatry.* 2001; **14**: 866–74.

5 Adams KB, Smyth KA, McClendon McKJ. Psychological resources as moderators of the impact of spousal dementia caregiving on depression. *J Appl Gerontology.* 2005; **24**: 475–89.

6 Caap-Ahlgren M, Dehlin O. Factors of importance to the caregiver burden experiences by family caregivers of Parkinson's disease patients. *Aging Clin Exp Res.* 2002; **14**: 371–7.

7 Chappell NL, Reid RC. Burden and well-being among caregivers: examining the distinction. *Gerontologist.* 2002; **42**: 772–80.

8 Oyebode J. Assessment of carers' psychological needs. *Advances in Psychiatric Treatment.* 2003; 9: 45–53.

9 Pinquart M, Sörensen S. Gender differences in caregiver stressors, social resources, and health: an updated meta-analysis. *J Appl Gerontology.* 2005; **24**: 475–89.

10 Pinquart M, Sörensen S. Gender differences in caregiver stressors, social resources, and health: an updated meta-analysis. *J Gerontology: Psychological Sciences.* 2006; **61B**: P33–P45.

11 Savundranayagam MY, Hummert ML, Montgomery RJV. Investigating the effects of communication problems on caregiver burden. *J Gerontology: Psychological Sciences.* 2005; **60B**: S48–S55.

12 Thommessen B, Aarsland D, Braekhus A, *et al.* The psychosocial burden on spouses of the elderly with stroke, dementia and Parkinson's disease. *Int J Geriatric Psychiatry.* 2002; **17**: 78–84.

13 Cousins R, Davies ADM, Turnbull CJ, *et al.* Assessing caregiving distress: a conceptual analysis and a brief scale. *B J Clin Psych.* 2002; **41**: 387–403.

14 Aneshensel CS, Pearlin LI, Schuler R. Stress, role captivity and the cessation of caregiving. *J Health Soc Behaviour.* 1993; **34**: 54–70.

15 Cohen CA, Gold DP, Shulman KI, *et al.* Factors determining the decision to institutionalize dementing individuals: a prospective study. *Gerontologist.* 1993; **33**: 714–20.

16 Colerick EJ, George LK. Predictors of institutionalization among caregivers of Alzheimers patients. *J Am Geriatric Society.* 1986; **34**: 493–8.

17 Gerritsen JC, van der Ende PC. The development of a care-giving burden scale. *Age Ageing.* 1994; **23**: 483–91.

18 Moritz D, Kasl S, Berkman L. The health impact of living with a cognitively impaired elderly spouse: depressive symptoms and social functioning. *J Gerontology.* 1989; **44**: S17–S27.

19 Isaacs B, Livingstone M, Neville Y. *Survival of the Unfittest: a study of geriatric patients in Glasgow.* London: Routledge & Kegan Paul; 1972.

20 Cousins R. A study of psychological distress in caregivers of Parkinson's patients. University of Liverpool. Unpublished PhD thesis; 1997.

21 Davies ADM, Cousins R, Turnbull CJ, *et al.* The experience of caring for people with Parkinson's disease. In: Percival R, Hobbs P, editors. *Parkinson's Disease: studies in psychological and social care.* London: BPS Books; 1999, pp. 154–98.

22 Young RF. Elders, families, and illness. *J Aging Studies.* 1994; **8**: 1–15.

23 Aarsland D, Karlsen K. Neuropsychiatric aspects of Parkinson's disease. *Curr Psychiatry Reports.* 1999; **1**: 61–68.

24 Chaudhuri KR, Healy DG, Schapira AH. Non-motor symptoms of Parkinson's disease: diagnosis and management. *Lancet Neurol.* 2006; **5**: 235–45.

25 Dubois B, Boller F, Pillon B, *et al*. Cognitive deficits in Parkinson's disease. In: Boller F, Grafman J, editors. *Handbook of Neuropsychology*, Vol. 5. Amsterdam: Elsevier; 1991: 195–240.

26 Ishihara L, Brayne C. A systematic review of depression and mental illness preceding Parkinson's disease. *Acta Neurol Scand*. 2006; **113**: 211–20.

27 McDonald WM, Holtzheimer PE 3rd, Byrd EH. The diagnosis and treatment of depression in Parkinson's disease. *Curr Treat Options Neurol*. 2006; **8**: 245–55.

28 Sano M, Mayeux R. Biochemistry of depression in Parkinson's disease. In: Huber SJ, Cummings JL, editors. *Parkinson's Disease: neurobehavioural aspects*. Oxford: Oxford University Press; 1992: 229–39.

29 Miller N, Noble E, Jones D, *et al*. Life with communication changes in Parkinson's disease. *Age Ageing*. 2006; **35**: 235–9.

30 Chesson R, Cockhead D, Romney-Alexander D. Quality of life with Parkinson's disease: views of Scottish consumers and providers. In: Percival R, Hobbs P, editors. *Parkinson's Disease: studies in psychological and social care*. London: BPS Books; 1999, pp. 93–130.

31 Qureshi H, Walker A. *The Caring Relationship: elderly people and their families*. London: Macmillan; 1989.

32 Meara J, Michelmore E, Hobson P. Use of the GDS-15 geriatric depression scale as a screening instrument for depressive symptomatology in patients with Parkinson's disease and their carers in the community. *Age Ageing*. 1999; **28**: 35–8.

33 Davies, ADM, Cousins R, Turnbull CJ, *et al*. *Perceived Psychological Change and Caregiver Distress in Caregivers for Patients with Parkinson's Disease*. London: Parkinson's Disease Society of the United Kingdom; 1998.

34 Pinquart M, Sörensen S. Associations of stressors and uplifts of caregiving with caregiver burden and depressive mood: a meta-analysis. *J Gerontology: Psychological Sciences*. 2003; **58B**: P112–P128.

35 Lyons KS, Zarit SH, Sayer AG, *et al*. Caregiving as a dyadic process: perspectives from caregiver and receiver. *J Gerontology: Psychological Sciences*, **57B**: P195–P204.

36 Oliver M. *The Politics of Disablement*. London: Macmillan; 1990.

37 Morris J. *Pride Against Prejudice: transforming attitudes to disability*. London: Women's Press; 1991.

38 Twigg T. Carers, families, relatives: socio-legal conceptions of caregiving relationships. *J Social Welfare Family Law*. 1994; **3**: 279–98.

20

Palliative care

MAHENDRA GONSALKORALE

Introduction

At the very outset, it is important to define the term *palliative care*. The WHO defines it as 'The active total care of patients whose disease is not responsive to curative treatment. Control of pain and other symptoms and of psychological, social & spiritual problems is paramount. The goal of palliative care is achievement of the best quality of life for patients and their families.'[1]

Parkinson's disease (PD) is a progressive degenerative neurological disorder and although significant advances have been made in our understanding of the disease and its management, there is as yet no curative treatment and those affected will deteriorate at variable rates with worsening disability and reduction in quality of life. Patients with PD therefore fall into the category needing palliative care. However, it is useful to make a distinction between applying a palliative care approach and providing palliative care. No one would argue that all PD patients would benefit from the application of the principles embodied in the WHO definition, i.e. the palliative care approach, but palliative care as such, especially the involvement of palliative care services, is mainly required in the advanced stages of the disease. There are very few publications on palliative care in neurological disorders.[2,3,4]

The palliative stage is heralded by a worsening of mental and physical symptoms with a progressively decreasing response to drugs and an increasing sensitivity to their unwanted effects. Mental and psychological problems become worse and carer stress becomes a major issue. Issues that need addressing include maintenance of nutrition, risk of aspiration pneumonia, risk of pressure sores, risk of contractures, pain management, increasing confusion and communication problems. There is often benefit from withdrawal of dopaminergic drugs. Urinary and bowel symptoms such as loss of bladder control and constipation are common. Management of the patient in their own homes becomes increasingly difficult and decisions may need to be made about where the patient should be managed and by whom. Finally, as the end approaches, it is important to manage the terminal phase leading to a dignified death.

A SPECTRUM OF PRIORITIES OVER TIME
Reassess diagnosis, treatment and support for patient and carers

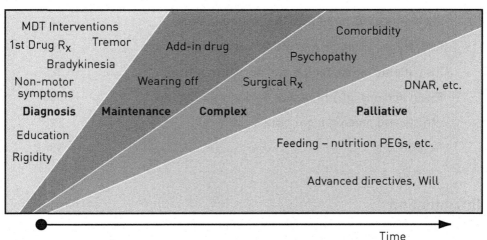

FIGURE 20.1 The stages of Parkinson's Disease.

Progression of PD and life history of PD patients

The four-stage paradigm for the life history of a PD patient was introduced as a pragmatic simple clinical scale which defines clinical needs, priorities and caring strategies. The four stages start with the diagnostic stage, progress through to the maintenance stage, the complex stage and end in the palliative stage.[5] This model is very useful but it must be remembered that these stages are not clearly demarcated. Many common principles are applicable at all stages, as, for example, a holistic and multidisciplinary approach. The model has now been modified to reflect this.[6] There is no accepted definition of when the complex stage ends or the palliative stage begins. A useful modification of this model may be to show some overlap between the stages and clearly indicate that the principles of palliative care apply at all stages but in different degrees (*see* Figure 20.1).

A difficulty arises because of the commonly held but incorrect view of palliative care as synonymous with terminal care. The WHO definition can also cause some confusion as it includes the statement 'not responsive to curative treatment'. Curative obviously implies cure but in the early stages of PD, drug treatment can be so effective that although the patient is not 'cured', he/she leads a virtually normal life and may not be psychologically prepared to accept the need for palliative care even in its broadest sense.

The WHO definition (heavily coloured by the dominance of cancer patients within a palliative care service) rightly places great emphasis on control of pain. In the palliative stage of PD, however, although control of pain is important, the need for relief from other major symptoms requires greater emphasis. It is important to stress that terminal care, although of great importance, is only one aspect of palliative care. The goals of help with psychological, social and spiritual problems will be paramount as in other diseases requiring palliative care. The achievement of the best quality of life for patients and their families is definitely important in PD.

Some aspects of palliative care

Palliative care is a distinct and growing medical speciality in the UK legitimised firstly by The Royal College of Physicians in 1987 and latterly in academic institutions with appropriate accredited programmes.

The key principles underpinning palliative care are:
- ➤ focus on quality of life, which includes good symptom control
- ➤ whole-person approach, taking into account the person's past life experience and current situation
- ➤ care which encompasses both the dying person and those who matter to that person
- ➤ respect for patient autonomy and choice (e.g. over place of death, treatment options)
- ➤ emphasis on open and sensitive communication, which extends to patients, informal carers and professional colleagues.[3]

Palliative care services

The major emphasis of palliative care services in the UK has been on cancer but, increasingly, other chronic conditions such as heart failure, severe respiratory disease and chronic neurological conditions are being recognised.[7] The National Council for Hospice and Specialist Palliative Care services recommends that 'every person with advanced, progressive and incurable illness should receive palliative care, appropriate to their assessed need'.[8]

In UK Hospices fewer than 6% of patients have non-malignant diseases and a small number of hospices treat only cancer.[9]

The most common connection between specialised palliative care services and a PD patient is when there is an incidental cancer diagnosis. Optimising PD medication could be an important aspect of affording the best quality of life for such patients. A co-operative approach between palliative care services and those who are managing the patient's PD will produce the maximum benefit to the patient. The specialist services that have been developed primarily for people with cancer are shown in Table 20.1.[10]

TABLE 20.1 Specialist palliative care services

Specialist palliative in-patient care in hospices or in specialist palliative care units
Specialist palliative community care provided mainly by teams of clinical nurse specialists to people in their place of residence – more intensive support for limited periods can often be provided by the Marie Curie Nursing Service and 'Hospice at Home'-type services
Specialist palliative hospital support teams
Specialist palliative day care/therapy
Education and Training in Palliative Care
Bereavement Support Services
The Gold Standard Framework (GSF) for managing cancer patients at home in their final year with a networked primary care team. The principles of the GSF with seven standards covering Communication, Co-ordination, Control of symptoms, Continuity out of hours, Continued learning, Carer support, and Care in the dying phase are eminently applicable to terminal PD patients.[11]

Progression of Parkinson's disease

How should we prepare patients to come to terms with the fact that they have an incurable progressive disease which in time will lead to a need for increasing care and support? It is probably not appropriate to discuss such issues in great detail in the very early stages of the disease apart from being very honest with those who wish to know more about their prognosis. It is reassuring to the patient to know that the service will respond to changing needs as the disease evolves. If a good relationship is established, then, over the course of time, serious issues can be dealt with in a sensitive manner. Those fortunate enough to have a PD nurse specialist have found them an invaluable resource in dealing with the clinically deteriorating patient.

Parkinson's disease is a progressive disorder. There are conflicting data on whether it affects life expectancy, some indicating increase in survival after the introduction of levodopa and some showing no change.[12-23] The rate of progression is extremely variable and the time taken to reach the palliative stage by progression from the complex stage is therefore also variable.

The following clinical indicators may give some indication of progress.
1. Tremor dominance at presentation with very little bradykinesia often indicates a more benign course.[24]
2. Early onset of falls is unusual in idiopathic PD and could point to a diagnosis of MSA and other PD syndromes which on the whole, have a more rapid course.[25]
3. Early onset of cognitive dysfunction indicates a more aggressive course and also the possibility that the diagnosis could be dementia with Lewy bodies (DLB).
4. Age of onset of PD is a significant determinant of cognitive impairment and clinical decline was significantly greater in subjects with disease onset after age 60 compared with young-onset PD.[26]
5. Hoehn & Yahr stage at presentation rather than duration of disease determines rate of motor progression.[27]

Although these indicators are helpful, most often it is extremely difficult to prognosticate on the rate of progression for individual patients and it usually takes years of follow-up to get some indication.

Mortality in Parkinson's disease

Patients and families often ask about the effects of PD on life expectancy. Mortality rates differ in published studies for a variety of reasons.[12-23] These include: co-morbidity, stage of disease at entry, diagnostic accuracy, and heterogeneity of PD with sub-groups with different rates of progression.

In one of the best-known population studies conducted by Hoehn and Yahr in the USA[24] in 1967, 28% of subjects were dead or disabled within 5 years; 60% of those observed in the first 5–9 years, 83% in 10–14 years, and 90% lived for 15 years. About 10% were found to run a benign course and were alive with little disability at 20 years after diagnosis. A more recent study in Australia, which followed patients over 10 years, showed similar results. In this study, 22% were dead or disabled within 4 years, 71% dead or disabled within 10 years and 10% followed a benign course.[28] The authors of the study concluded that despite levodopa, the mortality of people with PD – with the exception of very young patients – remains increased compared with that of the general age-matched population. A recent review suggests that mortality may not be affected by treatment.[12] The apparent reduction is seen in first years of treatment and may be related more to the degree of functional disability rather than the duration of treatment.

Initial reports when levodopa first became available suggested that life expectancy returned to near normal with this agent.[20,21,22] This is now thought to have reflected the benefit of levodopa early in the course of the disease in drug-responsive patients, who then 'caught up' in the mortality stakes by the early 1980s.[12,23]

Principles of management of the palliative stage

The National Institute for Clinical Excellence (NICE) has produced recommendations for Palliative Care in PD.[29] An important recommendation is that the palliative needs of PD patients should be considered at all stages of the disease. Early discussions would enable the palliative care stage to be better managed both from the patient's point of view and that of the carer. Relief of distress in patients and carers will require support from many agencies (such as social services, voluntary services, community health services and supportive organisations like the Parkinson's Disease Society) and from many professionals (such as doctors, nurses, therapists and clinical psychologists). The Parkinson's disease nurse specialist (PDNS)[30] is a key person in supporting the patient and the carers. Community services such as District Nursing for supportive home care, occupational therapy for assessment and provision of equipment and physiotherapy regarding advice on lifting and handling are invaluable.

Problems associated with the palliative stage (*see* Table 20.2)

As the prevalence of dementia in PD is high with estimates varying between 20% and 45%,[31,32] patients often come into contact with or are primarily cared for by Mental Health Services. The Mental Health Team will need to work closely with the medical/neurological team. Clinical psychologists have a major role to play in managing psychological challenges faced by the patients and their families. Unfortunately, the availability of this service is extremely variable in the UK. Its work includes the assessment of mood and well-being, and identification of factors impacting on mood and well-being; exploring the patient's current coping mechanisms and building upon these where necessary, and – most importantly – identification of the needs of carers and offering them support where necessary.

Increasing care needs may require a review of the best setting for individual patients. Most could be maintained at home but some may require institutionalisation. Ideally, a case facilitator or key worker should co-ordinate services.

Drooling of saliva, which is a major symptom from both the patient and carer points of view, can be helped by simple advice. Management may include advice to swallow more frequently, cautious use of oral anticholinergic drugs (caution in elderly subjects who may become more confused), injection of parotid and submandibular glands with Botox[33] and, in some cases, the use of external irradiation of the parotids. A recent study by showed that 1% atropine drops applied twice daily sublingually may be useful.[34] Atrovent spray (as used for COPD patients) has also been used.

Somatic complaints such as constipation, pain and continence problems will become more frequent. Autonomic dysfunction leads to urinary disturbances and orthostatic hypotension. Both could be made worse by medication and medication review is an important aspect of management.

Neuropsychiatric problems such as depression and anxiety are frequent but can occur exclusively during 'off' periods. Anti-parkinsonian drugs can cause hallucinations even in non-demented PD patients. Axial signs, such as freezing, postural instability or dysarthria become levodopa resistant. Sleep disorders include insomnia, hypersomnia and REM sleep disorders.

TABLE 20.2 Problems associated with the palliative stage of Parkinson's disease

Modality affected	Consequence	Complications
Mobility	Worsening mobility	Falls, fractures
	Increasing falls	Pressure sores, contractures
Speech and swallowing	Swallowing problems	Aspiration pneumonia
	Increasing dysarthria, dysphonia	Poor nutrition
		Drooling of saliva
		Communication problems leading to poor mood and carer stress
Psychological	Feelings of helplessness, worthlessness and guilt	Deterioration in quality of life
	Depression	Deterioration in quality of life and carer stress
	Anger, frustration and low morale	Poor nutrition
	Lack of motivation for feeding	
Autonomic	Bladder and bowel control	Urinary incontinence
		Constipation
General symptoms	Pain and fatigue	
	Sleep problems	
Lack of response to drugs	Poor symptom control	Deterioration in quality of life
Increased sensitivity to side effects of drugs	Propensity for mental side effects	Optimisation of medication becomes more and more a 'balancing act'
Cognitive	Increasing confusion	Deterioration in quality of life, carer stress

PD drugs should be reviewed carefully. Both underdosage because of negative attitudes to the patient as well as over-enthusiastic but ineffective and often harmful excessive dosage may need adjusting by a specialist. Reducing the dosage may produce some reduction of the functional status but the improvement in mental clarity is often sufficient reward. In some instances, PD patients appear to be deteriorating only because they have not been able to take their medication, and rapidly improve when drug treatment is restored. This may require temporary use of apomorphine or giving L-Dopa via a NG tube. Thus a sensible balance has to be achieved by individualised medication.

Regular monitoring of body weight is a good way of detecting poor intake. Many factors need to be addressed before considering nasogastric feeding or percutaneous endoscopic gastrostomic (PEG) feeding. Poor intake may simply be due to inability to feed without assistance. The patient needs to be assisted in a sensitive manner to eat without affecting his self-respect. Failure to eat may be due to unrecognised depression requiring treatment or it may be due to cognitive impairment, requiring assisted feeding and active encouragement to feed. Careful consideration must be given to exclude dysphagia and this must include non–PD causes such as a pharyngeal pouch. Dysphagia is a common and distressing problem, and patients are often acutely embarrassed by the dribbling and coughing associated with trying to eat, while their carers are often frustrated by how long it takes to complete a meal. Simple attention to detail such as presentation of food, and the social context in which meals are partaken of may resolve the problem. Dysphagia may be due to improper timing of medication and improper presentation and dose of medication.

Having examined all these factors, if nutritional intake is a problem, serious consideration must be given to the insertion of a percutaneous endoscopic gastrostomy (PEG). PEG feeding is indicated for those patients who feel hungry or thirsty or who are unable to consume sufficient calories to meet their metabolic needs. This may be delayed far too long and the patient becomes undernourished and feeble. There is a good case to discuss this with the patient who is in the complex stage and who is still able to state his/her wishes based on proper information on feeding options given to him/her. Improved nutritional status will result in a greater sense of well-being and should enhance patients' quality of life. Insertion of a PEG can be associated with significant early mortality and morbidity. The decision to use a PEG feeding tube requires an in-depth assessment of the potential benefits to the individual. There is no data on survival rates of PD patients on PEG feeds compared with those not on PEG feeds.

If a patient is acutely ill from an unrelated and treatable cause, subcutaneous apomorphine could be used on selected subjects if a nasogastric (NG) tube is not in place or cannot be used. NG tube feeding is unpleasant and cumbersome and is generally not well tolerated but may be needed as a temporary measure.

All patients in whom PEG feeding is proposed should be reviewed by a multidisciplinary nutrition team. (For a review of the risks of PEG see 'Scoping our practice', the 2004 Report of the National Confidential Enquiry into Patient Outcome and Death at www.ncepod.org.uk/2004report/PDF_chapters/PEG_Chapter.pdf)

End-stage problems and their management

Particular challenges faced are: maintenance of nutrition; prevention of aspiration pneumonia; prevention of pressure sores and contractures; increasing difficulty with communication; management of bowel and bladder, and increasing confusion and apathy. Bowel management by regular enemas or suppositories and bladder management by application of external sheath drainage in suitable men and proper use of incontinence pads in both males and females will be necessary. Only rarely should indwelling permanent catheters be introduced since inappropriate use leads to restlessness, discomfort and urinary tract infections.

Anti-parkinsonian drugs become less effective and there is increasing sensitivity to unwanted effects of drugs, often requiring reduction of dosage or withdrawal of drugs. Drug withdrawal should be gradual.

Confusion and agitation could be a reaction to infection, physical discomfort for any reason, or may be due to constipation or retention of urine. Pain and psychological distress may increase and carers require increasing support. Maintenance at home may become difficult even with statutory support and institutionalised care may be sought. The point at which this is reached can often be delayed with responsive and sympathetic support for the carer and respite admissions on a regular and planned basis. Some districts offer day care which is much appreciated by the carer. If crisis admissions can be prevented by anticipatory care, permanent institutionalisation can often be avoided. Respite admissions could gradually progress to permanent care with greater acceptance by the patient and family.

PD patients in residential and nursing homes

The cost of managing PD patients in residential and nursing homes is a major component of the overall cost. The annual direct costs for patients in full-time institutions may be nearly five times the cost of managing at home.

The process of admission and the subsequent care and review mechanisms are variable and often unsatisfactory. The terminal phase may not be managed. Some studies have shown disturbing facts regarding medication management, review processes and the recognition of PD in residential and nursing homes.[35]

Little is known about the skills of staff in relation to PD management. Patients receive little or no maintenance physical therapy. Specialist medical follow-up and supervision often ceases after admission to nursing homes.

The prevalence of PD in nursing homes is estimated to be around 5–10% of residents.[36] The presence of hallucinations/delusion is a risk factor for nursing-home admissions,[37] whereas motor severity and the presence of memory problems do not have the same impact on nursing-home placement.[38]

Dying and end-of-life care in Parkinson's disease

The commonest documented cause of death in PD is pneumonia. However, ascertaining the cause of death from death certification is unreliable. Other common causes given are cardiovascular causes and PD itself. Incidental causes such as carcinoma and peritonitis have also been described. Although cases of suicide have been described, there is no data to indicate how common this is. In some countries where assisted suicide is allowed, PD patients have made use of this service. Most deaths will ocur in hospital.

Patients dying from any disease need to do so with dignity. Some of the barriers to the care of dying patients are summarised in Table 20.3.[39]

TABLE 20.3 Barriers to management of dying patients

Barriers to 'diagnosing dying'	Effects on patient and family if diagnosis of dying is not made	Educational objectives for overcoming barriers to diagnosing dying
1. Hope that the patient may get better	1. Patient and family are unaware that death is imminent	1. Communicate sensitively on issues related to death and dying
2. No definitive diagnosis	2. Patient loses trust in doctor as his or her condition deteriorates without acknowledgment that this is happening	2. Work as a member of a multiprofessional team
3. Pursuance of unrealistic or futile interventions	3. Patient and relatives get conflicting messages from the multiprofessional team	3. Prescribe appropriately for dying patients to: • discontinue inappropriate drugs • convert oral to subcutaneous drugs • prescribe as required drugs appropriately, including for pain and agitation • prescribe subcutaneous drugs for delivery by a syringe driver
4. Disagreement about the patient's condition	4. Patient dies with uncontrolled symptoms, leading to a distressing and undignified death	
5. Failure to recognise key symptoms and signs	5. Patient and family feel dissatisfied	4. Use a syringe driver competently
6. Lack of knowledge about how to prescribe	6. At death, cardiopulmonary resuscitation may be inappropriately initiated	5. Recognise key signs and symptoms of the dying patient
7. Poor ability to communicate with the family and patient	7. Cultural and spiritual needs not met	6. Describe an ethical framework that deals with issues related to the dying patient, including resuscitation, withholding and withdrawing treatment, foreshortening life, and futility
8. Concerns about withdrawing or withholding treatment	All the above can lead to complex bereavement problems and formal complaints about care	
9. Fear of foreshortening life		7. Appreciate cultural and religious traditions related to the dying phase
10. Concerns about resuscitation		8. Be aware of medico-legal issues
11. Cultural and spiritual barriers		9. Refer appropriately to a specialist palliative care team
12. Medico-legal issues		

Care of the dying pathways

The development of care pathways for the dying patient attempts to address some of these issues. The care pathway piloted in Liverpool[39,40] identifies the following goals of care in the dying patient.

➤ Maintaining comfort.
➤ Review of medication and discontinuing non-essentials. As required, drugs are written up per protocol, e.g. pain, nausea, agitation.
➤ Discontinuation of inappropriate interventions, e.g. blood tests, antibiotics, monitoring vital signs. Document patient's not-for-CPR status.
➤ Addressing psychological and insight aspects.
➤ Assessment of patient's language of choice for communication.
➤ Dealing with living wills (advance directives).
➤ Religious and spiritual support for patient and family.
➤ Communications with family to identify how family or other people involved are to be informed of patient's impending death. Family or others involved given relevant hospital information.

A sensible approach would be to ascertain the views of the patient but this is often difficult or impossible because of associated cognitive impairment or difficulty in communication. Advanced directives ('Living wills') are often helpful and the practice of creating these is becoming more common in the UK. New laws on power of attorney will allow a designated advocate to act in the patient's interest in treatment and care decisions.

➤ Communication with primary healthcare team.
➤ Ensuring that the general practitioner is aware of patient's condition.

Finally, the plan of care is explained and discussed with the patient and his/her family and their understanding of the plan of care is clearly documented.

Ethical and medico-legal issues

Many ethical issues arise in the management of patients with advanced-stage PD. These include managing feeding problems (which mainly revolve around the use of nasogastric feeding and the use of PEGs), managing their medication (including drug withdrawal), and around cardio pulmonary resuscitation (CPR).

The General Medical Council (GMC) is responsible for advising medical practitioners on the medico-legal aspects and clear published general guidelines are available from the GMC.[41] Additional guidance is available from The National Council for Hospice and Specialist Palliative Care Services,[42] The British Medical Association (BMA)[43] and The British Geriatrics Society.[44]

REFERENCES

1 World Health Organization. Cancer pain relief and palliative care. Report of a WHO expert Committee. *WHO Technical Report Series*, No. 804.

2 Kristjanson LJ, Toye C, Dawson S. New dimensions in palliative care: a palliative approach to neurodegenerative diseases and final illness in old people. *Med J Aust.* 2003; **179**: S41–S43.

3 Proceedings of the Satellite Symposium 'Palliatve Care in Neurology'. Sixth ENS meeting; 1996, June 8. *Journal of Neurology.* 1997; **244** (Suppl.).

4 Ethics and Humanities Subcommittee of the American Academy of Neurology. Palliative care in neurology. *Neurology.* 1996; **46**: 870–2.

5 MacMahon D, Thomas S. Practical approach to quality of life in Parkinson's disease. *J Neurol.* 1998; **245** (Suppl. 1): S19–22.

6 Thomas S, MacMahon DG, Maguire J. *Moving and Shaping: a guide to commissioning integrated services for people with Parkinson's disease.* On behalf of the PDS UK Primary Care Task Force. Parkinson's Disease Society of the United Kingdom (2006). www.parkinsons.org.uk/PDF/Moving_Shaping_complete.pdf

7 National Council for Hospice and Specialist Palliative Care Services. *Reaching Out: specialist palliative care for adults with non-malignant diseases.* London: National Council for Hospice and Specialist Palliative Care Services; 1998. www.ncpc.org.uk

8 National Council for Hospice and Specialist Palliative Care Services. Strategic Agenda for 2001 to 2004. Principles that it believed should underpin the functions of planning, commissioning and delivery of palliative care services. www.ncpc.org.uk

9 Morris C, Gonsalkorale M. Palliative care and Parkinson's disease. *EPNN Journal.* 2004; **3**.

10 National Council for Hospice and Specialist Palliative Care Services. *Specialist Palliative Care: a statement of definitions.* Occasional Paper No. 8. London: National Council for Hospice and Specialist Palliative Care Services; 1995, October. www.ncpc.org.uk

11 Thomas K, Department of Health. *Gold Standards Framework.* London: Department of Health; 2005. www.goldstandardsframework.nhs.uk

12 Clarke CE. Does levodopa therapy delay death in Parkinson's disease? A review of the evidence. *Mov Disord.* 1995; **10**: 250–6

13 Poewe WH, Wenning GK. The natural history of Parkinson's disease. *Neurology.* 1996; **47** (Suppl. 3): S146–S152.

14 Louis ED, Marder K, Cote L, *et al.* Mortality from Parkinson's disease. *Arch Neurol.* 1997; **54**: 260–4.

15 Ebmeier KP, Calder SA, Crawford JR, *et al.* Parkinson's disease in Aberdeen: survival after 3.5 years. *Acta Neurol Scand.* 1990; **81**: 294–9.

16 Diamond SG, Markham CH, Hoehn MM, *et al.* Multi-centre study of Parkinson mortality with early versus later dopa treatment. *Ann Neurol.* 1987; **22**: 8–12.

17 Wermuth L, Stenager EN, Stenager E, *et al.* Mortality in patients with Parkinson's disease. *Acta Neurol Scand.* 1995; **92**: 55–8.

17 Uitti RJ, Ahlskog JE, Maraganore DM, *et al.* Levodopa therapy and survival in idiopathic Parkinson's disease: Olmsted County Project. *Neurology.* 1993; **43**: 1918–26.

19 Treves TA. Parkinson's disease mortality. *Adv Neurol.* 1990; **53**: 411–5.

20 Shaw KM, Lees AJ, Stern GM. The impact of treatment with levodopa on Parkinson's disease. *Q J Med.* 1980; **49**: 283–93.

21 Joseph C, Chassan JB, Koch ML. Levodopa in Parkinson's disease: a long-term appraisal of mortality. *Ann Neurol.* 1978; **3**: 116–8.

22 Hoehn MM. Parkinsonism treated with levodopa: progression and mortality. *J Neural Transm.* 1983; (**Suppl. 19**): 253–64.

23 Curtis L, Lees AJ, Stern GM. Effect of L-dopa on course of Parkinson's disease. *Lancet.* 1984; **ii**: 211–2.

24 Hoehn M, Yahr M. Parkinsonism: onset, progression, and mortality, *Neurology.* 1967; **17**(5): 427–42.

25 Wenning GK, Ebersbach G, Verny M, *et al*. Progression of falls in postmortem-confirmed parkinsonian disorders. *Mov Disord*. 1999; **14**(6): 947–50.

26 Diamond SG, Markham CH, Hoehn MM, *et al*. Effect of age of onset on progression and mortality in Parkinson's disease. *Neurology*. 1989; **39**: 1187–90.

27 Goetz CG, Stebbins GT, Blasucci LM. Differential progression of motor impairment in levodopa-treated Parkinson's disease. *Mov Disord*. 2000; **15**(3): 479–84.

28 Hely MA, Morris JGL, Traficante R, *et al*. The Sydney multicentre study of Parkinson's disease: progression and mortality at 10 years. *J Neurol Neurosurg Psychiatry*. 1999; **67**: 300–7.

29 National Institute for Health and Clinical Excellence (NICE). *Second Draft Guidelines for Diagnosis and Management of Parkinson's Disease in Primary and Secondary Care*. London: NICE; 2006, pp. 147–51. www.nice.org.uk

30 Morgan E, Moran M. The Parkinson's disease nurse specialist. In: Playfer JR, Hindle JV, editors. *Parkinson's Disease in The Older Patient*. London: Arnold; 2001, pp. 273–82.

31 Lierberman A, Dziatolowski M, Kupersmith M, *et al*. Dementia in Parkinson's disease. *Ann Neurol*. 1979; **6**(4): 355–9.

32 Brown RG, Marsden CD. How common is dementia in Parkinson's Disease? *Lancet*. 1984; **2**: 1262–5.

33 Mancini F, Zangaglia R, Cristina S, *et al*. Double-blind, placebo-controlled study to evaluate the efficacy and safety of botulinum toxin type A in the treatment of drooling in Parkinsonism. *Mov Disord*. 2003; **18**(6): 685–8.

34 Hyson HC, Jog MS, Johnson A. Sublingual atropine for sialorrhea secondary to parkinsonism. *Poster P-TU-194*. XIV International Congress on Parkinson's Disease; 2001 July 27 to Aug 1; Helsinki, Finland.

35 Bowman C, Caine S, Beer J, *et al*. A report of a survey examining the medical care of Parkinsonian nursing home residents in Weston-s-Mare. Submitted to *The PDS* in 1967.

36 Mitchell SL, Kiely DK, Kiel DP, *et al*. The epidemiology, clinical characteristics, and natural history of older nursing home residents with a diagnosis of Parkinson's disease. *J Am Geriatrics Society*. 1996; **44**: 394–9.

37 Goetz CG, Stebbins GT. Risk factors for nursing home placement in advanced Parkinson's disease. *Neurology*. 1993; **43**: 2227–9.

38 Aarsland D, Larsen JP, Tandberg E, *et al*. Predictors of nursing home placement in Parkinson's disease: a population-based, prospective study. *J Am Geriatr Soc*. 2000; **48**(8): 938–42.

39 Ellershaw JE, Ward C. Care of the dying patient: the last hours or days of life. *BMJ*. 2003; **326**: 30–4.

40 Ellershaw JE, Murphy D. The Liverpool Care Pathway (LCP) influencing the UK national agenda on care of the dying. *Int J Palliat Nurs*. 2005; **11**(3): 132–4.

41 General Medical Council. *Withholding and Withdrawing Life-prolonging Treatments: good practice in decision-making*. GMC guidelines. London: GMC; 2002. www.gmc-uk.org

42 National Council for Hospice and Specialist Palliative Care Services, Ethics Working Party. *Ethical Decision-making in Palliative Care: artificial hydration for people who are terminally ill*. London: National Council for Hospice and Specialist Palliative Care Services; 1997, August. www.ncpc.org.uk

43 British Medical Association. *Withholding and Withdrawing Life-prolonging Medical Treatment: guidance for decision making*, 2nd ed. London: BMA; 2001.

44 British Geriatrics Society. *Compendium of Guidelines, Policy Statements and Statements of Good Practice*. 'Nutritional Advice in Common Clincial Situations' (revised March 2006). www.bgs.ork.uk/Publications/Compendium/compend_2-5.htm

APPENDIX 1

Useful rating scales

Useful texts

Wade D. *Measurement in Neurological Rehabilitation*. Oxford: Oxford Medical Publications, Oxford University Press; 1996.
> This book is a useful resource for standard measures in the management of people with disability arising from neurological conditions.

Burns A, Lawlor B, Craig S. *Assessment Scales in Old Age Psychiatry*. London: Martin Dunitz; 1999.
> This is a compendium of more than 150 scales used in mental disorders of the elderly.

Lam RW, Michalak EE, Swinson RP. *Assessment Scales in Depression, Mania and Anxiety*. UK: Informa Healthcare; 2005.
> This is a useful compendium of assessment scales for mood.

Hodges JR. *Cognitive Assessment for Clinicians*. Oxford: Oxford Medical Publications, Oxford University Press; 1996.
> This small book reviews neuropsychological assessment and explains the principles behind the tests.

A brief review of some commonly used rating scales and references

Diagnosis

United Kingdom Parkinson's Disease Society Brain Bank Clinical Diagnostic Criteria

These are well-validated criteria used for research, trials and database. They may be difficult to apply clinically especially early in the disease, as they require evidence of progression and levodopa responsiveness. The presence of mixed pathology in elderly patients (e.g. vascular lesions giving an extensor plantar response) may lead to exclusion.

➤ Hughes AJ, Daniel SE, Kilford L, *et al*. Accuracy of clinical diagnosis of idiopathic Parkinson's disease: a clinicopathological study of 100 cases. *J Neurol Neurosurg Psychiatry*. 1992; **55**: 181–4.

Disease severity
Hoehn and Yahr (1967)

This is a basic five-point scale used in many studies, but is of little day-to-day clinical use. Mixes pathology with impairments and disabilities, and should no longer be used.

➤ Hoehn MM, Yahr MD. Parkinsonism: onset, progression and mortality. *Neurology*. 1967; **17**: 427–42.

Unified Parkinson's Disease Rating Scale – UPDRS (1987)

Widely used in research, and some sections useful clinically. Includes sections on mental function, daily activities, motor function and side effects. Useful for monitoring progress, but time consuming. Selective use of sections (e.g. motor function) can be useful.

➤ Fahn S, Elton R, Members of the UPDRS Development Committee. In: Fahn S, Marsden CD, Calne DB, *et al.*, editors. *Recent Developments in Parkinson's Disease*, Vol. 2. Florham Park, NJ: Macmillan Health Care Information; 1987, pp. 153–63, 293–304.

Parkinson's Aware in Primary Care

A new model for staging disease management and reviewing care needs in diagnostic, maintenance, complex and palliative stages. Easy to follow, and useful particularly at primary and secondary care interface.

➤ The Primary Care Task Force for the Parkinson's Disease Society (UK). *Parkinson's Aware in Primary Care*. Parkinson's Disease Society, 215 Vauxhall Bridge Road, London SW1V 1EJ, UK; 1999.

Side effects of medication
Complications of therapy section of UPDRS

Abnormal involuntary movement scale (AIMS). Good validity and reliability. Not widely used.

➤ Chien CP, Jung K, Ross-Townsend A. Methodological approach to the measurement of tardive dyskinesia: piezoelectric recording and concurrent validity tests on five clinical scales. In: Fann WE, Smith RC, Davis JM, *et al.*, editors. *Tardive Dyskinesia: research and treatment*. New York: Spectrum; 1980, pp. 233–66.

Activities of daily living
UPDRS
See above.

Barthel ADL Index (1965)
A generic scale in common use in geriatric medicine. Widely used and well validated.
➤ Wade DT, Collin C. The Barthel ADL index: a standard measurement of physical disability? *Int Disability Studies.* 1989; **10**: 64–7.

Nottingham extended ADL
Little published information or validation. Can be used as a postal questionnaire.
➤ Nouri FM, Lincoln NB. An extended activities of daily living scale for stroke patients. *Clin Rehab.* 1987; **1**: 301–5.

Schwab and England
Used as part of the UPDRS, giving a percentage disability. Subjective, and of little clinical use.
➤ Schwab RS, England AC. Projection technique for evaluating surgery in Parkinson's disease. In: Gillingham FJ, Donalson MC, editors. *Third Symposium on Parkinson's Disease.* Edinburgh: Livingstone; 1969, pp. 152–7.

Cognition
Mini Mental Test Score of Folstein – MMSE
Used as a screening tool. Usefulness in following progress in dementia in doubt. No frontal lobe functions assessed.
➤ Folstein MF, Folstein SE, McHugh PR. 'Mini Mental State': a practical method of grading the cognitive state of patients for the clinician. *J Psychiatr Res.* 1975; **12**: 189–98.

Cambridge Examination for Mental Disorders (CAMDEX)
Cognitive section revised (CAMCOG-R). A well-validated tool for screening for cognitive dysfunction, which is more sensitive to early change than MMSE. Revised format now includes more frontal assessment.
➤ Roth M, Huppert F, Mountjoy C, *et al. The Cambridge Examination for Mental Disorders – Revised.* Cambridge: Cambridge University Press; 1999.

Addenbrookes Cognitive Examination (ACE-R)
More sensitive to executive cognitive impairment in PD. Combines MMSE with clock drawing and frontal tests.
➤ Mathuranath PS, Nestor PJ, Berrios GE, *et al.* A brief cognitive test battery to differentiate Alzheimer's disease and frontotemporal dementia. *Neurology.* 2000; **55**(11): 1613–20.

Rivermead Behavioural Memory Test (RBMT-II)

This is a test of everyday cognitive tasks. It is easy to apply and widely used. It can be administered repeatedly using parallel versions.

➤ Wilson BA, Cockburn J, Baddeley AD. *The Rivermead Behavioural Memory Test.* Titchfield, Hants: Thames Valley Test Company; 2003.

Frontal assessment battery (FAB)

A simple and well-validated 10-minute bedside frontal lobe screen.

➤ Dubois B, Slachevsky A, Litvan I, *et al*. The FAB: a frontal assessment battery at bedside. *Neurology.* 2000; **55**(11): 1621–26.

Clock drawing test

A simple test of frontal and temperoparietal function. Scored using the Schulman scale. Validated in PD.

➤ Shulman K, Shedletsky R, Silver I. The challenge of time: clock drawing and cognitive function in the elderly. *Int J Geriatr Psychiatry.* 1986; **1**: 135–40.

Depression
Geriatric depression scale (GDS-15)

This is a well-validated and widely used scale for depressive symptoms. Validated for use in PD.

➤ Yesavage JA, Brink TL. Development and validation of a geriatric depression screening scale: a preliminary report. *J Psychiatr Res.* 1983; **17**: 37–49.

Other scales, including the Hamilton, Beck Depression Inventory and The Hospital Anxiety and Depression Scale can be used, but are not as well validated in the elderly and in PD.

Carers
Caregiver Strain Index (CSI)

Increasingly used, well-validated measure specifically designed to measure strain in the carer.

➤ Robinson BC. Validation of a caregiver strain index. *J Gerontol.* 1983; **38**: 344–8.

Quality of life
Parkinson's Disease Quality-of-Life Questionnaire (PDQL)

An easy-to-use 37-point scale specific for PD. Well validated, and used in longitudinal cohort study.

➤ De Boer AGEM, Wilker W, Speelman JD, *et al*. Quality of life in patients with Parkinson's disease: development of a questionnaire. *J Neurol Neurosurg Psychiatry.* 1996; **61**: 70–4.

Parkinson's Disease Questionnaire (PDQ-39)

Easy to use, disease-specific scale. Responsive to disease severity, and good longitudinal validation.

> Jenkinson C, Peto V, Fitzpatrick R, *et al.* Self-reported functioning and well-being in patients with Parkinson's disease: comparison of the short form health survey (SF-36) and the Parkinson's disease questionnaire (PDQ-39). *Age Ageing.* 1995; **24**: 505–9.

APPENDIX 2

Useful addresses and websites

AGILE www.agile.uk.org Physiotherapy and older people.

Association of British Neurologists. The ABN. www.theabn.org.uk

Association of Chartered Physiotherapists Interested In Neurology, ACPIN
www.acpin.net. Honorary Chair: Nicola J Hancock (Chartered Society of
Physiotherapy Special Interest Group).

Association of Physiotherapists in Parkinsons's Disease Europe (APPDE).
http://appde.unn.ac.uk/

British Geriatrics Society Special Interest Group in Parkinson's Disease.
www.pdsection.org.uk

British Geriatrics Society, Marjory Warren House, 31 St Johns Square, London
EC1M 4DN, UK. Tel: 020 7608 1369; Fax: 020 7608 1041. www.bgs.org.uk

Community Rehabilitation Team Network. www.rehabteams.org/index.asp

DeDRoN Research Network. Clinical studies group for Parkinson's disease.
www.dendron.org.uk/about/index.html

DVLA Swansea, SA99 1BN, UK. Medical Unit. Tel: 01792 783686. www.dvla.gov.
uk

European Parkinson's Disease Society (EPDA). www.epda.eu.com/

Forum of Mobility Centres. www.mobility-centres.org.uk/services/
drivingassessment.htm

International Tremor Foundation, Disablement Services Centre, Harold Wood
Hospital, Romford, Essex RM3 0BE, UK. Tel: 01708 378050; Fax: 01708 378032.
www.essentialtremor.org

Mobility Advice and Vehicle Information Centre (MAVIS), Department of
Transport, TRRL, Crowthorne, Berks RG11 6AU, UK. www.dft.gov.uk/
transportforyou/access/mavis/?view=Standard

Movement Disorder Society, 611 East Wells Street, Milwaukee, W1 53202, USA.
Tel: +1-414-276-2145; Fax: +1-414-276-2146; e-mail: info@movementdisorders.
org website: www.movementdisorders.org

National Council for Palliative Care – Neurological Conditions Policy Group. www.ncpc.org.uk/policy_unit/neuro_pg.html

National Service Framework for Long Term Conditions. www.dh.gov.uk/ PublicationsAndStatistics/Publications/PublicationsPolicyAndGuidance/ PublicationsPolicyAndGuidanceArticle/fs/en?CONTENT_ID=4105361& chk=jl7dri

National Tremor Foundation, Disablement Services Centre, Harold Wood Hospital, Gubbins Lane, Romford, Essex RM3 OAR, UK. Tel: 01708 386399; Fax: 01708 378032; e-mail: tremorfoundation@aol.com website: www.tremor.org.uk/

Neurological Alliance. www.neural.org.uk/

Neurosciences on the net – links to many sites and journals. www.neuroguide.com

NICE Guidelines PD. www.nice.org.uk/page.aspx?o=CG035

Occupational Therapy Specialists Section – Neurological Practice (formerly NANOT). www.cot.org.uk/specialist/neurology/intro/intro.php

Parkinson's Disease Non-motor Group. www.pdnmg.com

Parkinson's Disease Nurse Specialist Association. www.pdnsa.net

Parkinson's Disease Society of the United Kingdom, 215 Vauxhall Bridge Road, London SW1V 1EJ, UK. Tel: 020 7931 8080; Fax: 020 7233 9908; Helpline: 0808 800 0303; Monday-Friday: 9:30am to 9pm, Saturday: 9:30am to 5:30pm. e-mail: enquiries@parkinsons.org.uk website: www.parkinsons.org.uk

Primary Care Neurology. www.p-cns.org.uk/

Progressive Supranuclear Palsy. The PSP Association, The Old Rectory, Wappenham, Towcester, Northants NN12 8SQ, UK. Tel: General Enquiries – 01327 860299; Subscriptions and Donations – 01327 861007; Telephone Counselling Line (North) – 01939 270889; Telephone Counselling Line (South West) – 01934 316221. www.pspeur.org/

Royal College of Speech and Language Therapy. www.rcslt.org/ (They have a link under Parkinson's Disease to the PD Section.)

Sarah Matheson Trust for multiple system atrophy, St Mary's Hospital, Praed Street, London W2 1NY, UK. Tel: 020 7886 1520 Monday-Friday (9.30–4.30); Fax: 020 7886 1540; General enquiries: office@msaweb.co.uk website: www.msaweb.co.uk

Scottish PD pathway. www.pathways.scot.nhs.uk/Neurology/Neurol%20PD%20 23Sep05.htm

Stroke Association. Registered Office: Stroke House, 240 City Road, London EC1V 2PR, UK. Tel: 020 7566 0300; Fax: 020 7490 2686; Textphone: 020 7251 9096. www.stroke.org.uk

WEMOVE – Worldwide Education and Awareness for Movement Disorders. www.wemove.org

APPENDIX 3

Clinical algorithm

Source: NICE guideline CG035, www.nice.org.uk

Intervention for people with PD

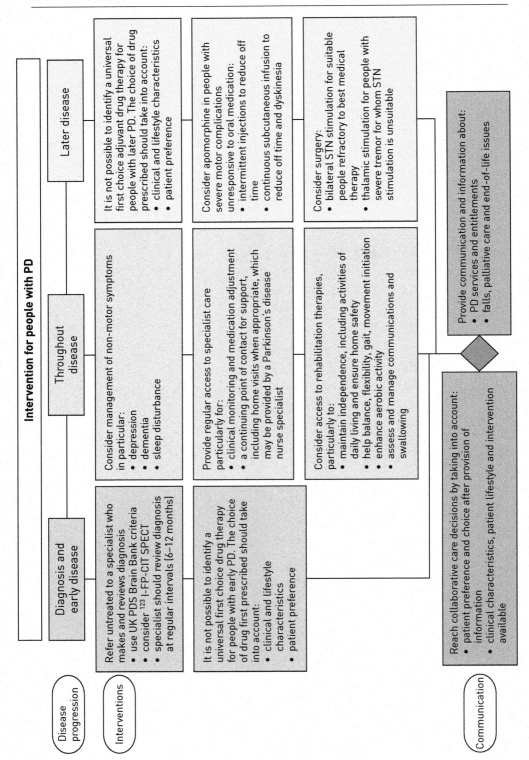

Disease progression

Diagnosis and early disease | Throughout disease | Later disease

Interventions

Refer untreated to a specialist who makes and reviews diagnosis
- use UK PDS Brain Bank criteria
- consider ^{123}I-FP-CIT SPECT
- specialist should review diagnosis at regular intervals (6–12 months)

It is not possible to identify a universal first choice drug therapy for people with early PD. The choice of drug first prescribed should take into account:
- clinical and lifestyle characteristics
- patient preference

Consider management of non-motor symptoms in particular:
- depression
- dementia
- sleep disturbance

Provide regular access to specialist care particularly for:
- clinical monitoring and medication adjustment
- a continuing point of contact for support, including home visits when appropriate, which may be provided by a Parkinson's disease nurse specialist

Consider access to rehabilitation therapies, particularly to:
- maintain independence, including activities of daily living and ensure home safety
- help balance, flexibility, gait, movement initiation
- enhance aerobic activity
- assess and manage communications and swallowing

It is not possible to identify a universal first choice adjuvant drug therapy for people with later PD. The choice of drug prescribed should take into account:
- clinical and lifestyle characteristics
- patient preference

Consider apomorphine in people with severe motor complications unresponsive to oral medication:
- intermittent injections to reduce off time
- continuous subcutaneous infusion to reduce off time and dyskinesia

Consider surgery:
- bilateral STN stimulation for suitable people refractory to best medical therapy
- thalamic stimulation for people with severe tremor for whom STN stimulation is unsuitable

Provide communication and information about:
- PD services and entitlements
- falls, palliative care and end-of-life issues

Communication

Reach collaborative care decisions by taking into account:
- patient preference and choice after provision of information
- clinical characteristics, patient lifestyle and intervention available

Index